Love is Simple, But W
Not

A pathway through the hum
of love and sex

The characters and events portrayed in this book are fictitious. Any similarity to real persons, living or dead, is coincidental and not intended by the author.

Self-published by the Aaron Institute, LLC

ISBN: 979-8-3293-3381-7

INTRODUCTION 13

SEX **14**

SEXUAL HEALTH 14

1-1. The Lessons Sex Wants to Teach Us 14

1-2. Growing Up a Sexual Being 17

1-3. Don't Look Past Sex
The positive effect of sex 18

1-4. The Place of Sex in Our Lives
Why we give sex "special" status 21

1-5. Did you mean intimacy or sex?
Exploring their differences 23

1-6. Talk About It, Talk About It
The importance of sexual conversation 25

1-7. Being a Good Lover 26

1-8. Sexual Maturity 28

1-9. Getting to It
The issue of initiating sex 29

1-10. "Always-Yes" Policy
An alternative to rejecting the partner 31

1-11. Sex in Later Life 34

1-12. Touching Instructions
Sexual guidance for success 36

1-13. Sex and Religion 39

1-14. Being Gay or Not 41

1-15. Sexting 43

1-16. Teaching our Children About Sex 47

1-17. Stress and Sex 49

1-18. Sounds of Loving

How we vocalize sexual pleasure 51

1-19. Warming it Up to Hot
Foreplay for heating up passion 53

1-20. Protecting Sex
Relationship adversity harms a sex life 55

1-21. Late Night Rendezvous
Is sex only for nighttime? 57

1-22. The Key to Great Sex 59

1-23. Considering Sexiness
How we define what is sexy 60

1-24. Emotionally Sexy
The role emotions play in our sexuality 62

PLEASURE **64**

2-1. The "Mmmmm" Word
A discussion of masturbation 64

2-2. The Clitoris: Tiny but Mighty 66

2-3. The Oooh in Orgasm
The ecstasy in orgasm 68

2-4. Pipeline to Pleasure
What we need to maintain arousal 69

2-5. G Wizz!
Exploring the G Spot 71

2-6. Making it Good, Even Great
Good sex versus not-so-good sex 73

2-7. Eroticism: What Turns Us On 75

2-8. Porn: Pros and Cons 77

2-9. Living Longer, With Pleasure
Sex supports well-being and longevity 79

2-10. Multiplying Your Pleasure
Attaining Multiple Orgasm 81

2-11. Fantasies
Exploring erotic imagination 82

WHEN SEX HAS PROBLEMS **84**

3-1. Delayed Take Off
The trouble of inhibited ejaculation 84

3-2. The Quest for Control
The problem of ejaculatory control 86

3-3. When Sex is Damaged
A discussion of past sexual trauma 88

3-4. The Sexless Couple
When sex has disappeared 90

3-5. Battling Bedroom Boredom
Considering sexual variety 93

3-6. Too Touchy
Too much sexual touch 94

3-7. Low Female Sexual Desire 96

3-8. Vaginismus: A Marriage Killer 111

3-9. The Unenthusiastic Partner
Regarding partners who avoid sex 114

3-10. Guilt of Pleasure
Considering how we view pleasure 115

3-11. Curing the Sexless Marriage 117

3-12. Failure to Rise
The challenge of erectile dysfunction 118

3-13. Battling Desire Discrepancy
When partners differ in sexual desire 120

3-14. She Targets Sex
Why a female partner may reject sex 122

3-15. Opposite Paths to Arousal
A key sexual difference 124

3-16. The Two Sides of Sexual Anxiety
How anxiety shows up in sex 126

3-17. Coping with the Porn Factor
Is porn good or bad? 128

3-18. Orgasm, Complicated
Orgasm's importance varies 130

SEXUAL PLAY **132**

4-1. Digging the Dirt
What is dirty can be erotic 132

4-2. Playing with Power
Using power and control erotically 134

4-3. The Multi-players
Discussing sex with multiple partners 136

4-4. Bound to Have Fun
Exploring the practice of bondage 138

4-5. A Threesome? Oh my! Why?
Including another sexual partner 140

4-6. Real or Fake?
The issue of faking orgasms 143

4-7. Play Nice! Take Turns
Equality, mutuality and satisfaction 145

4-8. More Than Just Lip Service
Focusing on oral sex 146

MEN & WOMEN **148**

5-1. A Man's Expectations 148

5-2. Women Don't Like Sex Part 1 150

5-3. Women Don't Like Sex Part II 152

5-4. The Male Zipper Problem
Why some men can't keep it zipped 154

5-5. The Erotic Nature of Men 161

5-6. The Animalistic Side of Men
Men's inner conflict about high sexual desire 166

5-7. #MeTwo: Considering Men 169

5-8. Sexual Desire and Men 178

5-9. For Men, there is no "one-size-fits-all."
Men are often confused by women 179

OUR BODIES **181**

6-1. Anatomically Unfair
The differences of intercourse 181

6-2. Politics of the Little Blue Pill
How pro-erection medicine alters a sex life 183

6-3. Time to Take Out the Garbage
The dangers of internalizing painful emotion 185

6-4. The Body of Love
The importance of physical love 187

6-5. For the Love of the Female Body
Between a woman and her body 189

LOVE **190**

7-1. Loving to Grow
Why we enter relationships 190

7-2. Loving Yourselves Promotes Passion
Self-esteem and love 192

7-3. Romantic Nourishment
A discussion of romance 194

7-4. I Love You, Please Change
Trying to change the partner 196

7-5. The Avoidant Partner
Partners who prefer distance to closeness 198

7-6. Enticing Love to Stay
Preventing love's deterioration 200

7-7. Anatomy of Commitment
Considering commitment 202

7-8. What Did You Expect?
Partners' unrealistic expectations 204

7-9. Choosing Love Over Power
Power blocks the flow of love 208

7-10. On the Road to Loving
Boundaries and limits when loving 211

7-11. Strength is Love's Vital Ally
Strength supports quality loving 213

7-12. Love, But Not Like
When our love is in conflict with feelings 215

7-13. Love's Gymnasium
Loving another deepens and heals our love 217

7-14. Careful Does It
The effect of small hurts on connection 220

7-15. Teaching You How to Love Me 223

7-16. Love is perfect
An exploration of love 225

7-17. Important, Special and Cherished
Maintaining special status between partners 227

7-18. Falling out of Love
Protecting the loving bond 229

7-19. Many Fish in the Sea, Sharks, too
The danger of sociopaths 231

7-20. Mothering Kind of Love
Men want a lover not a mother 234

7-21. Caring by Being Careful
Sensitivity to protect each other 236

7-22. Love, Who is it for?
Our notion of love is incorrect 239

7-23. Loving Our Partner, a Spiritual Discipline 241

7-24. When Love is Troubled 243

7-25. Simultaneity
Loving effectively at the same time 245

7-26. Love's Expiration Date
Invisible and unknown 247

7-27. Does He or She Deserve Love?
The tendency to withhold love 248

7-28. Better Loving Through Chemistry
Considering "chemistry" between partners 250

7-29. A thing called love
Why is loving so hard? 252

7-30. Loving yourself 253

7-31. Jealousy: Poisoned Love 255

INFIDELITY **258**

8-1. When Love is Given to Another 258

8-2. Protecting the Faithfulness 260

8-3. Repairing Trust 263

COMMUNICATION **265**

9-1. Do You Understand?
Importance of understanding your partner 265

9-2. Here Comes the Judge
The harm of judgement 267

9-3. The Language of Empowerment 270

9-4. Relationship Turn Signals
The necessity of consulting a partner 272

9-5. Communication: More Than Just Talk

The emotions which block communication 274

9-6. Offer Understanding Not Advice
The complexities of advice giving 276

9-7. When Wrong to be Right
The dangers of right/wrong debates 278

9-8. Assumed or True?
The negative impact of assumptions 280

9-9. The Power of Mind Reading 282

9-10. Conflict About How to End Conflict
Arguing about whose solution is best 284

RELATING **286**

10-1. Pain Runs the Relationship
The insidious power of unsolved problems 286

10-2. Teammates, Friends and Lovers
Three essential parts of your relationship 288

10-3. Veterans of Domestic Wars (VDW)
Shift from war-like to love 290

10-4. The Quiet Man
About non-communicative men 292

10-5. The Mirror Doesn't Lie
Partners as reflective mirrors 296

10-6. The Queen and the King
Give each other the royal treatment 298

10-7. Openness to Influence
The dynamic of influence between partners 300

10-8. Why Do We Marry? 302

10-9. Driving Each Other Crazy
Couples and driving, a source of tension 304

10-10. Pain in the Relationship
Coping with relationship pain 306

10-11. Just Not Feeling It
When our feelings and values conflict 308

10-12. No Time Like the Present
The habit of holding onto the past 311

10-13. Strong and Loving
Two essential qualities 313

10-14. Gridlock: It's Knot Love
Exploration of emotional gridlock 315

10-15. Honey and Money
Relationship and money 317

10-16. Powerful Understanding
Understanding can love powerfully 319

10-17. Valentine's Day Duty
The obligation of February 14 321

10-18. Honesty Between Us
A look at the value of honesty 323

10-19. Marriage: To Stay or To Go 326

10-20. That's Close Enough
Discrepancy of closeness between partners 329

10-21. Growing Together
Growth as a deep purpose of relating 332

10-22. Too Stressed Out
The deleterious effects of stress on loving 334

10-23. Stop the Hurt
The disproportionate effect of hurt 337

10-24. Fair Fighting Makes Togetherness Safe 340

10-25. Let the Games Begin…
The Games of Courtship 341

10-26. Touched by a Partner
The importance of physical touch 347

10-27. Saddled by Expectations

Unrealistic expectations in loving 348

10-28. Build-up of Toxicity in Relationships
Toxic emotions accumulate 351

10-29. Re-igniting the Flames of Passion
Surface efforts don't get it done 354

10-30. Making Love Throughout the Day
Importance of daily loving efforts 355

10-31. Vive la Différence
Resolving the gender difference 357

10-32. Kids Are Bad for Marriage 358

10-33. The Invisible Unspoken Contract
The tacit agreement partners make 359

10-34. Sooner, Rather Than Later
The eventual adversity of loving 361

10-35. Emotional Safety
Non-hurtfulness in a relationship 363

10-36. Conflict Need Not Damage Love
Problem-solving without hurtfulness 364

PERSONALITY AND EMOTIONS 367

11-1. Selfish versus Self-Full
Redefining the sin of selfishness 367

11-2. Emotional Hibernation
Withholding silently in pain 368

11-3. Never Quite the Same Again
A discussion of trauma 370

11-4. Becoming More Conscious
The mysterious unconscious 372

11-5. Nice and Strong
Strength as a core value of loving 375

11-6. At Work and At Home
Our differing personalities in each place 377

11-7. Bringing Fight to Fear
Challenging your fear 380

11-8. Letting Go of Anger 382

11-9. The Cage That Loves Us
How our limitations show up in loving 383

11-10. The Blind Spot
Our common emotional blindness 385

11-11. The Angry Lifestyle
The unhealthiness of internalized anger 388

11-12. The Dangerous Allure of Perfection
The dynamic of perfectionism 391

11-13. The People-pleasers
A unhealthy personality type 393

11-14. Strength is a Turn-On
The erotic nature of strength 396

11-15. Handling Anger While in Love
Taking the toxic out of anger 398

11-16. Living with Passion
Exploring intense aliveness 401

11-17. Our Disruptive Inner Three-Year-Old
Regulating powerful inner impulses 402

QUOTATIONS INDEX **404**

INTRODUCTION

These small pieces are inspired by the many courageous clients I have had over more than two decades. They have bravely sought to face and overcome their own pain, limitations, and struggles to grow and strive for their best in loving. Each piece is gleaned from observations I have made about repeated behavior patterns and from self-evaluation.

Additionally, having been married for more than three decades, my loving wife has generously provided me with many life lessons in how to love, how to love her and the meaning of marriage.

The short pieces are not intended to be scientifically rigorous and are not results of scientific studies, but are instead views of human emotion, behavior, and determination. Through love, sex, and relationships people practice to be their best and to reveal their deepest true nature.

This material is presented so that human love, in physical and emotional forms, is enhanced. The interplay of loving acts such as openness, conversation, time spent together, playfulness, and sex form a distillery to separate out what is not love, and to arrive at a purer love.

Each chapter originally was written as an article for a monthly magazine column I wrote over a fifteen year span. You may find that many topics and themes are repeated, but each repetition offers an opportunity to highlight a different nuance. Hopefully this strategy may lead you to greater self-awareness and improved loving.

SEX

SEXUAL HEALTH

1-1. The Lessons Sex Wants to Teach Us

Becoming a good lover and sharing ecstatic sexual experiences with your partner requires specific efforts. The benefits of these same efforts constitute life lessons which improve our lives far beyond the bedroom. All the lessons are really about love. Sex teaches us that while love is simple, it is not simple to master. Through sex, we are informed that loving one another is important and is optimized when balanced with loving ourselves.

Sex teaches us to get out of our own way. A lover who cannot escape the self-conscious thinking of a busy mind fails to get out of love's way. Blocking love's flow contributes to the development of dysfunction, disconnection, or mechanical sex. Relaxing and forgetting about ourselves enables us to be our best in both loving and living. Such a practice means we become less ego-oriented.

To practice getting out of our own heads, effort is well spent centering our awareness in our bodies during sex and beyond. Experiencing sex with our entire being can rock our world. Outside the bedroom, people whose awareness is mostly focused in their heads and on their thoughts are susceptible to anxiety-related problems which interfere with comfort, flexibility, and high sexual performance. When we are involved in an engrossing activity, we naturally forget about ourselves. In such moments, our awareness is centered in our body which is a necessary condition for having fun.

Loving ourselves is the main struggle. When we love ourselves completely, including our human limitations and our sexuality, we are well-primed to be a very good lover for our partner. Our bodies, too, deserve our love, which is achieved when we get beyond shame and self-criticism and arrive at self-acceptance. Our bodies are meant for love and health but not perfection. Being generous with ourselves positions us well to give generously to others.

Openness, which is necessary for relaxation, is a deep practice that improves our relationship with our partner, but also benefits the relationship we have with the very life that flows through our bodies and lives. Being closed, cautious, and fearful just won't do. For arousal, pleasure and orgasm to bloom, a lover must surrender in openness. Adopting an attitude of openness supports flowing instead of mechanical sex. The practice of openness builds personal strength and confidence as the lover tolerates increased vulnerability.

Being of service is a different way of loving. As a partner, spouse, or parent, we are called on repeatedly to be of service, even when it is not convenient. Just to be of service, sometimes we make ourselves available to provide sexual satisfaction, too. To give in the spirit of true service, whether it be sexual or not, forgetting about ourselves is required in order to succeed at giving in a manner that satisfies the recipient. Sharing our pleasure and arousal is a gift of service to our partner as well. True service is a selfless act that provides the other satisfaction, and how much we give is irrelevant.

Loving others through service must be balanced with loving ourselves. Because although it is true that each one of us is a complete individual, at the same time we are an indivisible part of the whole. In loving ourselves, our needs, too, must be met. Advocating for our own satisfaction, sexually and otherwise, builds emotional strength. All giving and no receiving generates resentment, which has the potential to block the flow of love. Balancing giving and receiving is a vital life lesson.

Breathing is essential for sustaining our lives, but rhythmic inhaling and exhaling usually occurs unconsciously. Conscious deep breathing has the potential to make sex even better by expanding pleasure to become a full-body experience. Conscious breathing facilitates deep relaxation and is advocated by most spiritual traditions as a way to maintain health and promote growth. Conscious breathing is a secret that magnifies pleasure, in part because it forces us to stay in the present. Staying in the present is a practice that amplifies the experience of each moment and, if practiced daily, brings the sacred into every moment of our lives.

As a team sport, sex needs partner coordination. Often dismissed as too basic to be considered, the important skills of sharing and taking turns are balanced well by successful lovers. Throughout our lives, as we are obliged work closely with many others to contribute and achieve our goals, the importance of our ability to share and take turns cannot be overrated.

Sex can be a celebration of life; it is the mystery of humanity being divided into separate individuals and genders. It is also the acceptance and love of having bodies, and including our bodies in loving the self and the partner. It is a celebration of life expressed in playfulness where joy and an innate child-like nature are shared with the partner. Humor, good-natured teasing, laughter and spontaneity all build this fun. Allowing our child-like qualities to migrate into other places in our lives colors the world with beauty.

When tag-teamed with love, sex is the teacher of many important lessons. Attending fully to the present by drinking in every moment and sensation permeates each gesture, word and touch with love. If practiced well in the bedroom, each lesson learned enables us to experience passionate aliveness outside of the bedroom.

> The more intimately you know someone, the more clearly you will see their flaws
>
> — *Anonymous*

1-2. Growing Up a Sexual Being

Who are we as sexual beings, and how did we get that way? Because sex is shrouded in mystery and veiled with taboos, questions about our sexuality rarely arise unless a serious and unavoidable sexual problem forces us to ask questions. Sexuality is a part of each and every one of our lives, whether we celebrate it or not. Even those who claim that they are nonsexual must admit that they would not exist if not for their parents' sexual act. The particulars of our sexual development contribute to how we view our sexuality, the kinds of feelings we have about sex, what turns us on, and how we choose to include or exclude sex from our life.

Because of the strange way we collectively regard sex, it is easy to incorrectly assume that how we personally developed sexually can be attributed basically to sexual influences. This is generally untrue; it is mostly sexually unrelated elements that have the greatest impact on our sexual development. In fact, our sexuality is mostly developed during the period of our lives that is least identified with sex: our our baby years and childhood. Both our sexuality and our eroticism, meaning that which we find sexually exciting and arousing, are mostly developed by the time we are six years old. The tendency to identify sexuality with adult sexual activities means that we fail to recognize sexuality in its less mature forms. As children, we had sexual feelings and eroticism, yet they were rarely manifested in what adults identify as sexual, except for curiosity-based exploration of our own body and the bodies of other children.

There are many factors that have a strong effect on developing sexuality, ultimately determining whether we become sexual beings who cherish sexuality or repress it, crave sex or avoid it, whether sex, for us, will be shame-based, dysfunctional, compulsive, or joyous. The following elements in our early family environments were significant in our developing sexuality: the presence of positive and loving touch; valuing emotions and emotional expression; the lack or presence of physical, emotional and sexual hurt/trauma; praise leading to a positive sense of self; balanced boundaries that kept us emotionally safe; positive comments and positive treatment of our bodies; the presence of an active and satisfying social life; parents who demonstrated love and respect for themselves, each other and you; parents who demonstrated a value for love and their own sexuality; parental permission for sex to be regarded as a healthy part of your life; and parental offering of sexual information.

As you can see, most of the contributing factors have little to do with sex itself. Parents should be aware of the importance of these factors in order to provide a happy and satisfying future for their child as he or she grows towards adulthood. If you find that your relationship with your sexuality limits your, or your partner's, potential for satisfaction, please do not fear; many people, with self-love and a concerted effort to grow, may overcome the sexual limitations caused by past negative factors.

1-3. Don't Look Past Sex

Most couples drastically under-utilize sex. If used to its fullest extent, sex may strengthen relationships, but most do not realize its high potential to triumph over individual separateness by unifying two people into a strongly connected and unified couple. As a vital part of loving relationships, sex remains challenging and controversial.

For many couples, sex is a source of tension, conflict and dissatisfaction. Sexless couples, who have been without sex for years, are too common. The love partners have for each other becomes more complicated when their bodies are included. An inescapable reality is that we are sexual beings, but collectively our sexuality is regarded negatively, like an unwanted stepchild.

In the public sphere, the topic of sex raises eyebrows, due to the discomfort it causes. Yet virtually every adult is or has been sexual. Generally, sex has been linked with sinfulness and carnality, an association that remains in the form of shame in present-day consciousness. Sex is frequently newsworthy, but when sex makes the news it is always painfully connected with abuse, violence, obsession, harm, adultery, pedophilia, teen pregnancy, disease, etc. These factors add to the accumulation of discomfort and unhealthiness associated with sexuality. The loving side of sex gets contaminated by this darkness.

Sex is critically important. It lies at the crossroads of our personal, emotional, spiritual, and governmental lives. If not for sex, you would not exist to read this article. It is responsible for the survival of our species, even though when most lovers engage in sex, it has little to do with reproduction, but instead is about connecting. Your identity is strongly influenced by your gender, a sexually significant factor. Our social networks are defined by our gender and are energized with the buzz about who may hook up with whom. Our legislatures create laws regulating where, how and with whom we can be sexual, if we are to receive societal approval. Our religious organizations, for centuries, have pontificated about the morality of how, when, where and with whom we may be sexual. In relationships that fail, sexual problems are commonly a contributing, but undeclared, factor. Sex is the hugest part of being human about which we remain ambivalent and uncomfortable.

The aforementioned issues cause sex to be a weak link for many couples. Because of its high potential for bonding and pleasure, sexual activity is disappointing to many partners because these potentials often fail to be realized. Romantic partners are often so uncomfortable with it that they do not even talk about sex with each other. In contrast, they may discuss a household project with ease, yet sex is also a "together" activity that requires coordination.

Marriage and love are not easy and, when troubled, sex is one of the first parts of a relationship to vanish. If the troubles remain unresolved, sex may never reappear, further weakening the connection of a loving bond. A manifestation of the atrophied state of sex in the modern world is that many mature adults have insufficient or inaccurate sexual information with which to form a satisfying sex life.

Developing a balanced, healthy attitude towards sex is difficult due to prevailing negative attitudes. In reaction to the veil of shame and discomfort which shrouds sex, we segregate this part of being human. By giving it "different" status, we confine sexual activities to very narrow circumstances, ensuring that it occurs infrequently. Sex is best if it is more a regular part of life, just like breathing or breakfast, rather than occurring only as frequently as an anniversary or holiday. For many this concept may sound sacrilegious, arousing the fear that having sex too frequently may rob it of its specialness. Sex should not be special, but love, that is shared best during sex, should always be considered special. If we regard sex as an ordinary part of being human, then we may have access to its full nourishing potential.

Sex is the kind of activity which strengthens a romantic connection and maintains and repairs it when infused with love and offered in an emotionally safe environment. Most long-term, committed couples greatly underestimate and under-utilize the power and potential of sex to make their relationship strong. Because of the inherent vulnerability of sexual togetherness, the possibility of healing and growth from sex are high. Yet most couples do not choose this kind of nourishment as frequently as would benefit them.

A beautiful ring is made up of a jewel and a setting. The jewel holds the value, but the setting frames it and keeps the jewel secure. Your love for each other is like the jewel; sex is the setting. Sex provides the right setting for you to love each other completely; in mind, body and spirit. Within your love relationship, have a lot of sex. It is better than arguing; it'll make your relationship stronger and is less expensive than a television streaming service.

> Sex is both a way of expressing a close connection, and also of building a close connection.

1-4. The Place of Sex in Our Lives

Sex, like no other part of our humanity, stirs our curiosity, fascination and repulsion. It causes controversy. Because sex can have power over us, provoking anxiety and obsession, we segregate it and give it "special" status in our lives. Yet sex cannot truly be separate, but must instead be tightly interwoven into every aspect of our individual uniqueness, because, in fact, it is not separate.

Sex is so powerful a force that many of us have difficulty coping with it. As with hunger, denying it will only be successful for so long. In our society we desire to keep sex safely at arm's length, causing it to be present in our lives in distorted and perverted forms.

Our sex parts are no less good than are our hands, but when another angers us, we equate them to a sex part. Have you ever heard somebody say in anger, "You are nothing but a hand?" Why do we choose to demean our genitals by associating them with people's hurtful or ignorant behavior? By doing so we demean our very genesis.

Sex is the source of tremendous ambivalence. Most agree that sex generates tremendous pleasure, though not all agree that such pleasure is moral. Most agree that sex is necessary, but also hold the opinion that it is not a suitable topic for discussion or education. We miss an opportunity to obtain the completeness that sex may provide when we reject it as unacceptable and view it with suspicion. Is sex a part of the devil's plan to lure us into sinful temptation, or is it a God-given gift that is part of a complete, good humanity? I believe we cannot achieve completeness until we accept and love all parts of ourselves.

More than just a physical activity, sex is an expression of our relationship to life itself. Sex is wonderful in that so much pleasure may be shared, but it is also about potentially seeking to fulfill our human incompleteness by gaining that which is missing, in the balance of our masculine and feminine qualities. Through sex and sexual energy this inner balance may be accomplished, but this necessitates accepting our sexuality as a positive and healthy part of our lives.

Sex and the sacred: the two must be linked. Sexuality is so powerful a force in humanity and our individual lives that, if befriended and combined with love, it can take us to the heights of spiritual potential. If rejected, sexual energy will close down our ability to reach our full human potential. By embracing sexuality as important and positive, the possibility of completeness is much closer to our reach, an achievement that is typically attributed to spirituality. It makes sense that Nature or God would make something that feels so good to be deeply important...a gateway to a deeper relationship with life.

Where is the place in our lives for sex? Nature or God intended for sex to be of primary importance, in part because the survival of our species is a priority, but also because sexuality is a route to grasp the sacred and heighten the potential of our lives.

{ Loving doesn't start until all the hurtfulness has stopped. }

1-5. Did you Mean Intimacy or Sex?

Sex has value, it is a good thing. When it is missing, romantic partners complain of dissatisfaction. The word "intimacy" is used euphemistically for sex...when the word "sex" is uncomfortable to use. The two are not the same. Intimacy is about the openness of emotional connection that lovers build.

Lovers say they want intimacy, but routinely they don't want its consequences: emotional complications, drama and loss of passion, and walls of disconnection. Intimacy often does not feel good, because it reveals those parts of us that are unwanted, incomplete, or filled with darkness. When lovers seek to build an intimate connection, they do not associate intimacy with these after-effects. Lovers want intimacy, thinking that it is good, but it shows us the ugliness within. Some are considered lucky in love, whereas most others are not. This is not how it works; it isn't about luck. Loving takes hard work and isn't always supposed to be fun.

Sex is not intimacy, though if partners are truly and deeply open to each other, sex can be intimate. Most sexual partners are not open to each other. Sex just becomes mechanical without an alive intimate connection. Many partners spend a great deal of time hiding from themselves and each other to avoid the pain of revealing fears, weaknesses and insecurities. The transformative effect of intimacy is simultaneously destructive and creative, but weaker partners shrink from its destructive side.

Closeness with another at first soothes loneliness, but as the relationship deepens, the old painful emotional residue from childhood is activated. Early in our lives, there was a time when we were impressed by our most intimate and influential relationships, which were those with our parents. Getting close to a loved one, which seems easy at first, creates an emotional echo of those older primary relationships. Intimacy is the activating agent which awakens old, unresolved emotions. The work of love is normal, though it may not look pretty.

The passage of time and the lengthening of a relationship's history deepens intimacy because partners grow mutually more familiar. Commitment speeds up intimacy, but also accelerates the pace at which old emotions are activated. Lovers get acquainted with each other's good, bad, and ugly qualities.

Not unusual is the partner who pines for a return to the early days when excitement, passion and ease of friendly relating characterized the relationship. But that was a time when the partners were actually less intimate, that is why it was easier. The partners knew each other less well. Partners could still believe each other's lies.

Our relationships demand that we constantly grow by deepening our capacity to love life, our partners, and ourselves. Developing and deepening intimacy forces us to be conscious of ever-deeper layers of ourselves. If we resist, our essence dies, and our relationships become either stagnant or bitter. The growth process within love relationships is one of accepting and loving every newly revealed part of ourselves. We share in an illusion that our troubles are down to our partners' poor characteristics, but the real struggle is with our inability to accept all parts of life, including our partner's shortcomings.

Our psyche and our partner will demand growth of our weakest quality first; but that same quality for us is also the issue that is the least pleasant task. The more painful an issue, the greater the likelihood that a partner will refuse to face it. When a partner refuses to grow, the essence of the relationship shrivels and dies.

Loving another and ourselves is the work of life. Intimacy is the openness and sharing required for that work to be done. The word "vulnerability" does not give adequate emphasis to the unfathomable fear it can foster. Being seen and known terrifies many, who flee from the sense of riskiness that intimacy provokes. Not until a lover loves and accepts him or herself sufficiently to be real in a relationship can the union of partners celebrate all that life and love have to offer. Not until a lover is fully exposed so all limitations are on display, and he or she is still accepted, can love bloom.

Intimacy is not sex, though sex can be intimate. A love relationship is the process of growing, and overcoming obstacles to love. It is hard, often uncomfortable work. The presence of discomfort is not a symptom of something being wrong, it is normal. Love relationships take a lot of work if they are to be vital, involving partners who are growing. Otherwise they are just miserable. This is what is real about intimacy.

1-6. Talk About It, Talk About It

Remember that dreaded conversation your parents were supposed to have with you, but probably didn't? Yeah, that one…about sex. While it is best for parents to summon the courage to address this difficult but vital topic with their children, most will try to avoid it out of discomfort and sheer embarrassment. If the content of family conversations were any indication of all that is real and important in the world, it would be logical to conclude that neither sex nor sexuality exists. This is the kind of environment in which most of us, now adults, spouses and lovers, developed our perspective on sex. Little wonder that the topic of sex is so full of embarrassment, discomfort and shame. The lessons of our families carry over into our marriages and love relationships, resulting in partners who stay safely clear of conversations about their sex lives.

Avoiding the subject does not make it go away, and the costs of doing so are potentially very high. Almost always, when an activity arouses anxiety, avoiding it not only makes the situation worse, but also means that an opportunity to grow emotionally is lost. The potential costs of a poor sexual relationship include putting up with an unpleasant or frustrating sexual experience for the rest of your life, chronic feelings of disappointment, regular feelings of pain, emotional disconnection from your partner, emotional distancing in your relationship, and finally divorce or break up. Of all the aspects of a love relationship, sex constitutes only a fraction, but if a sex life is troubled, this small part grows to infect all other parts of the relationship.

Sex is a team sport. As with any activity that involves more than one person, cooperation and coordination are essential for a successful outcome. Let the two of you be a team for your mutual sexual satisfaction.

Love relationships are intensely challenging. Emotional safety is the name of the game. By communicating your mutual sexual needs, the chances are increased that sex will become a part of your relationship where you can deeply relax and freely be yourselves. Optimally, you and your partner should be a team, in order to maximize your mutual pleasure and satisfaction. Your likes and dislikes in the sexual arena of your relationship are as telling about your individuality as your fingerprints. By sharing your preferences with your partner, you are expressing love by sharing yourselves, which is what a relationship is all about.

> It takes two emotionally strong partners to make one strong relationship.

1-7. Being a Good Lover

Getting it right in the bedroom has many benefits, especially in a long-term, committed love relationship, such as keeping the risk of an extra-marital affair low, experiencing deep closeness, seeing the look on your grateful partner's face, as well as giving and receiving the gift of pleasure. If you are a good and skillful lover, odds are you know it because of your partner's words and/or non-verbal reaction to your successful pleasuring. But if you are not such a good lover, it is likely that you will neither be told, nor will your partner's reactions be a full indication of your success or lack thereof. Lovers are notorious for avoiding ego-bruising messages, which say your skills could be better. Some lovers *really do* fake it.

What each individual defines as good sex can vary greatly. Getting to know what good sex means to your partner is an essential first step. A great way of learning about this is to ask your partner about his or her "peak" sexual experiences, and what characterized them. Also, inquiring about your partner's eroticism and embracing it is a way of practicing a deep form of loving acceptance.

Do not assume you are a good lover; ask if there are ways you could give your partner more pleasure. Gracefully giving your partner the opportunity to share openly about what could be better will win his or her gratitude so long as you accept the answer without defensiveness, but with an eagerness to learn and improve. During sex, vocalizing your pleasure is a way of sharing the best in you with your partner. Your "song" communicates to your lover when he or she is doing something well or poorly and teaches him or her about what you like best. Sharing your excitement vocally contributes to turning on your lover.

Sexual dysfunctions need not derail good sex. Ways of giving pleasure are limited only by your imagination; so don't insist that the two of you are limited to only one or two.

Openness to new variations battles bedroom boredom and is an attitude which is sure to please a more adventurous partner. A tense or inhibited partner can be a real turn-off. Talking about sex when outside the bedroom can significantly enhance the quality of your sexual experiences. Remember, sex is a team sport. The team wins when team members synchronize with each other.

> Consistent deliberate effort at first becomes easy and natural effort later.

1-8. Sexual Maturity

Sexuality is an aspect of being human that is fraught with shame. Through our culture we inherit numerous negative, shame-building messages about our bodies and sexuality. In order to develop into an adult with a healthy sense of sexuality; we must pass through a rigorous and complex emotional/physical/spiritual obstacle course in which many falter. Each one of us can achieve maturity by letting go of shame and accepting ourselves as good, healthy sexual beings.

To give you an idea of what healthy sexuality is, I suggest to you several guideposts along your journey which you may consider: first that sex is a healthy, vital part of the human experience. In saying this, I do not mean that all the ways people sexually behave are healthy, but that in each one of us, there is some form of sexual expression that is important and essential to our complete humanness. Pleasure is a right and a gift, that we may experience through our bodies and has no necessary link to feelings of guilt or shame.

Because of old beliefs and attitudes, it is difficult, though important, to accept that our bodies, including our sex parts, are good and deserve positive attention and praise rather than criticism and negativity. Sexual maturity blooms when we demonstrate that sex is an expression of the highest and best in us, and that shame has no place here.

We have matured when we have developed a sexual voice, evidence that we possess the strength to be responsible for our sexual experience, and that we choose to vocalize our sexual needs, and do so by lovingly offering instructions to our partner as to how our body works and how we need to be pleasured.

Maturity in sex means possessing the ability to share with our partner in a reciprocal manner, so that we express the strength to give pleasure as well as the strength to surrender in receiving it as well. It also means an ability to let go of ourselves by falling into relaxation, despite the inherent vulnerability in sexual sharing.

Sex and love are often linked, but the two are not the same. In mature sex, pleasure is given lovingly, so that the line between them melts away. As sex and love are blended when mature partners master the art of pleasure, so too, does sexuality blend into spirituality when the merging of partners overcomes the experience of separateness. Sex is not less than spirituality, but an essential and healthy beginning in the human journey of growth towards it.

{ The *natural* you
is the attainable and
healthy perfection. }

1-9. Getting to It

In your relationship what is that first gesture which begins your journey towards a passionate encounter? Is it a special glance? A look in the eye? Or perhaps a kind of touch? Each couple takes a different route to get there. In previous sections I have provided techniques for sex to become better, but what good are these suggestions if sex doesn't even happen? Taking the first few steps towards sex is an obstacle for some couples, and he lack of sex or sexual satisfaction places many couples at risk of a breakup.

Initiating sex is vital to lovemaking. It is not unusual that, by tacit agreement, one partner assumes the sole responsibility for initiating sex. Commonly a male partner owns this obligation, if only because he usually possesses greater sexual desire. If he attempts to signal that a moment of desire has arrived and his approach causes discomfort, a sexual encounter will not occur. The female partner, feeling emotional discord, is likely to defer due to "not being in the mood." Each advancing step towards greater sexual involvement must please, excite, arouse, soothe and relax the partner. If there is a pattern of discord in these approaches, the couple is at risk of becoming sexless.

Initiating sex must be sensitive to the "temperature" between partners. If partners are tense and cool, the initiator faces a tough task to heat things up enough that the passive partner may become warm and receptive. He or she may feel that this burden is too much of an obstacle to potential success, and that they are being set up to fail, and this may contribute to accumulating resentment.

Steps to initiate sex must provoke in the partner very specific responses; feelings of being desirable, valued, relaxed, safe, close, connected and excited, and linked to all this, the beginning of arousal. Any kind of negativity pours water on the flame of passion, by "turning off" the partner and causing disconnection. For a turned-off partner, the energy for arousal has been turned off and made inaccessible due to negative emotions that form a barrier. The initiating partner will succeed by being sensitive to the recipient's experience. Those couples who cannot agree on how sex should begin get lost in conflict over differences of manner and style. Their sexual disconnection is likely symbolic of a greater relationship disconnection.

Who initiates sex in your relationship? Is that process varied? Just as exciting sex is vulnerable to regularity, initiating it can also fall into a habit of repetition. Female partners routinely express a preference for a romantic path to passion, which expresses their desirability and value. This approach non-verbally exclaims, "You are irresistible; I must have you."

Male partners tend to prefer a direct, getting down to business approach. But what men seek is a responsive partner who actively demonstrates a welcoming receptivity, which non-verbally declares, "I am happy to be loved by you."

In those couples where one partner is the designated initiator, the risk of losing balance is ever-present. Most of us wish for our desirability to be confirmed. Female partners who routinely initiate are sharply aware of this, and quickly arrive at the point where reciprocation is demanded. Men, too, may want to be seduced, and there is nothing wrong with wanting to be wanted. When the responsibility for initiating is too one-sided, a couple's sex-life may become negatively contaminated with emotional toxicity that can harm an emotional connection.

The risk of rejection is a powerful force influencing the evolution of couples' sexual initiation process. This is especially true of male partners who, as a gender, tend to try and keep the risk of rejection very low, always wishing for a "sure thing." When a man finds a method that produces success, it is guaranteed he'll try it the same way again next time, rather than do it differently and risk a different outcome. After having been "shot down" several times, men and women are often tempted to stop initiating sex altogether, rather than face rejection again.

What is the motivation for the sexual initiative in the first place? Certainly, desire can arise from our own body's need, but it is better to instead let a desire to love and please your partner be the force behind initiation. Love is more than a feeling; it may be expressed by every look and touch. When sexual initiation frequently leads to exciting, pleasurable experiences in which you both feel loved, the path to passionate success will be shortened.

1-10. "Always-Yes" Policy

In many relationships, sex is a source of tension and conflict. In others, where dissatisfaction has been a chronic experience, emotional connection and sex get buried under layers of hopelessness.

There is no getting away from the reality that all partners are different, and sex is a place where those differences are likely to show up dramatically. In uneven environments, sex and sexual needs can be negotiated in a way that reduces tension, especially in couples where sexual differences are not extreme. This allows sex to function in the relationship the way it should; to demonstrate love, nourish and deepen the connection.

To shift sex from the "problem" column to the "strength" column, consider incorporating an "always yes" policy when it comes to giving sexual attention to your intimacy. This idea may initially provoke fear in some, especially in partners with lower desire, and may seem too good to hope for to partners with higher desire. Before you jump to conclusions, read on. Consider the way that parents regularly feed their children. If their child expresses hunger, parents will usually do their best to satisfy that hunger, even if the child does not always get the exact kind of food that he or she most wants (candy versus fruit). Sex is just another form of nourishment, but one that has been complicated with many factors.

By suggesting an "always yes" policy, the complications, politics, and power struggles are eliminated from this essential part of a love relationship. By cleansing sexual activity from tension and negative associations it may potentially be transformed from "just sex" into a method of loving. For instance, how would it be if there was an understanding between you and your partner that if either of you requested a hug, you would have confidence that a hug would be given? The same could hold true for your partner's time, or attention. How would it be if whenever you asked your partner for money, you could be completely confident that your partner would share money with you?

When joining with another in a love relationship, each one of us agrees to be of service. Providing money, safety, protection, security, dependability, love, cooking, housecleaning, or childcare are all varied ways to be of service to our partners. Being of service sexually is no less important than any of the others. Yet because of historical associations with hurtful imbalances of power, such as subservience, sinfulness and shame, it is hard to be sexually of service, especially for female partners, without negative associations of prostitution. In fact, sex is an important part of being human which is as much a part of the human spirit as any other aspect. By giving the person we love our time and attention, touch and sexual pleasure, we nourish them and make them strong. Being of service to our partner sexually is an important way to help make our relationships satisfying and stable, which is also a gift to ourselves.

It is unusual for partners to put the same value on sex, to have sexual desire at the same time, and want the same frequency of sexual activity. Along with the painful associations so many have with sex, these differences are very difficult to negotiate. If unresolved, this tension between partners quickly becomes toxic and infects much of a relationship. An "always yes" policy protects the relationship from this destructive influence. Suggesting that partners are committed to each other's life satisfaction and sexual satisfaction, does not suggest that either partner will be subservient and sell him or herself out. To be true to oneself, a partner must negotiate for a level of involvement that will not foster resentment, which would be equally as poor a choice as ignoring the partner's needs and allowing him or her to become resentful.

When it comes to sex, there is a broad range of ways to give and receive attention, touch, stimulation, and pleasure. These variations provide an opportunity for a partner to be more involved in the experience. The "always yes" policy means negotiating for a level of involvement that feels both comfortable and true to oneself. In the case of hunger and eating, there is a wide range of eating activities, each one fitting appropriately into a unique situation; snacks fit well in some circumstances while multi-course feasts are appropriate at others. Sometimes it feels right to give another person a snack while choosing not to eat. It is the same with sex; sometimes we are not comfortable partaking ourselves, but can still provide attention to our partner. When balanced with full participation at other times, this creates a relationship environment that may be tension-free. A sexually frustrated partner is unhappy and not fun to be with. Until sex is seen as a normal, everyday part of being human, it will be a weak link for many couples.

{ I love myself.

I'm not perfect, I'm human. }

1-11. Sex in Later Life

What is it about sex that spawns so many myths and misconceptions? Among the most common is that sex ceases as we get older. The prevailing youth-oriented, age-rejecting attitude is that as soon as a person ages past what we culturally-define as sexy, he or she ceases to be sexual. White hair is not considered sexy. But aging doesn't stop people from being human, and sexuality is a human trait, not just a trait of young people.

The myth tells us that as a normal middle-aged person matures in a healthy and proper way, interest in sex and the strength of sexual desire are supposed to gradually wane and gracefully fall away. But the myth isn't specific on when sexual interest should fall away; perhaps mature adults should no longer want sex once they reach 65, the retirement age? Fifty-five is beyond mid-life; maybe this is a good time for sex to stop. Certainly, sex after 80 is unthinkable. If you are younger than 40, at what age do you plan to retire your genitals? Sexuality has no expiration date.

The assumption is that older men's penises don't work, and older women have no interest in sex. Do older adults remain interested in sex? Just ask the staff in a nursing facility. Those who care for the elderly regularly witness the fact that some older people, even those who are significantly declining, remain sexual. In nursing facilities, special rules and privacy laws are necessary to protect seniors' freedom of sexual expression, because sexuality remains alive.

One sad truth contributing to the myth that sex disappears with age is that as relationships age many partners grow bitter and disconnected. In long-term relationships where partners do not solve problems, resentments and other toxic emotions accumulate. If not repaired, unhappy relationships cannot maintain the emotional connection vital to support a passionate sex life, and, in turn, couples are at risk of becoming one of a large number of sexless unions. It is far easier to attribute the lack of sex to more visible aspects of aging, such as physical decline, than it is to the invisible accumulation of negative emotion. The truth is that active sexuality helps to ward off the deterioration of aging more than aging trumps interest in sex.

If sex were just a physical act, then as the body ages and vitality declines, the assumptions about loss of sexual interest would make sense. But sex is far more than just a physical act. It is a means and method for delivering love; it is connection, care, loving touch and pleasure. Why would anyone, old or young, not want these?

The attitude that sex should only be associated with the young would be reasonable if its sole purpose was reproduction. My non-scientific opinion, based on conversations with hundreds of couples, is that people's choice to be sexual rarely considers reproduction, except to prevent it with contraception. Sex is more commonly associated with bonding, a need of both the young and the mature.

With aging, illness and physical limitations do affect an increasingly larger percentage of the population. Some people lose their full ability to function sexually. Illnesses, which contribute to suffering and decline, and the medications used to treat them, often interfere with desire and sexual functioning. Many mature adults do their best to remain active while adjusting and adapting. Instead of expecting perfect sex, limited adults prioritize the pleasure of care, patience, and warmth in their sexual play, in place of more physically-based performance considerations. In some ways, this shift from a physically-based to a more emotionally-based experience marks a qualitative improvement.

Older adults, as sexual beings, have advantages over their younger counterparts. Older bodies have long since departed from the unrealistic ideal, so more experienced people are free from body image concerns. Mature adults have had longer lives in which to accept and embrace sexuality, so the embarrassment factor is less potent. Knowing themselves well, mature adults are better able to relax. And finally, mature adults have had more practice and may be both more highly skilled as lovers, and also better able to enjoy themselves. For those of you who are younger, do not fret about losing your sex lives as you age. Don't buy into this myth. If you maintain your health, the quality of your sexual experiences may just improve as you age.

{ No amount of negativity will ever create a positive relationship. }

1-12. Touching Instructions

Sex is a team sport. Like any other team sport, the quality of communication between players determines the quality of the play. For the high number of couples who do not talk during sex, the quality of their intimate moments is lower than it might otherwise be. Without giving and receiving sexual instructions, dissatisfied lovers may remain so forever.

The obstacles to developing comfort in asking for what is desired are formidable. Openness is a primary relationship value and a necessary condition for love to flow. It is not unusual for a partner to be frightened by the vulnerability that sharing requires; when voicing a request, a lover is revealed and opens him or herself up to the risk of rejection. It is necessary to have knowledge of language, vocabulary and method to successfully speak up. When negative feelings build between partners, it may easily creep into the way they talk during sex, potentially "killing the mood."

For sex to be great, it demands that lovers master a lot of basic values: openness, taking responsibility for their own satisfaction, sharing, giving, receptivity, listening, relaxation, complete attention, and staying in the present. Having the capacity to use descriptive language requires comfort with bodies and sex parts.

Moods change, energy levels fluctuate, phases of relationships vary, and so do a lover's physical experiences and sensitivity to touch. In response to these variations, adaptation is needed for sex to be satisfying under a range of circumstances. Getting to a high level of arousal may be dependent upon drowning out the mental noise provoked by a stressful daily environment; providing the right kind of touch helps to bring one's attention front and center.

Voicing sexual instructions is an act of taking responsibility for your own experience. In doing so, you establish clear boundaries which help to foster the best kind of sexual experience: an emotionally safe one. Doing so communicates that "My experience is important enough that it must be understood and respected." Vocalizing needs and wants in and outside the sexual arena is a way to be a powerful partner. Being able to ask for what you want is the practice of "showing up." While uncomfortable for many, it is a stepping-stone on the path to overcoming discomfort, embarrassment and body shame. Partners who achieve success in this area know themselves and their bodies well.

Some guidance and instructions are vital, especially when an activity produces discomfort. When desires are shared delicately and responded to swiftly, such a moment is an opportunity for care to be shown. Giving good instructions may eliminate the necessity of having difficult and potentially damaging conversations. Within a couple's sex life, if a lover is directly praised when successful at pleasing, instructions will be less needed. Between lovers, communication during sex happens verbally and non-verbally. When partners generously vocalize their pleasure with sounds, less verbal communication is needed. But some partners, by being quiet, restrict the flow of important information and leave the other in the dark about mutual satisfaction.

Not all lovers are created equal, and some are less sensitive to touch, speed, pressure and motion than others. When sex play is not going well, both momentarily and chronically, negative emotions build. Couples challenged with sexual dysfunction are particularly susceptible. Giving instructions contains the danger of expressing built-up negative emotion in the form of criticism, anger, frustration, and blame. Tone of voice and inflection may subtly express these. When instructions are shared in this manner, there is a high risk of causing hurt, so high, in fact, that many couples abandon sharing instructions altogether to avoid the danger, or offer instructions by implying them instead. What instruction they do give may often be interpreted as, "You don't know what you are doing," or "You are not a good lover." Insecure lovers have difficulty distinguishing well-intentioned instructions from criticism of their sexual skills, but it is normal and helpful for lovers to guide each other.

To keep the possibility of a damaged sexual encounter low, follow these suggestions: check in with each other by making an agreement about including or excluding the giving of instructions; so that you are both on the same page. All instructions are best if expressed in a positive way. Instead of, "Not like that!" say "Can you please do that differently." Asking permission to give instructions can decrease the risk of hurt: "May I describe what I'd like?" Avoid commanding tones. Talk about what you like instead of what the partner is failing to do.

Using a past example may be helpful, "When you did this it felt really nice..." The less unintended hurt during sex the better. The goal is to maximize your mutual pleasure by becoming a synchronized team.

> In a relationship, you can do little good until you have learned to do little harm.

1-13. Sex and Religion

When you and your honey climb into bed with the intention of snuggling and sharing pleasure, do you also intend to bring the church under the sheets? Unintentionally and unconsciously, many people do. A strong link exists between religion and sex. Traditional religious organizations espouse behavior that is good, not bad and that is right, not wrong. Through the centuries, religious education has associated sex more with what is bad, wrong and sinful than what is sacred. Instead of being viewed as an expression of the divine, sex is regarded suspiciously as a weakness of the flesh. The result of this influence is that sexuality, a natural part of being human, is tainted with shame, guilt and ambivalence.

Two broad kinds of spiritual traditions characterize the journey to completeness: the masculine approach which declares that God is not here, and we must reject all that is not God to find Him. The feminine approach proclaims that God is omnipresent, in all things, and human completeness is attained by loving and embracing everything. Christianity, the religious tradition that forms the foundation of our culture, is predominantly a masculine way. It urges us to reject all things that are not God in order to become complete. Included in this rejection are the physical desires of sex and sensuality, described as temptations of the devil that may prevent us from spiritually developing. The current era of masculine-based traditions is fading, as is demonstrated by the decline in church attendance and frequent church closures. A feminine spirituality is blooming, as seen in the diminution of paternalism and the increase in influence of women both socially and economically. Through such a transition, sexuality is gradually becoming celebrated as necessary, healthy and spiritually important.

However, the residual effect of centuries of masculine-based teachings continues to linger. Guilt, shame, embarrassment and general discomfort characterize many individuals' deeply held feelings about their bodies and sexuality. Being a good, moral person seems at odds with being a passionate, enthusiastic lover. Deep within the minds and consciousness of many, an inner conflict binds them, preventing relaxation and producing inhibition. The tragedy here is that the inability to be free from such inner restraint puts many romantic unions at risk of dissolution.

A paradox is that most young people have not been raised in a structured religious environment, yet still they carry the burden of sexual strictures taught to older generations by traditional religion. The shame and discomfort surrounding bodies and sexuality has been passed on, while being disconnected from the complete teachings that contributed to growth and development. Sexuality and values will always be strongly linked, but if the two are inconsistent, then inner conflicts occur which undermine health and strong love relationships. The values which declare physicality, body-centered pleasure and sexuality to be carnal and sinful have become disconnected from their purposeful source. They have now become discarded fragments over which many people can stumble on their journeys of spiritual growth. In the current climate, people being free to love, mind, body and spirit, is a necessary capability for a strong and moral life.

It is vital to our social fabric and community strength that the couple, as the primary building block of families, is strong. If men and women are ashamed of their natural being, their inhibitions restrict them from openly loving themselves and their partners. Sex is not everything, but it remains a necessary part of being human; if any part of our humanness is rejected, we cannot be complete. The residual negative sexual values which contaminate our psyches prevent the healthy expression of our passion. If sexuality is associated with sinfulness, sex and love cannot not be combined. When denied their proper flow, sexual energies ally with darker forces and are expressed in immoral, destructive and perverted ways, an all-too common phenomenon that shows up daily in the news. Negative attitudes towards sexuality cause the term "sacred sexuality" to seem like a contradiction of terms.

What are your values? Have you inherited unhealthy views? It's a worthy task to scrutinize your values and attitudes and adjust them to ensure they are positive and healthy.

> There's only one corner of the universe you can be certain of improving, and that's your own self.
>
> — *Aldous Huxley*

1-14. Being Gay or Not

When searching a field of clover, happening upon a four-leaved one is considered good luck. The four-leaf clover is a rare variation, but common enough that it is worth the search. Homosexuality is somewhat of a rare variation of the ways of being human...it has always existed and is present enough that it ought to be considered normal, even though it is less common than heterosexuality. From the perspective of eroticism, homosexuality is simply one variation among many within the general human need to love and merge with life.

The tendency to regard homosexuality as an aberration is an outgrowth of our socially constructed and enforced artificial model of masculinity and femininity. In this model, men and women are socially encouraged to possess personal attributes that cause each gender to reside at an extreme and opposite end of a spectrum. If someone defies this categorization, they are at risk of being rejected. In reality, the difference between homosexuality and heterosexuality is not about that...it is erotically more akin to one person being attracted to brunettes, while another is attracted to tall people.

From an erotic perspective, making a category of those who are attracted to people who have the same genitals is a ridiculous endeavor, because eroticism naturally varies so broadly. Cultural and societal structures, which narrowly define genders and gender roles, are responsible for the judgement of which sexual choices are right and wrong.

Being gay is a blend of sexual and cultural factors. Gay culture has its own unique qualities, that are not the same as the eroticism shared by gay people. Equally, in heterosexual culture, there are masculine and feminine values that are supposed to define men and women. Football players manifest certain aspects of the masculine ideal; most men share some of these qualities but not to this extreme. Football players are neither representative of all men nor of male eroticism. We could say the same about beauty pageant entrants and all women. Gay culture also functions this way. It is not the same as homosexual eroticism, which is the real determinant as to whether an individual is homosexual.

Our erotic nature is formed both by our physical bio-chemical make-up and our early environment. These factors determine to whom we are attracted, as well as how we love them or are loved by them. Having an attraction to those of the same gender is not a personal choice. It is as much a choice as is our favorite color, the specific hobby from which we get the most enjoyment or whether we are born with a male or female body.

Homosexuality is not a narrowly defined category. Many heterosexual people have sex or fantasies of sex with others of the same gender, but still define themselves as heterosexual. Many people who define themselves as homosexual have heterosexual experiences. Others avoid the labeling because their eroticism is fluid and can be homosexual at one time, heterosexual and omni-sexual at others.

The kind of eroticism we possess is neither good nor bad but is just an expression of who we are. Redheads make up approximately 2% of the United States' population. Having red hair is neither good nor bad, though it may be fortunate or unfortunate depending upon the circumstances. Distinct erotic features are no different.

How common are gay people? They are more common than redheads or four-leaved clovers. Depending upon the study, between 3% and 10% of the US population identify themselves as homosexual. A 2006 New Zealand study concluded that those who have occasional homosexual interests form 20% of the population. However, a 2011 Gallup telephone survey indicated that US adults believe that gays make up 25% of the US population. From an erotic perspective, being homosexual is just another way of being normal. Instead of focusing on who and how a person loves, it is more important to consider *whether* a person loves and is loved by another.

1-15. Sexting

Until recently, sex has stayed neatly in its proper place behind closed doors. But this long-lived comfortable trend is now being disrupted. Sexting and other computer-based communication methods are eroding traditional values of privacy and propriety. Sexting, a word derived from the blending of the words sex and texting, is the use of texting and other computer-based means for the sending or receiving of sexual communication or sexually explicit images over the internet. It is a new and disruptive change agent.

Originally texting was most popular with young people, kids in junior high and high school. Eager to embrace new and different technologies, young people are also interested in sex and given to sexual exploration and experimentation. Young people naturally discovered how texting could support their sexual curiosity while also remaining hidden and seemingly private. With the popularity of electronic devices, especially smartphones, previously established boundaries between what is private and what is public are being subverted. Increasingly, private sex is falling into public view. Simple cellphones have transformed into ubiquitous, indispensable and sophisticated smartphones; even children have them to guarantee constant contact with their parents and friends. An unintended consequence of this rapid development is that poor judgement may be widely and instantly published with just the tap of a finger. Technology is changing the social landscape; yet with every new freedom comes increased responsibility.

When computers and the internet combined in the early 90s to create the tremendous change-force they have become, viewing sexual material was among its most popular initial uses. So, linking the internet to sexual activity is as old as the internet itself, especially considering that early computer users were disproportionally male. First it was phone sex; then it was cybersex, and now it is sexting. As numbers of female users have increased, so has the internet's use for relationship purposes, with the development of social media websites. When a new technology blooms, early adopters quickly discover ways to exploit its features for sexual purposes. This continues with newer methods of communication, such as texting, and audio/visual methods such as Skype and Facetime. The distribution of pornography and erotic material, or the enablement of sexual contact with partners or video-cam sex workers remains a substantial use of the internet and technology.

Recently, and for the second time, Anthony Weiner, a former gubernatorial candidate for New York, was discovered to be sending pictures of himself and his genitalia to a woman other than his wife. Past revelations of his sexting habit had destroyed his former candidacy to be a New York Senator. Despite the public betrayal of his wife, she has stood by his side. By his private and sexually compulsive behavior becoming public, Anthony Weiner unintentionally brought the issue of sexting into public discussion yet again. Texting and video chat provides ease of use combined with the illusion of privacy and anonymity. When water is dammed, it will always take advantage of any available opportunity to flow; sexual energy does the same. A large crack has formed in the foundation of ethics and morals which declare that sexual expression ought to be private. Many people, with a mobile phone conveniently located in their pocket or purse, are choosing to be sexual in ways and places that were previously unsuitable for such activity. Behaving in sexy ways in non-sexy places can be highly erotic. Sexual temptation has never been so high.

The rapid proliferation of mobile devices has enabled the migration of computing from the office desk to the living room couch to the bedroom; comfort fosters intimate communication. On the internet, where privacy is an illusion, the convenience, ease of use, comfort, and intimacy of sharing seem to frequently trump good judgement. Because mobile devices provide both audio and visual communication, they offer a high temptation of being employed for sexual purposes. A recent ad for an Android smartphone highlights the newly available sexual freedom; it features a husband leaving on a trip and his wife delivering to him a "private" video by bumping their phones.

Who is using mobile devices for sexual purposes? Generally, it is believed that it is only young people, who were the first to enthusiastically embrace texting to communicate with friends. On the contrary, it seems that now, everybody who is a technology user embraces the blending of technology and sex. The media has published numerous articles citing how children as young as 10 are shockingly expressing their sexuality by sending others nude and sexually explicit pictures of themselves. Studies have suggested that from 20% to 50% of middle school and high school age kids are sexting. Other studies have seemed to indicate that a large majority of young adults aged 18 to 30 are using mobile computing to enhance their sexual expression. While no exact numbers have been published regarding older adult and seniors' rate of technology adoption in their sex lives, it is likely that older adults who are sexually active and utilize technology also employ this method to facilitate sexual activity. Along with the erosion of traditional morals and values, sexting has forced us to realize that very young people are highly sexual...an uncomfortable reality that challenges our societal concepts of purity and innocence. Technology has unintentionally gifted us a window into others' sexual behaviors and shattered the illusions of the past, which were created by keeping sex hidden.

In many parts of our lives, computers and computer technology have magnified the potential for and effect of mistakes. Because computers, and now smartphones and tablets, operate so quickly, it has never been so easy to do something so erroneous so effortlessly as it is now. Sexual expressions are the tip of the spearhead of an impulsive moment. With just a soft, split-second tap of a button, an ill-conceived choice can be widely broadcast; regret is very long-lasting once the internet is involved. Our split-second decision becomes part of a permanent online archive. Sexting provides unparalleled freedom to make extremely poor choices. Additionally, the law has not kept pace with technology: the sexual images young people may send are still considered child pornography, and thus young texters, truly guilty only of poor and impulsive judgement, by sending sexually explicit self-portraits, may be at risk of prosecution.

Sexting often functions as sexual initiation. At times it may simply be a game of good old fashioned "playing doctor" or "I'll show you mine if you show me yours," with a technological twist. These are common and normal flirting, pre-foreplay activities through which partners ramp up their delicious excitement while proceeding towards the fulfillment of their sexual intentions. At other times, responsible, non-impulsive adults choose the available technology to fulfill their otherwise hindered sexual needs. Couples, especially those who are separated by required work-travel, bridge the gap of distance by using texting and video chat to maintain an erotic connection. Mobile technology perfectly fills the need to maintain intimacy and connection, despite physical distance between partners. Despite the seemingly private nature of electronic playfulness, most flowing data on the internet may be intercepted or may become public.

Neither sex nor technology is new. Yet the combination of the two dominantly defies old social orders and values. But such disruption is not new, the development of the internet has already disrupted how we get things done; how we write; how we are educated; how we do our banking; how we buy music; how we read books; how we communicate; and also how we have sex. Sexuality will exploit any means or methods available for its expression. Technology, such as texting, offers this opportunity, and sexting in particular gives us an unanticipated view into the sexual expression of many; it surprises us to learn how vital and insistent the force of sexuality is. It will not be denied.

> The way to a woman's heart is through her ears.
>
> — *Anonymous*

1-16. Teaching our Children About Sex

All parents are eventually faced with the daunting task of teaching their children about sex. Most approach the duty with much ambivalence, if not outright dread. After all, there are few of us are who are deeply comfortable with our own sexuality.

We live in a culture where sex is rarely approached in a healthy manner. Instead people tend to go to the extremes of regarding sex as either sinful or obsessive debauchery. If we are to teach our children well about sex, we would do them the best service by first becoming comfortable with our own sexuality.

Many of us recall how our parents addressed the awkward subject with us when we were young...they didn't! Sex has historically been such a taboo subject that it was best avoided, but you and I know that our children deserve better.

Children are naturally curious. They are open to their own eroticism, which is unrelated to but eventually develops into adult sexuality. Infants are easily pleased and pleasured by their own bodily explorations, including their genitals. This is normal. At times intense curiosity about the opposite gender and the opposite gender's body can be within the range of normal for children.

Children's developing sexuality is strongly affected by many non-sexual family behavior patterns. For instance, the degree to which touch is used in positive ways to express affection between family members translates later in a child's life to how they equate touch with pleasure. Messages about a child's body impact upon a child's future sexual confidence and security. Encouraging social contact both in and out of the home teaches a child that others are safe and, later in life, results in his or her ability to be close and intimate with another person.

Parents often ask what age is ideal for their child to be informed about sex and sexuality. There is no single answer for this as each child matures at a different rate. Between ages nine and eleven, children are generally ready to have a more complete understanding of sex. But the sharing of this information should not be forced upon a young person.

Children will bring up the subject of sex, at times indirectly, which will provide you an opening to the topic. By doing so, a child is signaling that he or she is ready to receive some sexual information. A parent, to test the child's readiness may ask the child their opinion, for instance, "How do *you* think babies are made?" or "What do *you* think your friends meant when they used the word sex?" If your child answers correctly, say so and permit them to ask more questions or to bring up the topic at any time in the future. If incorrect, let them know that the reality is different than what they answered. If interested, your child will continue by asking questions and will be receptive to correct answers. This can flow into a more detailed conversation thus providing your child with the information that he or she is ready to receive.

The goal is to be sex-positive, meaning to frame sexuality in a way that it is understood as a healthy, acceptable and necessary part of adult life. It is also healthy to convey that sex is more than reproductive, more than just physical mechanics, but also includes pleasure, intimacy, love, and responsibility. Children who are well informed about sex are more likely to make wise sexual choices when older, a lasting gift to both you and them.

> Worrying is the least productive activity and a great waste of time and energy.

1-17. Stress and Sex

We balance many responsibilities while maintaining healthy and productive lives. When we take on new tasks, we invite additional stress into our lives. When we take on too many tasks, our lives resemble a congested highway at rush hour; all jammed up. To further illustrate this, imagine a small balance-scale sitting on your kitchen table. Now imagine placing a 1000 lb. weight on one side and a 1000 lb. weight on the other. Question: what do you have now? The answer: a crushed scale.

This is an approximation of what many people do to themselves. They take on too much and somehow attempt to balance it all. And they still expect to have a satisfying sex life. The very conditions that are required for a pleasurable, nourishing and exciting sex life are destroyed by the high level of stress that is present. For many people, this state results from making many "good" choices, of living out the American dream, of having the house, the kids, the fancy car, and the vacations. These are all good choices but making too many good choices often leads to very bad results: deadly stress. Balance is essential but attempting to balance too much is dangerous. Instead, keep life simple.

Sex is usually the expression of two partners building an emotional connection. Partners cannot connect if each is emotionally unavailable due to unhealthy stress. Relaxation is a vital ingredient in good sex, which allows sex to be fun, pleasurable and nourishing. Most older adults have the benefit of more free time and thus have the opportunity to fully enjoy sex. Sadly, often their bodies have succumbed to the damage caused by chronic lifetime stress, preventing them from enjoying healthy sexual functioning. Stress has a direct effect on the health of the heart, which is responsible for pumping the blood to create a solid erection in men or contribute to the orgasmic experience in women. Weight gain is also a result of chronic stress. A man's large belly reduces the effective length of his penis, possibly robbing his female partner of the maximum pleasure of intercourse. Exercise can protect a body from the destructive effects of chronic stress and helps to maintain healthy sexual functioning as well.

Stress is terrible for sex in other ways too. Chronic stress is an intimacy killer. Creating a satisfying love relationship or marriage is difficult, but add to that a large amount of stress and it becomes almost impossible. Partners have differences, but stress intensifies those differences and increases the likelihood of destructive conflict. Bad relationships usually do not include good sex, because the emotional connection has been damaged. Many bad relationships are sexless.

By keeping life simple and making both your relationship and your partner's happiness a high priority, you protect your love life and your sex life from being destroyed by stress.

On each side of the scale: one pound makes balance, a thousand pounds crushes the scale.

1-18. Sounds of Loving

Passionate lovers know that lovemaking can be a noisy business. Vocalizing our pleasure during sex is an essential part of lovemaking for many reasons. Despite the reality that the oooh's and aaaah's of sex form the basis for many jokes, the following explores why these sounds of love are so vital.

For sex to be good, partners must be relaxed. To get deeply relaxed, proper breathing is necessary. This is demonstrated in various spiritual disciplines such as yoga where deep breathing is encouraged in order to obtain deeply relaxed meditative states. Deep breathing in sex also aids partners, if relaxed, in being more conscious of their bodily sensations. Expressing pleasure in sounds also magnifies the pleasure, making a sexual experience fuller. Vocalizing pleasure forces a partner to breathe more deeply. In order to sing well, professional singers are trained to breathe deeply. Lovers, too, must breathe deeply to sing well the songs of pleasure and love. Sexual songs help lovers to lose themselves in that delicious sexual trance that is possible only in good sex. Being self-conscious is uncomfortable. When we are having fun, we have forgotten about ourselves...this is true of good sex as well.

Sexual pleasure and arousal are dependent upon awakened energy in the body, evidenced by the heat of our aroused body parts once lovemaking begins. If the sexual energy is confined to our sex parts, our excitement and pleasure will be limited. Expressing the excitement and pleasure in sounds, with accompanying deep breathing, sexual energy is drawn from previously limited physical locations, through now-opened gates, to flow all around our bodies, with the effect of producing a larger, full-bodied arousal instead of a pelvic-only excitement.

Expressing our pleasure in sound is a form of communication that allows an exchange of very important sexual information between partners. A partner learns from the other's sounds about the effectiveness of his or her pleasuring efforts, and they provide indirect instructions about what works and what doesn't. Listening carefully to our partner's song guides us in our creative endeavor to drive him or her crazy in new and successful ways.

Lovers influence each other in a deepening spiral of excitement. As lovemaking builds in intensity, the song lovers sing contributes to the deepening of passion. As one partner voices pleasure, the other grows more excited in response to the partner's sexy sounds, which, if well-expressed, then turns on the first partner even more, in a deepening cyclical pattern. By being generous with the expression of pleasure, we offer our excitement as a gift to our lover.

Nothing comes without a cost, and singing the song of pleasure also has costs. Lovers know all too well, that expressing oneself vocally can remove privacy; something that a sound-screen of music may preserve. Our song is as unique as we are; thus expressing it shares our deeper self with our lover. For some this feels too vulnerable and therefore revealing. Overcoming such fear is an opportunity for growth. Lovers who withhold their song and their breath can miss out. Silent lovers dampen their own pleasure while failing to fully relax; this robs the other of the pleasure of shared excitement and feelings of satisfaction that comes from being a good lover. Not much turns a lover on more than a partner's excitement. The sounds of love create a non-verbal conversation of love which offers the excitement of openness and intense, shared sexual pleasure.

> There is no pillow
> so soft
> as a clear conscience.
>
> — *French Proverb*

1-19. Warming it Up to Hot

Sometimes partners disagree on what makes up good foreplay. Female partners commonly complain of insufficient foreplay, but some men, too, wish for more. The debate may include a discussion about how long it should last, and which methods of pleasuring should be included. Often this discussion is truly framed by issues of arousal. Among the reasons for the importance of foreplay are the significantly different rates of arousal of men and women.

Men tend to become aroused much more quickly; within a few minutes (longer as men age), whereas women generally take more time to reach full arousal, typically between twenty to forty minutes. Because of the longer time required to grow to full arousal, the female partner is more likely to complain about inadequate foreplay. The shorter length of foreplay for men is reflected in their interest in skipping all foreplay due to their quick readiness to engage in intercourse. For her full pleasure, high arousal and excitement are necessary. Negotiating this difference well so that both partners arrive at readiness for intercourse is one important function of foreplay.

The touching, caressing, squeezing, kissing, and stimulating of the early phase of lovemaking are excitement-building efforts. If an eager lover moves too fast and begins something that builds excitement or intimacy too quickly, an assertive partner will signal that slowing down is needed. If such a request is not respected, discomfort will increase, along with the potential for emotional disconnection and a damaged sexual opportunity. This is can be the case when direct stimulation is applied to an erogenous zone before a partner is sufficiently aroused.

The foreplay phase of a sexual experience serves several functions, one of which is to help the partners gradually invest in the sexual experience, thereby facilitating the simultaneous development of two seemingly contradictory states, excitement and relaxation. Relaxation is not easy for many lovers to achieve during sex because of the inherent physical and emotional vulnerability that sex requires. Early pleasuring activities also help partners graduate to increasingly deeper levels of intimacy. This is no small task because intimacy does not come without vulnerability, an experience that raises fear and anxiety. More than a few partners avoid sex for this reason. The foreplay pleasuring helps to ramp up closeness slowly so partners can adjust to this increased level of emotional risk. Partners who are uncomfortable with the vulnerability of sex may seek to avoid foreplay as a way to shorten the entire sexual session, thus more quickly eliminating discomfort.

A session of foreplay also tests the level of intimacy each partner will allow. Intimacy is a test of openness; how much will a person allow? Openness is limited by the discomfort of fear; we become afraid of being hurt. Openness is also the absence of protection, a state in which vulnerability is complete. During foreplay, a negotiation occurs between partners as to the depth of intimacy which will be permitted.

The sexual differences between men and women are far less obvious than their physical differences. Many lovers will only come to appreciate these differences once they are explored and explained, a bit of communication that many women aren't comfortable giving and many men resist hearing. Each gender tends to assume that the other is similar, leading to potentially destructive negative assumptions. The kinds of sexual play that begin a sexual encounter negotiate these differences, thereby allowing partners to use them as a cause for celebration. Foreplay sets the tone and tempo of the sexual drama the way a good introduction gets our attention so we can fully lose ourselves in a good movie.

1-20. Protecting Sex

Sex does not exist as a separate and independent part of our love relationships, instead, sex resides within our relationships' context. The loving and hurtful ways of partners either support an active and satisfying sexual relationship or interfere with it. While this may seem obvious, too many partners unrealistically expect that sex will be unharmed by control battles, anger, conflict and all other negative influences.

Fostering an environment of emotional safety between partners is of key importance both to make the relationship healthy and to support the presence of a passionate, high-quality sex life. Imagine what partners have together as a precious ring; their love expressed for each other daily is the setting; the most pleasurable, intimate moments are the jewel. Good sex is maintained by all that is loving outside the bedroom; to endure, it must be protected from outside stresses and strains.

The boundaries that exist between partners emphasize the reality that each of us is separate, even though we unite in the union of a relationship. This paradox is acutely true when we are sexual; the boundaries of separateness must be honored carefully in the bedroom because, by doing so, this protection safeguards the possibility of sexual merging. Establishing clear, well-defined boundaries keeps partners safe from potential hurts, such as unmet expectations, disappointments and misunderstandings.

Well-established boundaries keep the sexual arena protected from fear and anxiety, as well as other uncomfortable emotions that can easily derail the highly-prized smooth flow of passion during sexual moments. Forming agreements and understandings about the way partners communicate and relate creates emotional safety. To do so may be challenging; many people are uncomfortable talking about sex, which truly is less uncomfortable than experiencing the disappointment of poor sexual experiences. If partners can depend upon each other to take full responsibility for their own sexual experience and satisfaction, then the connection between partners becomes much simpler and hence easier to successfully negotiate.

When you and your lover are sharing pleasure, how do you balance your desire to please your partner with getting your own sexual needs met? How are your requirements communicated? If a different kind of touch or attention would be better, are you likely to tell your lover, or do you hope that he or she properly interprets your facial expression and thereby gets the hint? If one of you gives instructions, is this likely to cause hurt or conflict? The potential for a negative incident during a sexual session injects an unwelcome visitor into your play in the form of tension and anxiety, the enemies of deep closeness, high excitement and high pleasure.

To increase the chances that each encounter will be remarkable, build an understanding with your lover that says: I will speak about my needs and I trust that you will speak about yours. If I want something in particular, I will ask for it. Promise to ask your partner questions about his or her experience instead of wondering powerlessly and risking proceeding unsuccessfully based on tenuous assumptions. Agree to communicate kindly and carefully. Make the promise that if you desire specific attention or pleasure, you will ask for it. Give permission to provide each other with instructions about your body and pleasure, but also discuss how those instructions are to be shared to avoid hurt.

Such agreements do initially challenge the comfort of some couples, especially those who avoid talking about sex. The roles into which partners habitually gravitate, such as sexual-event leader or passive follower, may be shaken up by these practices, but this cost is well worth the increased potential for pleasure and satisfaction. Without these rules, disconnection, negative assumption, conflict and disappointment are hiding just under the bed in every intimate encounter.

1-21. Late Night Rendezvous

Many couples choose the late night as the default time for sex. For most lovers, late night is probably the worst time for this important bonding activity. The last few minutes before sleep coincide with our lowest energy; sleeping is the reason we are in bed in the first place. Sex requires energy; good sex requires lots of energy! As a habitual practice this may be dangerous to your relationship. Regularly having sex when you are tired can all but guarantee that your sex life will fall into uninteresting routines that are vulnerable to dysfunction. As couples age, this likelihood is heightened. Only one incident of dysfunction can cast a long shadow of sexual troubles.

The reality is that in the early part of most relationships, sex is marked by high heat, passion and frequency, but slows and reduces in quality and importance as time passes. Relegating sex to the last moments of the day may be one contributing factor in this trend. Too many couples already populate the swelling "sexless marriage" category.

Keeping sex varied and exciting is vital. Changing up the times of your pleasure will help to inject some fun, but also provide the all-important energy needed for good sex. The early morning is an excellent opportunity, when privacy may also be available, obtained by setting the alarm a few minutes earlier. This is when the world is quiet. You aren't a morning person, you say? If you make yourselves receptive, you may find that sex and its arousal are more effective than coffee at waking you up. This way you will start your day with pleasure! How about a bathroom tryst beginning with a shared shower? This is a way to make your daily preparations more fun. How about an interlude of afternoon delight? Have you considered a before-dinner romp? Is an occasional lunch-time quickie ever possible? All these times in your day are far superior to the late night for satisfying your need for a deeper connection.

For partners who differ in their amounts of sexual interest, because one partner is hopeful and eager to sexually engage, while the other is equally eager to avoid that eventuality, tension is injected into the late night when relaxation should be fostered. Relaxation is an essential factor needed to prepare for restful sleep. For some, a sexual experience not only arouses them in excitement but also arouses their energy, so that afterwards sleep is unobtainable. This is not a great way to ensure being well-rested the next day.

Here are some reasons why couples choose the late night for sex, though none of them eliminate the destructive influences of this choice:

1. The opportunity for sex is afforded by evening togetherness.
2. For couples with young children, the late-night provides an occasion with privacy.
3. An orgasm is a wonderful stress relief which functions for some as a sleep aid.
4. For some, the evening is a time when lovers have "wound down" sufficiently for sexual desire to surface.
5. For others, the anonymity and therefore safety of darkness is available to make sex less anxiety-provoking.
6. If sex is not desired by one partner, procrastination efforts reach the end of the line in the late-night.

Of course, the argument that nighttime is the only available time when both you and your partner are together is often probably true. Currently, our lives are pushed to the limit with stress and demands. It is not just our sex lives that may benefit from choices that keep our lives very simple. The late-night choice proclaims that sex is the lowest item on your priority list. Giving it the crumbs of energy by making time for sex only when everything else, important or not, is complete, all but guarantees that your sex life will eventually wither, dry up and evaporate. Saying “no” to nice but unnecessary commitments can improve the quality of our lives overall and provide us with more time for essentials. We all want good relationships; maintaining yours by giving it the nourishment that it needs will reward you with that increasingly rare phenomenon...a happy, and long-term relationship.

1-22. The Key to Great Sex

A lot of people say they want great sex. There are tricks to being a great lover, many of which are not ready to be printed here. Among the more basic but nonetheless vital keys to great sex is relaxation. Disappointed? Relaxation doesn't sound very sexy. Great sex is also fun sex.

Try to recall different times when you were involved in activities that were fun for you. During these times, did you laugh at all? If you were having fun, you were probably relaxed, because having fun and being relaxed often go together. Contrary to popular belief, sex is more emotional than it is a physical activity. Our emotional state dictates the flavor of our experience and strongly affects the level of our performance, regardless of whether we are involved in a sporting competition, a job interview, a social gathering, or a sexual session with our love partner.

If stress or anxiety are present, our awareness of our bodies and sensitivity to the moment are dulled. It appears to our partner that there is simply "less of us" than if we were relaxed; just as if the volume of a beautiful song were turned very low, it would be more difficult to appreciate. If, during sex, we are worried about performing well, about satisfying our partner, about how our body looks, about our job, the kids, or, even worse, if we are disconnected from the present by thinking about problems, or mundane things like formulating our grocery shopping list, then our sexual experience will be neither relaxed nor fun. In this state, our bodies are less responsive and our experience of pleasure is likely to be muted. Our partner is sure to be aware of his or her loneliness in the sexual experience. Sex is an emotionally challenging activity during which the achievement of relaxation, especially for those who do not always delight in this kind of closeness, is difficult. If achieved, relaxation is a necessary key to fun and great sex.

1-23. Considering Sexiness

Wet from the shower, her petite foot stepped softly upon the plush bathmat. As she dried herself off, the lithe woman deliberately avoided glancing at her reflection in the bathroom mirror. Most others would consider her shape sexy, her appearance attractive; she truly does not. Those times when she does look at herself, she cannot hold back from harshly criticizing her thighs, tummy, breasts and butt. She finds herself lacking in beauty and sexiness.

What is "sexy?" Who decides? Sexiness is flaunted by the attention-craving media and used ceaselessly by advertisers to motivate us to buy their products. Sexiness has both cultural and individual definitions. In a potent way, the over-arching cultural definition of “sexy” rides roughshod over our personal preferences, disabling accurate self-appraisal and destroying the positive self-esteem of many. The culture says sexy is young, female, busty and usually blonde. This is important because ninety-nine percent of us are frequently and painfully reminded that this is an ideal to which we fail to measure up.

In a desperate attempt to more closely resemble this narrow ideal, many resort to risky surgeries, extreme diets, and expensive styling to tweak themselves. The quest to be sexy often dominates over the need to be healthy. The surface identities of many of us float on a sea of shame. When a person does not believe that they look beautiful or sexy, they conclude that they have little value. The effect of this phenomenon is that many feel so painfully insecure that intimacy, openness and vulnerability become hurdles that are too high to clear. As a result, love relationships cannot be tolerated.

The cultural phenomenon of sexy is built from men's visual appraisal of feminine desirability, women's intensely high valuing of beauty, and the innate hunger to be desired. The rush to be sexy leaves most of us far behind, feeling unsexy, and hugely inadequate. The less confident people are in their own intrinsic value, the greater their need to cultivate desirability and sexiness from shallow external qualities.

Lost in our relentless drive to place the newest perfectly sexy woman upon a pedestal, is the less dramatic reality that sexiness is truly an inner attitude of strengths and confidence. The fixation upon physical attributes carries with it the high cost of emotional disability which prevents loving and closeness. Feeling flawed, many are uncomfortable with any intimacy that they fear could reveal their insecurity and subsequent shame to another. If feeling sexy or beautiful is a precondition for both love and sex, because of this cultural phenomenon, many people will not abundantly enjoy either love or sex.

The prevailing definition of sexy says that those of us older than thirty-five have no business even trying to fulfill this ideal; older bodies are not sexy bodies. If you depend upon your physical appearance to feel valuable, then aging means losing your identity and value. This is a very painful loss; hence mature women refuse to reveal their ages, or lie jokingly at their birthday celebrations that they just turned nineteen. In long term relationships, especially for aging partners, sexiness must make the transition away from physical appearance and onto more enduring strengths if desirability is to remain alive.

People possessing a good sense of humor are seen as intensely attractive, even if they are not conventionally beautiful. A courageous act may elevate an ordinary-looking citizen to sexy hero status. When displaying deep love, care for another, or the strength it takes to allow vulnerability, a person may suddenly become very sexy in another's eyes. Kindness, caring, intelligence and confidence elevate each one of us to the realm of sexy and desirable. Touching the heart by showing sensitivity and consideration can transform another into an admirer.

In private, in the confines of a cozy bedroom, sexy is the partner who allows complete openness during intense sexual excitement. Sexiness may be shown by fully surrendering to a partner and being confident in love, while courageously expressing enthusiasm. Character strengths are sexy.

We should not deny external beauty, but nor should we get so fixated upon it that we lose sight of the deeper universal strengths that earn admiration. Few of us have god or goddess-like good looks or perfectly shaped bodies, but, despite our imperfections, what makes each one of us sexy is our capacity to love others, ourselves and life.

1-24. Emotionally Sexy

Sex is automatically regarded as a physical activity. Missing from this consideration are the emotions, which potently impact each sexual drama. Two constantly-engaged processes make up our moment-to-moment awareness; the first is the mind with its intellectual, rational cycle of thoughts; the other is our emotional process, demonstrated by a constant flow of feelings in reaction to the influx of ever-changing events. The emotional component of our being strongly influences how we experience situations, by coloring our perceptions. Our emotions also represent the main influencing factor when making choices. The way our emotions sway our experiences facilitates or blocks our ability to be relaxed, which enhances the flow of life force within our bodies. Just like non-sexual actions, sex, physical pleasure, and orgasm are the products of flowing life forces within our bodies.

Think about it...if you are experiencing uncomfortable emotions, your experience is dulled; you are slowed in your reaction time; your productivity level drops; your energy level is lower; your quality of life is poorer. The energy within your body is slowed by negative emotion the way electric current is slowed by a resistor. This is instinctive; when feeling bad, many romantic partners will say “no” to a sexual invitation, with the quip, “I’m just not in the mood.” In other words, the lover’s energy is just not flowing, or it would take too much effort to get the flow of energy started.

Over long periods of time, emotional habits and living out of balance cause a very slow, often undetected, accumulation of negative emotions, such as depression, frustration, resentment or anxiety. Chronic stress also causes many people to build defenses, manifested as an emotional wall against the sexual partner. Low self-esteem, poor self-image and discomfort with one’s body all are symptoms of the presence of these negative emotions. Resentment towards a partner may also be a potent negative force, blocking the flow of passion. Unlike thoughts, emotions cannot simply be switched off. Emotions are slow to change; slow to heal. Just as it is difficult to light a fire with damp wood, negative emotional build-up prevents "the fire" of good sexual desire, response, arousal, and orgasm. People who have significant internalized negative emotions are likely to experience sex as an activity in which they do not "feel" what they should in terms of pleasure, and often do not perform up to their own or their partner's expectations. Negative emotions contribute strongly to developing sexual problems and the stubbornness that prevents healing.

Partners who have experienced trauma, sexual or otherwise, may experience lingering negative emotion which prevents them from sexually functioning at all. Past hurtful experiences often interfere with feeling safe during sex, which is among the most vulnerable of activities. Calming anxiety is the key to good sexual pleasure and performance, not just for traumatized lovers, but for all of us.

The opposite of anxiety is relaxation. During sex, all positive aspects of sex are facilitated when we are relaxed and open to the flow of life energy in our bodies, thus opening the channels to connection, arousal, pleasure and orgasm. Relaxation is an ever-deepening state in which pure being is the extreme, a state in which old emotions are healed. Very deep relaxation temporarily frees us from all emotion. Being emotionally healthy helps us to be sexually healthy. The reverse is also true; participating in an active, healthy sex life helps heal unhealthy emotions by making us more aware of them, but also by opening us up to what is beyond them.

PLEASURE

2-1. The "Mmmmm" Word

Our relationship with ourselves is no different than any other love relationship; sex can be a way to express love. Pleasuring ourselves is one way to nourish a positive relationship within. Yes. I am writing about masturbation. Shocked? Strongly associated with shame and embarrassment, masturbation remains a hidden act, intensely private, which is rarely spoken of or admitted; yet it is widely, commonly practiced. The derisive nicknames: jacking off, jilling off, diddling, spanking the monkey, choking the chicken and so on, point to the associated shame, and the reason masturbation is kept a secret.

Unborn babies have been observed pleasuring themselves in utero. Infants and young children naturally explore their genitals, a practice often discouraged with the slap of a parental hand. Masturbation is a normal part of human sexual development, and if discouraged it can have long term negative effects on adult sexual health, such as increased likelihood of future sexual dysfunction and dissatisfaction.

A quote attributed to the famous sex researcher William Masters, of Masters and Johnson, reads,"99% of men masturbate and 1% lie about it." After questioning 3019 women, Shere Hite, who completed a large study of female sexuality in 1978, found that 82% of the female respondents masturbated at least occasionally. Such research suggests that sexually pleasuring oneself is not just normal but is common. It is only in public discourse that masturbation is rare.

Giving ourselves sexual pleasure facilitates a positive connection with our bodies and our sexuality. Some view it solely as a substitute for partner sex. Yet many experience masturbation as a distinct and vital activity which stands alone, giving each of us a sense of control over our sexuality and pleasure. The healthy frequency of solo sex ranges broadly from twice daily to twice annually. Both ends of the spectrum may represent a point of health. Masturbating frequently is unhealthy if it interferes with daily responsibilities, harms personal health, is compulsive, or replaces or forms a barrier to a healthy sex life with a partner. Infrequent self-pleasuring signals a health problem if it represents shame about one's body or sexuality, is due to an absence of sexual desire or accompanies a dissatisfying sex life with a partner.

Benefits from self-pleasuring are many and varied, such as the development of sexual skills and body-awareness that can be used to guide and educate a partner in creating sexual success. It may facilitate greater sexual abilities, such as increased female orgasmic potential or improved male ejaculatory control. In fact, masturbation is a practice encouraged by sexual health professionals as a way of helping sexually dysfunctional individuals to become functional. Women who do not give themselves self-love are less likely to be orgasmic. Some use self-pleasuring purely and simply as a method of stress reduction. Since being single does not mean that sexual desire stops, masturbation helps those who do not have an available sexual partner to cope.

Do you and your partner include masturbation in your intimate experiences? Many couples do not because of its strong negative stigma, considering self-stimulation as too intimate or embarrassing to even share with the lover. It may, nevertheless, be a new, intimacy-deepening activity to add to your sexual repertoire.

The most noble service masturbation provides, however, is helping relationship partners who possess widely varying sexual needs, otherwise known as a discrepancy of sexual desire. There would be a much higher rate of break up between such couples, who are often wracked with conflict about how frequently sex should happen, if masturbation did not help to fill the void created by the difference between the high sexual need of one partner and the low interest of the other.

Masturbation is a healthy, simple, no-cost, pleasurable, loving gift to yourselves. When combined with orgasm, which it almost always is, it is very good for your health, so long as it is free of shame. It can be argued that if we were not meant to give ourselves sexual pleasure, we would have been born with shorter arms!

2-2. The Clitoris: Tiny but Mighty

Descending far down through the dense and deep forest thicket, further down into the canyon cleft, there is a rise. Under that rise and hidden beneath a protective layer rests a silver pearl. She is the princess, waiting to be awakened.

She is the clitoris, the tiny little secret, and the main organ of female sexual pleasure. No other quarter inch spot on a human body, male or female, is more tightly packed with nerve endings, making the clitoris intensely sensitive and capable of providing great sexual pleasure. Because of her location on a woman's body, the clitoris has no direct reproductive purpose, unlike a man's penis. Stimulation of the clitoris is the way to female arousal and orgasm.

Lack of information, misinformation and myth cloud the reality of the clitoris. Even in mid-life, some women are unaware of the clitoris as the center of their body's capacity for sexual pleasure. Many male partners are uninformed about the role of the clitoris in female pleasure and arousal, and both partners are often uninformed as to the vital role of the clitoris in achieving orgasm and its lack of involvement during intercourse, leading to unrealistic sexual expectations and resultant disappointment regarding pleasure, orgasm and sexual confidence.

Outside the body, the clitoris is tiny, but internally, its size rivals that of a man's penis. During the development of a person in utero, the same cells develop into either a clitoris or a penis, depending upon influential gender hormones. Both organs are equally capable of providing its owner with great pleasure.

Yet there remains huge differences between how each functions, especially for reproductive purposes, contributing to misunderstanding of the clitoris. Many men assume that the clitoris, or something similar resides inside the vagina, causing intercourse to be equal in experience and pleasure for the female partner. This is not so, it is proven when comparing the number of women who orgasm during intercourse to men, which is about 30% to 100%. For most women, intercourse does not lead to orgasm, because the clitoris is located outside their vaginas.

Tightly packed with thousands of nerve endings, the experience of pleasure when stimulated may still vary. When using a light with a dimmer switch, even though the light is on, the brightness of the bulb may vary depending upon the dimmer setting. Similarly, the sensitivity of the clitoris' nerve endings vary depending upon many factors, including attitude towards sex (negative emotion has this same dimming effect on the clitoris' sensitivity). Stimulating an unaroused clitoris may cause discomfort. A woman who is unable to relax, who is preoccupied with worry, or experiencing any negative emotion will notice that her clitoral sensitivity is "dimmed" or it may even be unresponsive.

Male partners find confusing the fickle nature of the way a woman is pleased, and the receptiveness of her clitoris. Unlike men, who are generally less dynamically influenced by their emotions, and therefore experience less variation in sexual response, women may vary greatly in how they like to be touched, stimulated and stroked. The clitoris being so small, under varying conditions, some partners are challenged to both locate it and provide a touch which is pleasing for that unique moment.

Given the variability of the clitoris, it is wise for a woman's partner to be receptive to her guidance and instructions, and for the woman to be brave enough to offer them. A useful method for teaching a new partner is to place the clitoris owner's hand over the partner's hand to demonstrate the kind of motion, direction, pressure, speed and intensity of touch desired, and whether or not such method of stroking should be varied or maintained to maximize pleasure.

Tiny but mighty, the clitoris is the pathway to intense pleasure in your female partner. Through listening to her and learning, mastering the variety of touches and strokes is one way of showing deep love.

2-3. The Oooh in Orgasm

At the pinnacle of each sexual experience, tension and high excitement release into pleasure-filled waves of bliss for an experience called "orgasm." This release is so highly sought after that many do not consider a sexual experience complete without it. Both the rapidly-growing multibillion-dollar pornography industry and the thriving sex toy industry depend on the value people place on heightening their orgasmic experience.

People need ecstasy and bliss. An ecstatic experience is one in which ordinary awareness gets a boost from something much larger and deeper within us. The experience of orgasm is one way to obtain these incredibly strong feelings, which many crave so greatly that they fall into self-destructive activities that provide only a hint of these peak states. People drink alcohol and take drugs to satisfy their need for ecstasy. Bliss can be experienced with making an exciting purchase while shopping, or tasting food that is "just divine" or "out of this world." Winning at a sporting event or on a gambling bet provides a little bit of bliss. Most unhealthy dependencies are formed out of the desire for ecstasy and bliss. Ecstasy is also experienced in orgasm, but orgasm itself is very healthy.

During an orgasm, physiological changes occur that promote health and well-being. Levels of serotonin and important chemicals increase in the brain. This causes us to feel good and healthy, while also reducing depression. Levels of oxytocin, known as the love hormone, also increase, resulting in feelings of love, calmness and relaxation. Endorphins are released upon orgasm, increasing our tolerance of pain, and studies show that men who have regular orgasms have a low risk of prostate cancer. So in addition to feeling good, orgasms are good for our health.

Obviously, orgasms are different in men and women. In men, orgasm is almost always linked to ejaculation, a vital event for the reproduction of our species. With women, an orgasm has no direct link to any reproductive benefit except for pleasure, which encourages sex. Another large difference between the genders is that men do not learn to have an orgasm; instead, they usually experience it spontaneously during puberty through what is called a wet dream. On the contrary, women have no such spontaneous event and must consciously learn to become orgasmic. While most are capable of learning, some women never do. Sadly, the lack of orgasm can negatively affect women's self-esteem and the quality of their love relationships. Despite efforts to develop orgasmic ability, not-yet-orgasmic women often do not practice self pleasure frequently enough or for long enough duration to achieve success.

Orgasm is among the healthy ways to include an ecstatic experience in your daily life. The potential for orgasm is built within you.

2-4. Pipeline to Pleasure

Our bodies are made in such a way that, if they are healthy, sex will be pleasurable. For those who do not like sex, odds are that it is not pleasurable, and it follows that then there will be no desire for it. While the causes of discomfort with sex are many, this article will focus on what helps to make it a pleasurable experience.

The largest single factor determining whether sex is pleasurable or not is a lover's ability to relax, a mantra which I have repeatedly expressed. To produce sexual pleasure, the need for relaxation extends to all parts of our being, increasing in importance as we age. To be receptive and ready for very good sexual experiences, our minds, emotions, bodies, and love relationships must all be aligned. Even though a lamp is plugged into the wall, it doesn't mean that it is turned on. Flicking the switch is a deliberate choice, as is being receptive.

Think of a water pipeline formed by segments of pipe. In order for the pipe to deliver water, all the segments of the pipe must be connected, aligned and open, otherwise the water will not flow. From a sexual perspective, we function similarly: for sexual energy in our bodies to flow and create arousal, the "segments" of our minds, emotions and bodies must all be aligned in receptivity. If misaligned, arousal will not occur, or will only rise to a limited degree. For a person who doesn't get turned on, he or she is likely to say, "I don't like sex." or "I don't know why people think sex is such a big deal."

Some partners complain that preparations for a sexual encounter require getting over a difficult emotional "hump." Once beyond this hurdle, they feel free to fully enjoy the experience. Many agree that this is like going on vacation; the preparations of packing and arrangements are tedious, but once at their vacation destination, most are glad they went. The analogy represents the efforts to "align" the emotional segment of the pipeline by identifying and neutralizing the negative influence of difficult emotions. Old and negative beliefs about sex may be emotional obstacles. Emotional pain left over from past wounds can also interfere.

The mind represents another pipeline segment. From a sexual standpoint, the mind can be a huge obstacle, unless it is empty or erotically focused with sexy thoughts. Such thoughts promote arousal. Distracting thoughts and worries all block arousal and represent a segment out of alignment. The mind takes its lead from the prevailing emotions...if negative emotions are present, the mind will stray. To align the mind, it must be made still, which may be accomplished by being fully present to all sensations in the moment.

The body, too, needs to be in a receptive state. Our bodies are a storage receptacle for our rejected, unintegrated emotions. A person's body is available for pleasure and arousal if emptied of tension. Clues that it is not receptive include responding to touch with ticklishness, discomfort, startling, or by tensing up. A tense body is a pipe segment misaligned for the flow of sexual energy and thus arousal may not be achieved, limiting the possibility of pleasure.

The final segment of this pipeline is the emotional connection between partners. If partners are well-connected in love, relaxed and feeling safe, their openness can invite an exchange of arousal, which may energize an upward spiral of excitement, lifting both partners to great heights of pleasure. This happens when our minds, emotions and bodies are relaxed while also aligned for a single sexual purpose...to be open, to love and to feel pleasure.

> Drugs and alcohol make you feel *real good...* while they destroy your life.

2-5. G Wizz!

Unknown to many lovers is the mysterious and marvelous G-spot. Named for the German gynecologist Ernst Gräfenberg, but already previously known for centuries by ancient Taoist and Tantra sexual practitioners, the G-spot is located inside a woman's vagina. If stimulated properly by a lover, it can provide a lucky woman with exquisite pleasure. Within the fields of sexology and female reproductive health much debate has been raised by the phenomenon of the G-spot. While its physical existence remains unproven by many studies, and is merely suggested to be real by others, it has been emphatically claimed as truly existing by many women. The fact that no single study has confirmed specific proof that a physical G-spot actually exists, suggests that the intense pleasure associated with G-spot stimulation may be caused by a combination of physical, emotional, and energetic factors, not easily measurable. Adding to its allure is the female ejaculation or expulsion of a, usually clear, fluid from the urethra, occurring simultaneously with an intensely powerful orgasm. Studies have confirmed that the ejaculate is different from urine.

Both G-spot orgasms and female ejaculation are likely to be of interest to adventurous lovers who prefer intense ecstatic experiences. Not only may succeeding at achieving these heights of sexual fun offer satisfying thrills, but the great openness and vulnerability required by sharing of such profound experimentation provides women with feelings of liberation, while also deepening the bond between partners. G-spot stimulation also provides the potential for healing old wounds, especially those of a sexually traumatic nature, because old, painful emotions may be stored in this part of a woman's body.

The G-spot is located one to two inches inside the vagina on the front wall, under or behind the pubic bone and generally behind the clitoris. It is stimulated best with a partner's fingers, inserted when the female partner is on her back with the partner's palm facing up and fingers stroking the G-spot location with a "come here" kind of motion. However, specially curved vibrators are available that are designed for G-spot stimulation. Locating this sensitive spot, which may be felt as a rough and raised patch on the vaginal wall, may take a bit of trial and error, as well as good communication between partners. Simultaneous clitoral stimulation may be helpful. Emotional safety and unflagging positive support provided by a woman's sexual partner are necessary elements, as a woman must relax and let go completely to experience such a profound release. Pressure by a partner will only prevent success. As with any new sexual activity, time and practice are necessary to develop comfort, competency and success.

A common obstacle for many women is that initial G-spot stimulation causes the sensation of needing to urinate, which can raise the specter of an embarrassing moment. This is because of the G-Spot's proximity to the urethra. A natural tendency for most women is to tense up in reaction to this sensation. Success will arrive when despite this fear, a woman relaxes into it. With patient tolerance, getting beyond this discomfort may yield great rewards. Spontaneous ejaculation during orgasm is not unusual early in a young woman's active sex life. However, uninformed and inexperienced, most women react with horror that they urinated during an intimate moment. Uninformed about the phenomenon of female ejaculation and its normality, most women are unable to distinguish between urine and ejaculate. Forever after, such women remain sexually on-guard for fear of repeating this kind of embarrassing moment. The vigilance they enforce can harm their sexual excitement and pleasure while also blocking the high intensity of future orgasms with ejaculation.

Female proponents of G-spot stimulation and ejaculation, especially those who teach others how to develop this capacity, claim that every woman is capable of learning to achieve orgasms with ejaculation. Sexologists express concern about the notion that some women may achieve G-spot orgasms and ejaculation, but others will feel pressure to succeed at this new sexual benchmark, and feel like a failure if they don't succeed. You must realize the important truth that all love-based sexual pleasure and orgasms are good, and that not all women need to pursue G-spot orgasms or ejaculation to be good enough. Should a woman be open to this exploration, the benefits may include healing, empowerment, a potentially deeper connection with her partner, and a whole lot of pleasure.

2-6. Making it Good, Even Great

Sex is automatically regarded as a physical activity. Lost is that mind, body and spirit must be included if romantic partners are to fully love each other. If delivered sincerely, love causes a partner to relax and open up in receptivity. Conversely, if love is withheld or insensitively given, a partner may shut down as a means of self-protection. In the form of sexual activity when bodies are included in loving, sex may be either good or bad, satisfying or dissatisfying. Bad sex fails to bridge the gap of separateness between partners; without sex achieving "good" status, love relationships remain vulnerable because the bond has not been nourished. The promise to share deeply connecting moments of ecstasy remains unfulfilled.

What is good sex? Though not exactly the same for each lover, a general set of characteristics contribute to making sex good rather than bad. Achieving this nebulous goal is not always easy, because sex resides in the land of taboo and is often tainted by shame. Sexual problems may not be easily discussed or resolved. In the game of baseball, players must together coordinate their efforts, so if the ball is thrown to first base to get out the opposing player, it must be thrown to the right spot in the right way at the right time for the play to succeed. Sex, likewise, is a team activity. Partners make it good by coordinating their efforts to give that which is best at the right time and in the right way.

Good sex requires mutual partner satisfaction. For some couples, this may be as simple as each partner experiencing orgasm, a bar set rather low. Partners with higher expectations seek lengthier, more pleasure-filled sessions. The degree to which partners feel close and deeply well-connected is another consideration as to whether sex is of high quality. Lovers being open and relaxed creates this possibility. At its best, the connection of sexual partners escalates into a merging where partners forget about themselves, and all separateness is lost in a blissful fog of pleasure.

What fosters such ecstasy? Partners who give generously, lack inhibition, and are non-judgemental are open to learning about the other's sources of sexual pleasure. In good sex, partners become a well-coordinated and well-lubricated team for mutual satisfaction. Communication during sex, if shared carefully, offers guidance for dynamic adjustments so sexual play matches the mood of the unique moment. Talking gently back and forth ensures that each lover gets the touching right. Partner sensitivity facilitates this success. If each partner has the confidence that he or she will be unhesitatingly listened to and responded to, the sexual arena is made safe. Safety enables relaxation, a necessary requirement to open the gates of bliss.

Good sex is free from mechanical actions that suggest that partners are not open to the present moment. Being in the present means that togetherness is fully alive. When partners are completely present, the potential for connection and nourishment that comes from loving touch is at its highest. Deeply satisfying experiences are also free from conflict and power struggles. A parallel exists between sex and communication; being understood feels satisfying, whereas argument and misunderstanding is frustrating. When another "gets us" it feels good. In the sexual arena, having someone "get us" is no different.

There is little is more exciting than a totally turned on partner. Generously exhibiting and expressing excitement will infect the other with high arousal, much the way one candle may light another. Good sex includes high excitement. When both partners are expressive, and each, in turn, excites the other, the intensity of sexual play grows higher and higher in an upward spiral of intense arousal. For many lovers, letting their play go a bit beyond the border of what is regular into new territory, going where they have not gone before, adds to higher excitement. The potential in sex is for love to be expanded to unimaginable heights, which is unfortunately far beyond the expectations of most lovers. Good sex is a loving adventure that can leave both partners grateful and breathless with wonderment.

> In a love relationship, strength is not how much you can lift, it is how much you can love.

2-7. Eroticism: What Turns Us On

Deep within the recesses of who we know ourselves to be, unresolved conflicts reside, which first developed when we were small children. We cling to these conflicts dearly. We regard them as deeply personal and intensely intimate. Such internal dilemmas guide us when we choose the content from our unlimited imagination to populate our sexual fantasies with choices perfectly tailored to suit our erotic needs. Situations are erotic when they cause us to be sexually excited and aroused.

Many people have buried their eroticism so that the impulse to create a fantasy does not exist for them. It does in fact exist, but lies outside of their conscious awareness. A myriad of social pressures, of should-haves and could-haves, of rights and wrongs, have strongly influenced many to repress their eroticism so that they may join those who are regarded as being acceptable and "good enough" by others.

As children, being small and surrounded by powerful and able adults, the threat that our needs would not be met was ever-present. The resulting childish conflicts are simple; to gain the power to overcome powerlessness, to gain control to overcome feelings of being out of control, and to gain certainty in order to overcome uncertainty. That is why so many sexual fantasies are dramas of power, in which we may delight in our powerfulness or powerlessness, or we may free ourselves by overcoming laws or limitations. The sources of our sexual excitement are so deep and near our center that they are sources of tremendous vulnerability; hence we label them as too deeply personal to commonly be shared, often even with our life partners. Yet sexual fantasies are not uncommon, and their plots can even be seen as formulaic.

When we are with our lover, hopefully in a sexual garden of delight, playfulness is valuable. Eroticism and sexuality are adults' play. We play at creating scenarios that include body, mind and spirit while exploring ways to resolve these deep conflicts so as to feel free. By doing so intense pleasure is produced.

Passion in our love play is the brass ring in what is universally called "good sex." In order to experience the full possibilities of joining with the one we love, without exception, all of our self must be shared. By first knowing and then revealing our eroticism we truly make ourselves vulnerable, but also open ourselves to levels of love that are widely sought after and deeply valued. Knowing our own eroticism is essential to value ourselves and our sexuality.

2-8. Porn Pros and Con

Pornography is not just negative. In the case of guns, it's how they are used that makes them dangerous. The analogy continues with cars; cars help a great many people, but if used carelessly, people may be killed by them. Pornography is often the focus of negative attention because of moral considerations, but pornography has flourished in part because sexuality is such a huge and important part of our lives as human beings.

The mere presence of such a large variety of pornography only underscores sexuality's vitality and importance. Unless we fully accept our sexuality in a healthy and positive way, it will always surface in our consciousness and our world in distorted, perverted, and unhealthy ways.

It is the tendency in the media for topics to come to attention when they grow to become problematic; however, during times of normality issues go unnoticed. Pornography is used by many individuals in ways that are not damaging to either love relationships, personal morality or healthy sexuality, but these situations tend not to be worthy of concern.

It is completely true that pornography and sexuality have a dark side and that much of the sex industry lives within this dark side. It is also true that sexuality is tremendously important to all of us, and has a large, but untapped bright side in our social consciousness.

Much of the problem with pornography is that it is used by a great many people to gain sexual pleasure and satisfaction while avoiding intimacy. As a result, as a sex therapist, I see many couples without an active sex life and an emotional disconnection while one partner, often the male partner, masturbates frequently while using pornography. This is certainly a negative phenomenon and allows coupled individuals to avoid addressing a challenging difficulty. However, there are also a large number of married spouses who find a large discrepancy in the level of sexual desire between the partners. The use of pornography in this situation by the higher-desire spouse actually aids the couple's intimacy by avoiding the build-up of destructive tension between partners. Of course, this only works when the use of pornography is open and accepted by the lower-desire partner.

A huge problem associated with pornography is porn addiction, also referred to as sexual compulsivity. Because sex is pleasurable, a disproportionately male tendency is to seek sexual pleasure to calm issues linked to anxiety, stress and self-esteem. People who use porn for this purpose become increasingly isolated and emotionally trapped in a compulsive cycle of pleasure-seeking.

Yet I recently learned about a study in which the researchers looked at the use of pornography and found a causal link between the use of pornography and a reduction in sexually related crimes such as rape.

Of the many couples I have talked to while providing treatment, it is not unusual for them to have utilized some form of pornography, whether it be images, videos or literature, to enhance their sexual experiences. Some have utilized porn in order to learn and practice different forms of sexual activity, to increase excitement and variety.

Many of my patients who struggle with their sexuality have needed to understand their own eroticism in a better way. The use of pornography aids their exploration and helps them to understand their own eroticism.

At its best, pornography is fantasy created in one of a variety of media. Fantasy is an extremely healthy activity which allows each one of us to experience things that we desire, or about which we are curious, while at the same time not taking any risks or challenging real-life limitations, boundaries and laws. It is a freedom that is essential to our well-being.

Certainly, at its worst, pornography debases our morality, our spirit, our soul, and our sexuality. There is no doubt that the darkest aspect of our sexuality leads to sexual slavery, darkness, and the lowest form of human expression. It is up to each one of us to use our strength and our love to express our sexuality in a way which raises up the level of our entire humanity.

> We grow a little every time we don't take advantage of another's weakness.
>
> —*Bern Williams*

2-9. Living Longer, With Pleasure

Our very active media generously offers us guidance about what is healthy and what is not. Yet all too often it seems that the advice says that, in order to be healthy, we must give up something we enjoy. I am not going to do that. Instead, I wish to tell you about a way to experience more pleasure while also living healthier, longer lives. Have more sex! Sex is extremely healthy for our bodies and emotions and also protects our marriages from the many destructive forces spouses encounter. Unlike other ways to maintain our health and marriage, it is pleasurable.

A collection of studies from 1972 to the present offer strong evidence that sex is healthy and that having regular sexual activity and frequently experiencing orgasms protects our health and promotes our well-being in a wide variety of ways. One example, that will come as good news to those of you who deeply value an attractive appearance, is a ten-year study which found that people who engage in sex more frequently tend to appear more youthful than those who have sex less often.

For those people who wish to delay death (most of us!), several studies, including a longitudinal study of 918 middle-aged men, found that the men who experienced more frequent orgasms reduced their risk of death by 50% compared to those who enjoyed less frequent sexual pleasure. The same study specifically linked frequent of sexual intercourse with a 50% reduction in the risk of death by a coronary incident. Does this mean more loving strengthens one's heart? The study does not conclude this exactly, but it may be so.

It appears that having more sexual pleasure also means experiencing less pain. Several scientific studies have concluded that enjoying sexual pleasure, including orgasm, can increase a person's pain threshold, effectively reducing the subjective discomfort a person feels. If we agree that a higher quality of life is related to feeling less pain, then sexual activity is an effective method to obtain this higher quality of life.

Ever said no to your partner's wish for sex due to a headache? A 2001 study found that orgasms reduced the pain of a headache more quickly than did medicine. A similar, but different study found that having an orgasm relieved some of the pain of migraines. So next time, do not let that headache deter you!

Other studies have concluded that sexual activity benefits women's reproductive health, making the menstrual cycle more regular, reducing the severity of cramps and reducing the risk of developing endometriosis, while also lowering the risk of breast cancer. For men, frequent ejaculations lower the risk of prostate cancer. By enjoying regular sex, both genders have ensured a lengthening of their sexually active lives, thus confirming the saying, "Use it or lose it."

Having more sex is emotionally beneficial. Studies have found that frequent sex is good for your mental health, protecting against depression. I am sure it will come as no surprise to you that sex has positive effects on love relationships, improving the qualities of intimacy and relationship satisfaction. Given that sex is one of the issues that is most often a point of conflict between spouses, making your sex-life satisfying is one way to ensure that your marriage will be long-lasting.

Regular sex lengthens our lives and makes them less painful, healthier, and of higher quality. If you wish to learn about the benefits of sexual health and the studies referenced in greater detail, go to the article entitled, "The Health Benefits of Sexual Expression," online at: http:// www.plannedparenthood.org /resources/research-papers/ sexual-expression-6358.htm.

2-10. Multiplying Your Pleasure

Attaining Multiple Orgasm

It is easy to get the impression that multiple orgasms are a phenomenon only accessible to certain lucky women and sexual Olympians, and unavailable to ordinary citizens like you or me. It is also widely believed that men are barred from enjoying the increased intense pleasure of multiple orgasms. These conclusions are not matched by reality. Experiencing more than one orgasm in a single sexual session is possible with routine and consistent practice of simple exercises over several months. Both men and women are equally gifted with the capacity to expand their pleasure beyond a single climax.

Sound like an exaggerated claim? It is not. Our nervous system is like the electrical grid which powers our homes, but instead of electricity, excited sexual energy flows within the "wiring" of our bodies to produce sexual pleasure. It takes a lot of energy to create heat, as evidenced by your electric or oil bill during the winter. When a person is sexually attractive to us, he or she is said to be "hot." When we get physically aroused, we feel heat in our bodies, usually near our genitals. This heat is the byproduct of a lot of energy, which can be used more efficiently to create greater pleasure than most allow themselves.

The ability to experience more than one orgasm depends upon how we circulate this heat, or sexual energy, not just in and around our sex parts, but throughout our entire body's nervous system. To do this well requires that we eliminate the obstacles that interfere with the energy's transmission. Negative emotions, shame, discomfort with one's body, or negative feelings about sex all block the flow of sexual energy, which is vital to increased pleasure and the possibility of multiple orgasms. The more deeply relaxed we are, the greater the pleasure to which we have access. Having full awareness of our sexual response adds to our comfort and the depth of relaxation. Deliberate and consistent practice places such benefits within reach.

Men have equal capacity for multiple orgasms, but, unlike

women, they must first master the task of separating orgasm from ejaculation, an achievement that few men know is possible. Most men will feel a shiver down their spine at the thought of those embarrassing moments when failure to control the timing of their ejaculation saddles them with feelings of masculine failure and inadequacy. Ejaculatory control problems are the most common sexual dysfunction. Training to achieve multiple orgasms begins with practices that build the kind of control about which most men only dream.

Why would a person wish to develop this capacity? Increased pleasure alone might not justify the effort, but beyond the pleasure are other significant benefits. By circulating the highly nourishing sexual energy throughout the body, all organs are nourished, greatly adding to physical health. For men, this results in a sexual experience that is energizing and increases their ejaculatory control. The greatest benefit, however, is when both partners have developed the ability to have multiple orgasms, and enjoy a dramatically deeper connection, both during lovemaking and well beyond.

2-11. Fantasies

In our fantasies, where our creative abilities are unlimited, we can fly, be very rich and powerful, be loved completely and have the greatest sex imaginable. Fantasy serves our sexuality well. Imagination, the engine of fantasy, is like an empty movie set within which we, as the writer/producer, can place anything. What and who we choose to populate our fantasies with is at our own, completely free discretion. The way we design our fantasies strongly reveals our need for love, desirability, power, safety, and freedom.

Our sexual fantasies are strongly linked to our eroticism, the part of us which reacts to certain elements and situations with sexual excitement and arousal. Our erotic part is primal and does not know boundaries, yet serves as the director of our fantasy productions by guiding us in our choices about what kind of fantasy serves us best for our purpose at any given moment.

A strong fantasy life helps us grow emotionally, sexually and spiritually. In a fantasy, we are able to defy the rules of right and wrong by possessing the freedom to overcome real-life obstacles. In this imaginary domain, risk-free experiment is possible within sexual scenarios that are forbidden and unobtainable in the real world. Within the confines of fantasy, we may safely work out painful emotional challenges. The need for sexual novelty in many long-term relationships is frequently unmet; many marriages are saved by the palliative effect which fantasies offer to provide sexual novelty without risking infidelity.

A valuable aspect of fantasy is the facility to create excitement and foster arousal where insufficient stimulation is present, an unfortunate condition existing in the sex lives of too many couples. Our culture and committed relationships demand loyalty to many limiting factors that are not shared by our sexuality and eroticism, both of which are not nearly so selective. Fantasy helps us, especially people with greater sexual desire, to manage this difference while lessening the destruction to social order. Finally, our ability to fantasize provides us with the opportunity to test out ways to be sexual in a "trial run" mode before inclusion in real-life sex play.

Many people have trouble relaxing during sex, a symptom of a busy mind that cannot be slowed down and which interferes with achieving high arousal. Using fantasy is an effective strategy to harness the busy mind with an activity that not only does not block excitement or arousal, but adds to it. Our fantasies are like an erotic fingerprint that tells us exactly what our deeper needs are and what growth we should best pursue. Each time we fantasize, we are building an environment in which our need to grow is met by practicing ownership of the missing ingredient.

Yet our sexual fantasies do not belong to the domain of our intellectual mind, so the tendency to judge our fantasies is ill-placed. Fantasies are neither good nor bad; they are solely an expression of our inner state and need. When we judge them, we lose the opportunity to learn something about ourselves. Our fantasies of violent scenarios, ones that cause us inner moral conflicts, are normal and signify that necessary emotional work to integrate past injuries is in process.

Do we need to feel desirable? Does an inner sense of powerlessness cause you to fantasize about being powerful? Are your fantasies populated with people who adore you? Your fantasies speak most clearly about who you are and the direction of growth you need the most. Pay attention to these inner dramatic creations to learn more about yourself.

WHEN SEX HAS PROBLEMS

3-1. Delayed Takeoff

The plane sat still on the tarmac. Inside, the passengers waited impatiently, hoping that takeoff would happen soon. Hundreds of details must always line up perfectly for a plane to take off. When would the air-traffic control tower finally send the message, "Cleared for takeoff"?

Some men are like that...they do not take off, or take a very long time to do so. Other men cannot finish at all, no matter how hard they try. Just like the passengers on the plane, if that plane doesn't take off, irritability and frustration will result. If not corrected, the difficulty or inability for a man to ejaculate can have troubling effects on the man, his partner and their relationship.

Delayed ejaculation, manifested by a struggle to ejaculate, is a sexual problem that doesn't get much press. Premature ejaculation, the more common and well-known difficulty, is its opposite. Both are regarded as problems of controlling the impulse; they represent a man's limited ejaculatory choice. With premature ejaculation, men have difficulty preventing ejaculation from happening before they are ready, while delayed ejaculation is when a man cannot do so when he wishes. Generally, men find it challenging to last long enough before ejaculating to fully please a female partner, as women are slower to gain arousal and orgasm. Because of the value of being a long-lasting lover, delayed ejaculation can seem like a blessing of endurance.

Deeper within, if a man knows that he cannot easily finish, he will approach each sexual encounter with trepidation. Contrary to popular belief, men, too, fake orgasms. Men who cannot ejaculate sometimes fake orgasms to lower the pressure between themselves and their partners caused by this problem. Feelings of embarrassment, shame, inadequacy, and confusion accelerate once the man's partner identifies that there is a problem. Some men begin to avoid sex to reduce the associated uncomfortable feelings. Men, often unaware of their feelings, may be unable to locate the emotional source of this dysfunctional development, producing feelings of powerlessness. A cycle of performance anxiety commences in which, during intercourse, a man tries increasingly hard to succeed. Vigorous effort is not always welcomed by a female partner whose arousal is declining. The unfortunate paradox is that the harder a man tries, the more elusive his success will be.

The knot of this problem grows tighter when the partner reacts in a hurtful or defensive manner. Female partners receive their man's orgasm as evidence of his attraction, coincidentally confirming her desirability and skill as a good lover. But when his orgasm does not arrive easily, or at all, a female partner tends to conclude that she does not turn him on. The partners' feelings and reactions may cause both the problem and a solution to grow exponentially more complex.

With each session of sexual togetherness, the negative impact of the problem builds incrementally. Men attend to problems uniformly by applying more effort, which is not helpful in this situation. Consider a bicycle wheel that is out of round. The more the imperfect wheel is used, the more out of round it becomes. Similarly, sexual partners react to each other by making adjustments to avoid discomfort and to fix the problem. If their efforts do not reduce anxiety or tension, the problem worsens.

As with many sexual dysfunctions, approaching sexual togetherness in a more relaxed manner comprises an important part of the solution. Many women who cannot climax, or who must try hard to get there, are similarly challenged. Relaxing is simple, but finding and removing the obstacles which prevent relaxation is more complex. The sources of anxiety are many. They may be hidden, and they may arise from very old, long-forgotten issues. Don't despair, however, because once uncovered, the obstacles to overcoming delayed ejaculation may not be hard to resolve. As always, a loving approach by both partners will help speed the flight towards success. Cleared for takeoff!

> We grow a little every time we don't take advantage of another's weakness. —*Bern Williams*

3-2. The Quest for Control

A woman faces a dilemma when her man regularly finishes the job before she reaches satisfaction. Either tell him of her unfulfilled need and hurt his feelings, or feign satisfaction and fume silently. Neither option is a good one. The easier choice is one taken by many women; pretend the experience was good enough and make the problem go away quickly but temporarily: It will only crop up again next time.

Men who cannot control the timing of their ejaculation are usually not fooled. Within, he is pained by his lack of lasting power. Within his deluded thinking, he may convince himself that she does not notice. Her pretense of satisfaction temporarily grants his wish, but they both really know the truth.

Poor ejaculatory control, formerly called premature ejaculation, is the most common sexual problem. A man who suffers from lack of control may not know how common it is, since men do not routinely talk openly about sex, let alone share their sexual problems. His worst fear is that his inability to satisfy his female partner will result in rejection.

Female partners, questioning whether they value sex too highly, ask themselves, "Can I accept that I will have no sexual satisfaction for the rest of my life?" But it is a real concern; long-term relationships may be fatally damaged by this chronic sexual problem and its fallout. Men who do not possess the control to fulfill their partners often feel deeply ashamed and inadequate. Some will actively avoid all intimate situations so as not to risk them becoming sexual.

Failure to develop control is not caused by any specific condition. Some men learn control easily while others do not. However, anxious men are far more likely to have this limitation, as are those uncomfortable with sex and closeness. The problem manifests physically, though its source is usually emotional. Growing up in environments in which sex and emotional closeness were viewed negatively contributes to the development of this problem. Each successive failure to last long enough undermines confidence while simultaneously emphasizing a growing fear that the capacity to last longer will never develop. The more pressure a man puts on himself to succeed, the deeper the problem's roots grow, and the more firmly he is caught in the grip of malicious performance anxiety. Each new time he witnesses disappointment on his lover's face, his shame increases.

Performance anxiety is a cycle in which each successive failure reinforces that ejaculatory control is unobtainable. The common reaction is to face every new sexual opportunity with fear of failure. The cycle solidifies into a self-fulfilling prophecy. The longer such a negative cycle is in place the stronger it grows.

Some female partners will reasonably take a man's lack of control personally. She may mistakenly conclude that she is not sufficiently attractive or doesn't turn him on. Some worry that an unrevealed relationship problem lurks within the male partner's psyche. These assumptions are overwhelmingly not true. The actual problem lies within the man, though she may help with the solution. As sex is contaminated by negative feelings, over time, both partners may start to avoid it, a pattern that is dangerous for a relationship's well-being.

Ejaculatory control problems are not permanent; though they may take significant effort to overcome. One challenge for men is to become conscious of the forces that fuel this problem in the first place. Feeling better about sex and himself will be vital. Growing more aware of the negative emotions which interfere with the awareness of physical sensations is one stepping-stone on the path to greater control. While ejaculatory control is the man's problem, the solution is best achieved when the path of resolution is traveled as a couple; so that the solution can strengthen the relationship as well as the man.

3-3. When Sex is Damaged

An unfortunate reality is that many romantic partners have been harmed by past sexual abuse. Statistics suggest that this problem is huge; roughly 33% of women and 25% of men have been violated during inappropriate sexual experiences early in their lives. The impact is huge as well; these men and women suffer a shattered sense of self, anxiety, and deep shame, preventing them from possessing a healthy sense of sexuality. Often saddled with sexual dysfunction, traumatized individuals struggle to form satisfying love relationships because their sexuality has been damaged.

Many people who have been hurt actively avoid sex. They want the love of a partner, but are limited by pain in their capacity to share completely. Their partners feel starved of the kind of intimacy that is a normal part of a romantic relationship. A tension-producing cycle of frustration and disconnection is formed. For some of these wounded people, because of their repressed pain, sexuality disappears into an emotional blind-spot, rendering it non-existent and simply irrelevant. So when their partner pleads with them to share sexual pleasure, the wounded one might defensively reply, "Why is sex such a big deal? I think you have a sex problem; it is too important to you."

Most react to early sexual abuse by becoming inhibited. For them, sex has become associated with painful shame and guilt. Many victims, if they can remember their past, blame themselves, fearing that they invited the hurtful sexual advances of the perpetrator, who violated their personal boundaries. It is not unusual for them to become unable to confidently define their boundaries, adding another cause for sex to feel unsafe. Paradoxically, others who have been hurt react to traumatic sexual experiences as if a switch has been flicked on instead of off, by being hyper-sexual. As adults, these people easily fall into a destructive cycle of sexual compulsion, who, in their pain, repetitively re-enact the original trauma with a long parade of new sexual partners. Whichever way the switch is positioned, sexually traumatized individuals are in pain and have difficulty maintaining relationships with healthy, balanced sex lives.

The partners of these individuals, starved of loving touch and passion, are hard-pressed to offer the compassion and understanding that is most supportive, especially when a traumatized mate blocks every attempt to obtain physical intimacy or emotional closeness. It can be dangerous territory; an unanticipated sexual overture or comment may trigger intensely negative emotions such as rage or flashbacks. Others, despite past abuse, permit sexual encounters, but emotionally "go away" during sex, a phenomenon which partners may interpret as rejection and which is called dissociation.

Imagine if you ate at a local restaurant and got food poisoning causing a violent stomach sickness that lasted for several days. How eager would you be to eat at that same restaurant again? Just the thought of eating there again might cause you feelings of revulsion. Sexually abused individuals may have this reaction to sex. It takes great courage and effort to heal. If you have been hurt, my heart goes out to you. It can never be your fault.

Sexual predators, most of whom have been abused themselves, selfishly prey on those who are vulnerable, such as children, to soothe their own discomfort. Perpetrators use coercive, subtle power to obtain what they want, without regard for the victim's well-being. In contrast, healthy sex within the context of an adult romantic relationship is not about power, but about love. It is an activity in which the partner's well-being is intentionally nourished. For individuals who have been hurt sexually, hurtful power and nourishing love have become fused so that sex is emotionally contaminated.

When sex is troubled, love relationships are at risk of getting polluted with tension. Sex can be both a way to love and a way to heal old wounds. Sexuality is a healthy part of being human; when wounded, bravery and strength are needed to restore its healthiness.

3-4. The Sexless Couple

Too many love relationships fall into a state of sexlessness. They are empty of passion. While exact statistics are difficult to obtain, anecdotal evidence suggests that a high number of couples let months, years and even decades pass without lovemaking. Missing from their relationships is the satisfaction, health and relationship benefits an active sex life provides. Most romantic partners reminisce about the early days of their togetherness when passion and lovemaking were thrilling, urgent and alive. When romantic partners are troubled, sex quickly disappears. Angry and disappointed partners don't want to get close to each other.

As a component of a relationship, sex promotes a deepening of the love bond. As a positive source of pleasure, connection and way of expressing love, sex may furnish a relationship with a vital resiliency that protects the relationship from many adverse life circumstances. Sex is a healthy activity that supports physical well-being, a healthy blood-pressure level, a strong immune system and a positive emotional balance, such as protection from the onset of depression. Dr. Daniel Amen, of PBS fame, in his book "Sex on the Brain" cites studies that indicate that men who have regular and active sex lives live longer than men who do not.

For the strength and longevity of love relationships, sexlessness is dangerous. A high proportion of those who divorce indicate that sex was a problem that contributed to the marriage's end; sex plays an important role in marital satisfaction. Sexuality is a fragile, but vital part of love relationships, vulnerable to many widespread deleterious factors. Within most relationships, partners have difficulty talking about sex. When the quality of sexual loving is poor, the risk for sexlessness is high.

If sex is less than satisfying, a partner is not likely to begin a conversation about dissatisfaction or propose changes for improvement due to shame, embarrassment, discomfort, and risk of hurting the other. Common are the couples who never succeed in addressing issues of dissatisfaction. When a high difference in sexual desire exists between partners, it leads to sexlessness if unresolved. For the high-desired partner, a sexless union is a fountain of continuous resentment from which a return to loving form is difficult. Other common negative factors that contribute to sexless relationships are low self-esteem, unresolved past trauma, sexual trauma, body-image challenges, sex-negative religious training, low sexual confidence, anxiety, and sexual misinformation. Child-bearing can also be a cause.

Sexless couples are not solving their problems. Chronic abstinence suggests that chronic problems remain unresolved. Among the most important strengths happy couples possess is to be a skilled team for problem-solving. Every couple has a few perpetual problems, those thorny issues which defy every effort at a solution. Barring a complete fix, the next best approach to a stubborn problem is to use strength to choose to prevent the problem from having the power to degrade the quality of life and love. This may be achieved by forgiving, forgetting or letting go. It is not easy, but better than the bitter, passionless alternative.

Sexual dysfunction is a significant contributing factor in the development of sexlessness. Unresolved dysfunctions result in sex becoming more uncomfortable than pleasurable and therefore not worth the effort. Watching television has a lower risk for negativity than a potentially disappointing sexual experience and represents a safer choice for evening entertainment than lovemaking for sexually troubled couples. The acute embarrassment of a sexual problem results in the avoidance of sexual activity as a first-line reaction. Unlike a physical health problem or injury, for which a trip to the doctor is not unusual, seeking help for a sexually based problem risks deep humiliation, and thus may be resisted for years. Sexlessness can become the status quo.

Fear can be a powerful negative force. Fear and its lesser manifestation, anxiety, play an instrumental role in the development of patterned sexual avoidance, sexual dysfunction and sexlessness. Sex is high on the list of anxiety-provoking activities because complete openness is the ideal. Many people cannot tolerate either the high level of vulnerability associated with sex or the lesser amount required to be emotionally open to the partner. Fear is integral to the ineffective resolution of problems, such as when hurtful anger erupts or a partner is unwilling to make changes. Fear-based missteps lead couples down the bumpy path that dead-ends in sexlessness.

Sexlessness does not just happen and usually does not develop by choice. Some couples suddenly fall off sexually after a large conflict or a failed sexual encounter, but for most, it is a slow, gradual slide into a passionless pit of sexlessness. After emotional disconnection and the building of emotional walls to create distance and safety, the frequency of sex slows and ultimately disappears. Partners may not even notice when sex fell inactive; for those couples, lack of intimacy just became normal.

Along with the death of sex, also dies the force for healing and bond-strengthening which sex provides. The golden glow couples enjoy after successful physical loving is a bit like a light in the darkness. We are not fooled; sex is not absolutely necessary; we can live without it. We can live without love, music, beauty and delicious food; bread and water will keep us alive. But within a loving couple, passion and sex bring quality of life, build good feeling and goodwill, and support a giving attitude; these make our loving connections strong and positive.

3-5. Battling Bedroom Boredom

McDonald's built an empire by cooking the exact same burger billions of times. By eliminating variety, McDonald's ensure that customers can be certain what they will get at each visit. While effective in the burger business, uniformity does not work when it comes to a couple's sex life. Long-term partners easily fall into patterned routines which degrade sexual excitement. When each sexual experience is the same, boredom results. High excitement is one of the factors which makes sex pleasurable. Routine sex is the bane of long-term committed relationships and intensifies a relationship's vulnerability to infidelity.

In a common relationship aging process, partners eliminate activities that produce anxiety or discomfort. Sex play that used to be fun, edgy or even kinky is abandoned as relationships age. Partners settle into comfort with each other. Couple after couple vote for emotional security over excitement. What is routine can feel safe and secure, but it is also walled off from the variations and risks inherent in life. Safety provides freedom from fear of failure or embarrassment.

Excitement is generated by novelty, surprise, and breaking barriers. Naturally, as relationships age, partners grow to know each other very well; not just the good about each other, but also the bad and ugly. The difficulty of negotiating partner differences causes partners to seek the safety of emotional distance. Routine sex allows partners to enjoy sexual pleasure without the vulnerability that comes from openness; but it also produces a sleep-walking kind of mechanical, disconnected sex.

Risking a journey outside your comfort zone by trying new ways to give and receive pleasure, causes emotional growth, a deepened connection, and greater aliveness. A way to wake up your sex life from a sleep-inducing routine is by initiating a positive, non-critical conversation with your lover, in which a desire for change is expressed. Creating change unilaterally, without your partner's agreement is likely to backfire. Three great books may guide your exploration by detailing hundreds of ways to give pleasure. “The Guide to Getting it On," by Paul Joannides is an excellent compendium of everything sexual. "The Joy of Sex" is the classic sex manual by Alex Comfort. Finally, "The Illustrated Perfumed Garden," adapted from a16th century text, illustrates dozens of intercourse positions. A warning here: several of the positions may nourish your chiropractor's career as much as it helps vary your sex life. Together with your partner, looking through these books can inspire a conversation about what each of you may be willing to try next. Pursuing variety does not mean that you discontinue setting personal limitations. On the contrary, it is normal to "draw the line" somewhere by excluding acts that you find objectionable. Yet expanding your comfort zone will always cause some discomfort, so expect it, but doing so will reward you with growth. Try to be open to something new.

Increasing the variety of your sex acts is not the only way to battle bedroom boredom. The amount of excitement partners feel when stimulated is in direct proportion to both how deeply relaxed each partner is and the depth of the loving connection they share. When together, if you and your partner are intensely, meditatively relaxed, the same old sex acts will be sparked with a highly charged, positive intensity.

Two ancient spiritual traditions, of Tantra Yoga and Taoism, offer methods to incorporate deep relaxation into sex play, thereby dramatically deepening partner connection. At the same time, sexual excitement is greatly enhanced. When experiencing ourselves deeply, boredom is eliminated, and satisfaction is expanded. Exploring such techniques potentially heightens sexuality into the realm of the spiritual where the quality of life both in and outside the bedroom is improved.

A quest for greater sexual excitement is really a desire to feel more alive. Sex is a great place to start.

3-6. Too Touchy

Many women are curious as to why their male partners sexually grab and grope at them, often at inappropriate times. A little playfulness is fun, but more than enough can be infuriating. The same holds true for ill-timed sexual innuendo. Rather than creating moments of endearment, irritation is provoked in reaction to the unwelcome attention. So many women vent, "Even though I tell him to stop, he keeps doing it!"

Men's persistent behavior defies logic because it decreases the chance that they will obtain satisfaction. Instead of warming up the female partner, it annoys her. The combination of a chronically sex-seeking man and an agitated female partner produces a negative dance which fuels a relationship downward-spiral. Couples have difficulty extricating themselves from this pattern.

Men seek to feel loved, to feel valued and to be closely connected. Generally, men's way to build this connection is through sex. With a singular focus, most men automatically seek sexual activity. If unsuccessful, they just try more of the same, but harder. Many do not consider less direct options. Women, if not feeling close, experience these attempts as insensitive to their needs and as unwelcome pressure.

Sexually-based comments, innuendo and touching by men expresses that they have unmet needs. Lack of sexual satisfaction, poor emotional connection with their partner, inner insecurities or some combination of these promotes this relentless behavior cycle. Men are likely to experience all their emotional needs as sexual, though if examined closely they will find that the feelings are not sexually based. Loneliness, disconnection, feeling unimportant, stress, insecurity, shame and anxiety are all distressing. Men will naturally seek soothing through interaction with their intimate partner. However, to openly express these feelings violates the masculine code of expression, which is to avoid admission of vulnerability, sensitivity, and weakness. To pursue sex escapes this bind for men because it demonstrates virility.

In a man's development, his emotional maturation coincides with a time of sexual development, often fusing emotion and sexual feelings. As a result, many men have difficulty differentiating between them. Among men who are constantly sex-seeking, it is common to find old emotional wounds that provoke feelings of insecurity and anxiety. To him, sex feels like the proper activity to soothe and heal these uncomfortable feelings. Unfortunately, seeking sex for self-soothing does not result in the female partner feeling loved or desired. Additionally, repetitive bids for sex build up the female partner's view of the male partner as needy, a weakness that sours attraction and puts out the fire of the female partner's sexual interest. Men who behave this way are likely to be in relationships that are not as close and secure as they desire, and their chronic inappropriate requests for sex simultaneously help to make the relationship less connected. Bids for sex are a way for men to express that they want more closeness and want to feel secure in their female partners' love, but women are turned on by their partners' strengths, not weaknesses.

The way out of this dissatisfying pattern requires adjustment from both partners. Once the male partner stops his negative habitual behavior, it is best that he switches the kind of attention he gives to his female partner to loving, non-sexual attention. He must be able to identify when a real sexual opportunity exists, complete with sufficient privacy, time and emotional connection, and initiate sex only at these times. His effort is best simultaneously joined by the female partner opening her emotional and sexual receptivity. If she is sexually unavailable, her lack of receptivity will contribute to the male partner's insecurity, fueling again his constant bids for sex. To escape this negative cycle, an active sex life balanced with a loving connection will be essential. With these simultaneous efforts, love can exist outside the bedroom without being contaminated by bids for sex.

3-7. Low Female Sexual Desire

Many women complain about having little sexual desire. Such women tend to feel bad about themselves because of what they may perceive as a personal inadequacy; often just another item added to their list of self-perceived shortcomings. While speaking to an area gynecologist, he voiced the fact that he and other women's healthcare physicians frequently hear this complaint from their female patients. The following is an exploration of the many causes of low sexual desire, lack of desire and outright avoidance of sexual activity altogether. This article makes many generalities which may be true for some, but not all women.

The basis of this chapter is that sex is a healthy part of the human experience, for both men and women. This article is also based on the belief that sex is integral to the human experience and need not be linked with shame. Most relationships include some form of sexual expression and activity, and an overwhelming majority of healthy partners expect, desire and even need some form of sexual activity to occur for the relationship to remain vital, satisfying and healthy.

But what causes this phenomenon of low female sexual desire? It is impossible to pin down what is a normal level of sexual desire, which exists within a broad range. Some healthy women feel that sex is not very important while other healthy women desire some form of sex daily. Most women fall into the middle to lower end of this range.

It is possible that a woman and her partner will have wide and potentially disruptive differences in their levels of sexual desire even while the levels of desire in both partners reside within the "normal" range. The friction between a woman with low sexual desire and her high-desired partner can threaten the very existence of their relationship. It can be the source of much pain and frustration. Several distinct factors contribute to women having the subjective experience of having little sexual desire.

Lack of Desire vs. Sexual Opposition

What seems to be "low desire" may not even be low sexual desire. Having a desire for sex is obvious in that it results in clear action of seeking out sexual activity, but the lack of such desire may actually be a wish to avoid sex, but for legitimate reasons. The two are often confused. A woman may call her inner experience "lack of desire," rather than distinguishing between these two distinct conditions. Low desire is characterized by devoting little or no effort to make a sexual experience happen, accompanied by little interest in doing so. A woman with low desire may not have an interest in sex, but also may not be strongly opposed to it either. Whereas not wanting sex is not a *lack of desire*, but instead is about an outright opposition to a sexual experience. The opposition may be expressed as a direct, “No, I don’t want sex,” or less obvious, passive maneuvers to render the possibility of a sexual experience unlikely.

Female Sexuality is Not Male Sexuality

There may be an assumption by a woman and/or her partner that she should feel sexual desire in the way that a man does. The temptation to view female sexuality through the same lens by which male sexuality is viewed can be destructive and create inaccurate conclusions as to what is healthy female sexuality, a practice which at times both men and women are guilty of. Just as male genitalia are obvious and “out there,” male sexuality is more openly expressed, direct and advertised. The result is that male sexuality has become the norm of sexuality as a whole, with which female sexuality is sadly and harmfully compared.

One assumption that exists about female sexual desire is that it should be similar to male patterns of desire. An example of the male paradigm adopted by or expected of women is displayed in television shows such as Desperate Housewives and Sex in the City where women have high sexual desire and assertively act upon it. For many women, this does not accurately reflect how they experience their own sexuality but may function as a nice fantasy.

It is not easy for men to understand their female partner’s sexuality. Men are much more likely to view their sexuality and their desire as a distinct and separate part of themselves, whereas for women, it is more usual that her sexuality and desire is a part of herself that is intricately woven without distinction into her sense of self and all other aspects of her life. Unlike men, who are more likely to use sex as an activity to relieve stress, most women experience sex as something that can be embraced when all else feels right. So a difficult situation, such as stress, problems, feeling overwhelmed, or low self-esteem, may cause a man to have increased sexual desire while it can cause a woman to have a lower desire.

Many men experience desire that interrupts them throughout the day as a strong longing, urging and hunger. For many women, this experience is just not present, and this is not abnormal or an indication of a problem. Instead, a feeling of well-being, of self-satisfaction or of closeness with her partner, may result in a woman being receptive to a sexual experience. But unlike a man, many women are not likely to experience anything like desire until *after* the sexual experience is underway and her body has become aroused. It is then that many women feel desire. The expectations of many have the order of events reversed. If a woman believes it should be the other way around, just her own self-criticism may be enough to cause avoidance of sex. Being criticized by her partner for not having "his kind of desire," can also be enough to dampen her receptivity.

Reasons for Opposition to Sex

It makes sense that a woman might not want to be sexual at all if the physical or emotional discomforts outweigh the pleasures. Most of the reasons listed below as to why a woman would be opposed to being sexual fall into that category. Many are emotion-based causes for opposition, yet these may not be obvious to a woman or her partner.

- The level of a woman's self-esteem has a direct bearing on her sexuality. If she does not feel good about herself, it is likely that she will not want to make herself vulnerable by allowing another to experience what she fears is an intrinsic lack of worthiness.

- A woman may hold beliefs that sex is dirty, bad or sinful, but be largely unaware that such beliefs are present. Such beliefs are often subtly fed to women in their upbringing since female sexuality remains tinged with societal ambivalence and shame. An early family environment lacking in positive touch, support and encouragement, the modeling of love and affection, and information about the healthiness of sexuality trains a girl to avoid closeness and positive touch; as a woman, she may feel uncomfortable with her body and her sexuality. An early family environment that also included shaming, criticism, and disrespect will have an even more profound effect on developing unhealthy attitudes towards or avoidance of sex.

- At the extreme are damaging experiences of emotional, verbal, physical, and sexual abuse. Women who have been abused, which accounts for an estimated one in three, may not have the capacity to trust another or feel safe enough to let a partner as emotionally close as sexual activity demands. If her traumatic experiences remain unremembered, or undisclosed, a partner may incorrectly assume that the woman has no desire for him, whereas the truth is that emotionally, she is uncomfortable with vulnerability.

- Many women are unhappy with their bodies, feeling that they do not possess the beauty or sexiness that a woman's body "should." Some women are uncomfortable with their vulvas, a possible contributing factor to the overall discomfort of the sexual experience. It is not uncommon that a woman has never viewed her vulva, and holds the belief that her vulva is an ugly, unappealing, even dirty part of her body. Having discomfort with her vulva, a woman may avoid letting her partner get close, especially for oral or manual stimulation.

- Since a woman's sexual receptivity may be emotionally and relationship-based, the quality of the relationship between a woman and her mate can have a direct effect on her openness to being sexual. If the relationship is troubled, or of poor quality, a woman may not desire sex with her partner. The accumulation of negative emotions, such as anger and resentment, in a long-term relationship tend to extinguish the flames of sexual desire causing a woman to avoid being sexual.

- In general, men seek to build a close connection with their female partner through sex. Generally, women build this connection through non-sexual means, such as sharing, non-sexual touch and affection, spending time together, talking, gaining understanding and mutual support. In relationships, both partners make the effort to build and maintain a connection, but because partners often go about this task in differing ways, tension and conflict can arise. If the male partner is strong in his efforts to be sexual but is not attentive to his female partner's method of building an emotional connection, her interest and desire to participate in his methods, through sex, will probably diminish.

- In general, negative emotions negatively affect the quality of a relationship between a woman and her partner, and negatively affect the sexual relationships between partners. Conflicts exist in all relationships, whether those conflicts are expressed or not. All relationships include unresolved differences between partners. The question of the degree to which those unresolved differences contaminate the goodwill between partners or not is significant both for the health of the relationship and also for its impact on the partners as lovers. In long-term relationships, where time has allowed for unresolved conflicts to fester, and for negative emotion, such as anger, resentment, bitterness, etc., to accumulate, these negative emotions can effectively kill sexual desire and eliminate sexual activity from a relationship.

- If there exists any tension between a woman and her partner regarding sex, then the sexual arena can become polluted with negativity. Included in this is a partner's request for sexual activities to which the female partner is opposed. If she worries that her partner will request these unpopular sex acts, she may opt to not be sexual at all so as to avoid facing a situation in which she either says "no," or puts herself in an undesirable sexual situation in which she would be selling out her own preferences. Pressuring a woman to be sexual in ways that are uncomfortable for her may contaminate sex and cause it to lose value for her.

- If the sexual experience is painful for a woman, she may seek to avoid sexual activity. Not all understand that if a woman is healthy, sex and intercourse need not be painful. Yet without this understanding, some women think pain is a normal part of sex and subsequently choose to just "grin and bear it." Doing so may cause cumulative physical harm and sexual problems for both partners. Healthy sex need not be painful.

Power Dynamics and Desire

A facet of relationships can be a competition, battle or negotiation for power. One place in which a battle for power can be waged is in the sexual relationship between partners. In a healthy relationship, power is shared and divided in an equitable manner. In unhealthy ones, power is used in ways that do not benefit both partners. Sex can be a medium of exchange in the relationship, or it can be an arena in which power is displayed. If power is unevenly distributed between partners, especially in the extreme, the female partner may lose sexual desire. If she owns most of the power, she may lose respect for her male partner and subsequently not desire him. If he has too much power, in her powerlessness she may feel bad about herself, have little self-respect or have resentment towards her male partner; either situation can produce a lack of sexual desire. A woman who feels she has no choice but to be sexual, whether or not she wishes to share herself, will lose desire as her sense of self and sense of her body are not being respected.

The Power to Choose

Children cannot own power because they do not possess the judgement or cognitive skills to make responsible choices. In a healthy environment, children are given small amounts of power by their parents so as to practice using it in constructive, successful ways without risking too much harm in the process. Adults who, as children, have not been allowed to practice using power, grow up without developing the capacity to make good choices, to make choices at all or to vocalize their needs.

Such individuals were typically parented by adults who were controlling or abusive...parents who were unable to let go of their own needs in order to address their child's needs. If a girl's needs are never considered, that girl will grow up to become a woman who will also ignore her own needs, or be unable to assess or value her own needs, including sexual needs.

Women who grew up in these kinds of family environments are unlikely to possess the kind of personal power commonly associated with adult maturity, such as emotionally participating in a relationship or sexual partnership as an equal partner. For such a woman and her partner, her behavior may look a lot like lack of sexual desire, but is probably less about lack of desire than it is about sexual avoidance, in which avoiding a sexual encounter is an automatic reaction, an attempt to side-step discomfort. Such avoidance is not a conscious choice, but a reflexive reaction, much the way a person will duck without thinking if they see something flying at their face.

Having power includes the power to make a choice, but for a woman who grew up in a family where she was given little power to make choices, owning this kind of power is not a choice. Emotionally, for this woman, having power is not an option, and is not considered. This emotional position, however, significantly affects the woman's relationship with her partner, and the sexual relationship. So much of a relationship is determined by how partners negotiate their differences and how each negotiates to get her or his needs met. A woman who does not own her power cannot be a partner in negotiation. To have a position in a negotiation, a partner must own power. A woman who cannot own power will avoid such negotiation, will not take a stand on an issue, is not likely to speak up for herself, if confronted is likely to either emotionally break down, become silent, or explode in a defensive eruption; all of which prevent negotiation from occurring and a resolution from being reached.

This lack of power shows up in the sexual arena when the woman cannot voice any choices or preferences for sexual activities. She may participate passively in sexual play for her partner, but does not experience the interaction as being for herself. Her partner's request for sex is likely to feel to her like a command, about which she has no choice, and in which she must please her partner or be a bad partner, but the power to voice an opinion in the matter does not exist.

Many other women are able to own their power, but still feel they have no choice in the matter of being sexual or not. Many women, in relationships with high or very high-desired partners, feel that they must constantly choose between two undesirable options: have sex and feel bad about themselves while avoiding conflict, or say no to sex and be saddled with an angry, pouting or abusive partner. A saying I have heard is: "If she cannot say "no," then she cannot really say "yes." Feeing that she does not have a choice in being sexual has a high chance of producing in a woman no desire for sex.

For many women, stress is a large, negative influence that interferes with sexual receptivity. The feelings of being overwhelmed and exhausted may cause a man to seek sexual release as a way to rid himself of tension, but for many women, it is not sex which nourishes as much as other activities. This is especially true of mothers of young children. It is not unusual that the situations which cause stress are also factors that interfere with partners spending time together. While for most men, sex is the way to reunite and re-establish a connection, the opposite tends to be true for most women who need to re-establish an emotional connection first before sharing themselves sexually. So for women living in very stressful environments, the lack of a sense of connectedness may look like a lack of sexual desire.

Boundaries

The more emotionally strong a woman is, the more she can define her boundaries, set limits, assert herself, while also being emotionally open to others and her partner. A woman who is not emotionally strong may not have her personal boundaries defined at all and routinely allow others to violate her: what stronger people would experience as poor judgement. The weakness of her boundaries prevents a woman from being able to have the power to assure her own personal, emotional safety. The closer two people become emotionally, as with partners in a love relationship, the more effort and the greater sense of self it takes to keep these boundaries distinct. If a woman's sense of self is not strong, she may have the experience of losing herself and her identity within the relationship.

Boundary considerations are heightened during sexual encounters between partners because it is during sex that two people have the potential to emotionally and even physically merge. If a woman's sense of her own self is not well defined or strong, sexual experiences can be anxiety-provoking and uncomfortable, causing such a woman to avoid the potential discomfort by avoiding the sexual experience.

Partners sometimes make assumptions instead of obtaining the correct information that direct communication provides. There is no arena within love relationships that is more negatively affected by this tendency than in sex. Because sex is often tainted with shame and embarrassment, partners commonly avoid direct talk about sex. Yet sex is a team sport. Just like all other team sports, the chances of victory are increased if the players communicate well. Assumptions are boundaries that have not been well defined. If sexual needs, desires, interests, preferences, dislikes and curiosities are never discussed, sex can be an activity complicated by uncertainty; a state which may cause a woman lack of interest.

Quality of Sex

The quality of the sexual activity between a woman and her partner can affect her desire to be sexual. Men and women are certainly not eager for bad sex. Because of the tendency for men to not understand female patterns of arousal and the tendency of many women not to voice their needs while ignoring their own body's signals, the chances for highly pleasurable sexual experiences are not as high as they could be. Because women respond to stimulation and reach arousal much more slowly than do men, it is not uncommon for couples to engage in intercourse before the female partner is ready, resulting in a sexual disconnect between partners, an occurrence which prevents the female partner from experiencing as much sexual pleasure as possible. If this pattern develops, a woman may experience a lack of interest in engaging in a sexual encounter in which her needs and high pleasure are not incorporated into the timing of the sexual play. This can occur without her conscious knowledge, instead, she just has a feeling of "I'd rather watch TV."

Sensuality and Pleasure

Lack of desire or lack of interest in sex does not mean that a woman has no interest in pleasure. When non-sexual pleasures are considered, such as a delicious meal, fragrant perfume, or the feel of a skilled massage, for example, it may be evident that a woman's sensuality is very much alive, even if the potential sensual pleasure in sex is nullified by other factors. A woman who lacks sexual desire does not always lack interest or enjoyment of pleasure. In fact, she may pursue non-sexual pleasures. The pleasures that are possible in a sexual experience are often dismissed by a woman who opposes sexual activity because the possibility of pleasure is blocked by emotional or relational factors.

Having developed a pattern of opposing sex, these tendencies may continue beyond the existence of underlying causes. In other words, opposition to sex may be its own cause, having gone unchallenged in the pursuit of growth. If the causes have been eliminated or outgrown, acknowledgement of the potential for sexual pleasure can be a path towards embracing sex as a healthy and important part of being female.

Women enjoy pleasures such as delicious food or making a purchase or spending time with friends, but bodily pleasures may be a distinct category of pleasure which has been tarnished by guilt or shame. Subtle cultural and religious messages have influenced the sexual development of women, pronouncing bodily pleasures to be sinful and immoral, and female sexuality to be suspect. Many women hold themselves back from sexual pleasure for this reason, even if they are not conscious of these subtle learnings. Yet the female clitoris has no functional purpose other than physical pleasure and is central in the increase of arousal to the culmination of orgasm. The presence of the clitoris proves that female sexual pleasure is normal and natural. Especially religious traditions have discounted the importance of the clitoris, which is outside of the vagina and therefore does not play a direct role in conception and reproduction.

Having Sex When Desire is Not Present

Since it is more common that the male partner is the "higher-desire partner," many women share themselves sexually when they have little interest in doing so. While treating women for sexual difficulties, I frequently hear from my female patients, "I had sex with him just to get him off my back." The pattern of engaging in sexual activity when no real interest is present potentially builds resentment, which can deepen a woman's lack of interest in sex. Also, a woman sharing herself when she truly does not wish to causes an internal disconnect between a woman and her body, her emotions, and her self-respect. This is because her fundamental needs during the sexual experience, and possibly in the relationship, are not being met. In a relationship where there is a large difference in desire between partners, participating in sex, even when there is no desire to do so, can be an act of generosity and love, that is if the participation is not due to control by the partner, or threat of anger. The test as to whether sharing oneself sexually even without desire is harmful is whether resentment results.

Other factors that contribute to low sexual desire are health problems and medications. Poor physical and/or mental health contributes to a lack of interest in sex. Physical problems limit the kinds of activities possible, making sex more complex and the politics of sex more complex, thus increasing the moments when choosing not to be sexual is easier, especially when tired.

Among the symptoms associated with depression are low energy, fatigue, lack of interest in the usually desired pleasures, lack of motivation, and lack of desire for sex. Depression is not always easily detected, even by the depressed person. Depression can be mild and chronic, which to a woman can become just a normal part of her everyday life experience.

The Ability to Relax

Relaxation is necessary not only for a high quality of life, but also as a necessary ingredient to enable us to have fun, to laugh and to have good sexual experiences. The ability to relax is not always easy to come by, especially in our fast-paced, high-tech contemporary lives where demands are high, and time seems short. Much like a rubber band that has been stretched for a long time and can no longer snap back to its original size, many women maintain fast-paced lives for so long that they can no longer relax. Good sex requires a significant ability to relax. Many women complain that they feel unable to slow their minds down during sexual experiences. If there is something about sex that is problematic for a woman, she might have trouble concentrating on the sensations provided by her lover's stimulation in her body and find herself thinking about non-sexual matters. This may also be true if she is anxious about sex itself. The discrepancy between the pace of daily life and the much slower pace of a sexual experience can cause an internal disconnect. Sometimes women seek to speed up the sexual experience, both to better match her internal pace, but also if she is uncomfortable with being sexual, to get the experience over quickly. If a woman is unable to relax, the sexual experience can produce discomfort simply by heightening her awareness of her inability to relax and of the potential pleasure she is incapable of experiencing at that moment.

Lack of Information and Unrealistic Expectations

Even in this age of great availability of information, women and their partners may still lack the right information and knowledge about sex and female sexual functioning. Male partners do not always understand the importance of clitoral stimulation for a woman's sexual pleasure the achievement of the female partner's orgasm. A woman, even if she is aware of this, may not tell her partner. Many couples are uncomfortable speaking about sex and avoid doing so to minimize the risk of hurting one another's feelings or to avoid feelings of embarrassment. Both men and women may expect that female orgasms should occur during intercourse, an activity during which direct clitoral stimulation does not occur. Statistics reveal that most women do not reach orgasm through intercourse. Unrealistic expectations can make a sexual experience disappointing. They may contribute to the female partner not desiring the kind of sexual experience she and her partner routinely have.

Complexity

At its best, sex is an interaction between partners that is both natural and simple. The more that negative differences between partners pollute the essential simplicity, the more undesirable the sexual experience can be for both partners. If sex is complicated by negative emotions, sexually related conflicts, a high frequency of problems, dissatisfactions, and risks of disappointment, then sex becomes overly complex and loses its allure. A woman may react to this situation before her male partner, especially if she is the lower-desire partner. To her partner, she may seem to have a lack of sexual desire.

Sexual Problems

Sexual problems are unfortunately common, and tend to become more common as women age. Among them are difficulties of becoming aroused and difficulties with achieving orgasm. Both problems, if not attended to, could be an obstacle to a woman having sexual desire. Some of the previously mentioned factors, such as anxiety or being sexual without desire can interfere with arousal. Medications also can inhibit arousal. But if a woman engages in intercourse prior to being fully aroused, the experience may be uncomfortable and ultimately painful...potentially forming a vicious cycle of decreasing sexual desire.

Failure to reach orgasm can be one element in a negative cycle that includes or causes low sexual desire. Some women have never achieved an orgasm and are unsure about what it is. Many other women have routine difficulty in achieving orgasm. Roughly one-third of women have never experienced an orgasm at all and approximately two-thirds rarely experience orgasm through intercourse, when direct clitoral stimulation is not present. Most women can learn to experience orgasm. Many women and their partners are unaware of the reality that these statistics bear out. Unrealistic expectations regarding orgasms can lead to frustrations, disappointments and even accusations. Reaching orgasm can be nearly impossible for most women if strong negative emotions, such as anger, depression or anxiety are present. It is an unusual woman who is eager to enter a sexual experience in which disappointment is assured.

Medications can reduce the possibility of orgasm. In situations where a woman knows that orgasm is unlikely, and/or if there is pressure from her partner because her orgasm is important to him, it may result in the woman having very little desire to have a sexual experience at all.

Many medications have a negative impact upon sexual response, such as interfering with arousal, evidenced by lack of lubrication, but also interfering with the ability to experience orgasm, thereby reducing the quality of, and indirectly resulting in lack of desire for, what may be perceived as a less-than-satisfying sexual experience. Many women are not aware that birth control pills may have the negative side-effect of lowering a woman's sexual libido because birth-control pills can cause testosterone levels to fall. If unaware of this truth, a woman may needlessly blame herself for her lack of sexual interest. Anti-depressant medications are notorious for reducing sexual desire. Many medications have a negative effect on sexual functioning and response.

Among the health considerations are hormone levels. Just as it does for men, the hormone testosterone plays an important role in female sexual desire, a factor for menopausal women in particular. If a woman has a low level of this vital hormone, she may then have a lack of desire for sex. For general well-being, including a healthy level of sexual desire, proper balancing of the levels of all hormones, estrogen, progesterone, and testosterone is optimal.

While not being the largest component in a love relationship, sex is an essential ingredient in most love relationships. Low female sexual desire disrupts that essential ingredient, and, if uncorrected, can and does create great damage to many marriages and love relationships. This article has detailed many of the factors which contribute to a woman's opposition to and/or lack of desire for sex, but by no means has it explored all of them or done so in the most detailed manner. Female sexuality is highly complex. Any attempt to understand why a woman has a lack of desire or avoids sexual activity must start with respect for and consideration of each woman's uniqueness. A sex-positive approach, using the healthiness and normality of sexual activity, can be a useful starting point in the exploration of the cause of low or no female sexual desire.

3-8. Vaginismus: A Relationship Killer

The fictional couple, Sharon and Bill, met at a party and were married ten quick months later. Sharing values of restraint and the purity of romantic love, the two held off on making their relationship sexual. Soon after meeting, Sharon had stated strongly to Bill that sex before marriage just wasn't within her ethical or moral framework. Bill understood. His feelings were so strong for Sharon, and having been raised in a moderately religious family, her need to wait before exploring sexuality seemed reasonable. Plus he wished to demonstrate that his love was pure and not based upon lust. Neither partner had a lot of sexual experience, though Bill had had a few previous sexual partners. Despite several prior boyfriends, Sharon had always chosen to remain chaste.

The challenge began during their honeymoon, after which the marriage remained unconsummated. Of course, Bill had been eager to share himself with Sharon, after having waited painfully for ten long months to enjoy the fulfillment of sexual pleasure. He wanted to be patient with her, yet it was apparent that when a sexual opportunity arose, her anxiety and discomfort grew. He was excited when she invited him in to share the experience of intercourse. Much to Bill's dismay and confusion, penetration could not occur; even after several attempts, during each of which Sharon cried out with feelings of sharp pain. Bill was confused and disappointed. Sharon felt deeply embarrassed. Being mildly uncomfortable with sex to start with, and not wanting to re-experience the traumatic moment, the two simply avoided both sex and talking about it for years. This story is not as unusual as you may think.

Sharon and Bill silently suffered with this shameful secret. Bill, conflicted in his intense frustration, did not want to force Sharon to do anything that caused her pain. Because of her many loving gestures, he felt confident in her love. She had hinted to her gynecologist that there was a problem, but the doctor gave her worry little importance and suggested that she and Bill use a lubricant. The doctor mentioned in a dismissive tone that during the internal exam, nothing unusual had been observed. Feeling ashamed, embarrassed, and deeply inadequate, she felt unable to press the issue with her doctor. Bill and Sharon allowed the sexual part of their marriage to remain unattended until years later when Sharon stumbled upon an article about vaginismus, an emotional condition resulting in the chronic spasming of a woman's pelvic-floor muscles, effectively preventing her vagina from opening.

To understand this more clearly, consider the example of

common muscle pain that so many people experience in their shoulders. In reaction to stress and tension, many people involuntarily and habitually tighten their shoulder muscles. If tightened chronically, these muscles eventually grow tired, tight, and produce a painful burning sensation. The shoulder pain sufferer over time will have lost the ability to consciously relax these muscles. Women with vaginismus suffer the same condition; however the muscles in question are located in their pelvis.

The cause of vaginismus is emotional though it manifests with physical symptoms. A woman may have anxiety and fear about the vulnerability that sexual activity produces. Women with histories of sexual abuse or trauma are more likely to experience the painful symptoms of vaginismus. During a marriage, accumulated emotional hurts and distrust may be an emotional precipitant for vaginismus, which can show up along a spectrum of intensity. For instance, some women just experience discomfort, such as pain or a burning sensation only at the moment of penetration, while others feel the pain, dull or sharp, throughout intercourse. Still others, like Sharon, are prevented altogether from having intercourse.

Untreated, this problem is a marriage killer; vaginismus is very treatable, yet it is often a mystery to the sufferer, the partner and the medical professionals women depend upon for healthcare. This is true, in part, because the source of the problem is emotional, the symptoms are physical, but without any obvious physical signs suggesting a problem. If not for the tremendous embarrassment of sexuality, and the discomfort that even the medical community has with sex, many women and many partners would be spared much pain and shame. A great resource for this not-so-uncommon difficulty is the website: www.vaginismus.com. Successful treatment will come from a sex therapist, a professional trained in the emotions which impact sexual health.

Change is constant.

Growth is a choice.

— John Maxwell

3-9. The Unenthusiastic Partner

The unintended pain caused by an unenthusiastic sexual partner can be substantial enough to harm or even end a relationship. What does "unenthusiastic partner" mean? It means a partner who is uncomfortable sharing themselves sexually. An enthusiastic partner is eager and excited to participate in sex and is uninhibited regarding full involvement, comfortably giving and receiving pleasure while also freely expressing the pleasure he or she experiences from being touched, caressed, and stimulated.

The unenthusiastic partner is inhibited and may avoid sexual activities. He or she is a passive partner who rarely, if ever, initiates sex and is passive during sex play. The unenthusiastic partner responds only to the other's orchestration. An inhibited sexual partner rarely has a "sexual voice," the ability to verbally express a desire for specific pleasure or a change in pleasuring activities. Yet he or she may be readily able to vocalize his or her dissent...to say "no" to sex or particular sex acts, a tendency which is sure to frustrate the more eager sexual partner. The quality of the sex with this kind of partner is poor, and probably dissatisfying to the more eager partner.

Other tendencies an unenthusiastic partner may exhibit include a variety of creative methods of excuse-making in order to ward off sexual advances by the other. Such excuses often have a hint of legitimacy, but cover up an irrational mixture of fear, anxiety and discomfort. The unenthusiastic partner may hesitantly have sex, but do so with only meager involvement. One behavior pattern of the hesitant partner, particularly the female partner, that can be a source of confusion, is that if she is willing to be sexual, she may wish to bypass all foreplay activities and engage immediately in intercourse. Initially, this may be mistaken for eagerness, but upon closer examination, it will be revealed that this strategy helps to keep the sexual encounter as brief as possible. A final tendency comes under the category of procrastination. The unenthusiastic partner will reject the other's initiation, saying that the time will come later, but will then provide a semi-legitimate excuse at that later time to avoid engaging sexually.

Consider the analogy of a tennis partner who shows up on the court, but who will not run and will only hit the ball back if it is hit directly to him or her. He or she shows no enjoyment for the game yet insists that he or she is "playing" fully. The unenthusiastic partner is likely to be saddled with sexual challenges, such as the inability to relax or the inability to achieve orgasm, having ejaculatory control problems if male, and being uncomfortable with his or her body. While no longer a term currently in use, the unenthusiastic partner may earn the description of being "frigid."

Encouraging greater sexual enthusiasm from this partner is no easy task, and a challenge that may achieve success only after patience and lengthy, careful effort. Only a loving approach will meet with any success...other efforts, such as those laced with control or anger will only backfire, causing the inhibited partner to become even more avoidant. Steady, loving, respectful pressure may bear fruit over the long haul, while also letting the hesitant partner know that sex is healthy and important; that he or she is loved, desirable and valued, and that you will never give up or back down. Sex is not the biggest part of a love relationship, but without a satisfying sex life, the loving bond of a love relationship is vitally diminished.

3-10. Guilt of Pleasure

How often do you hear somebody admit they don't like

sex? Probably not too often. The media frequently trumpets sex as commonplace, wonderful, and tremendously pleasurable. So it may seem strange that for many folks their experiences are far different. Some, and not even a small number, feel disappointed that their sexual experiences don't measure up to such high expectations. Physical limitations prevent some people, others fear closeness, but still more are prevented from enjoying sex due to the guilt they feel about experiencing pleasure.

For hundreds of years, the placement of sex in people's lives was determined by religious organizations. Churches informed the populace about what was sinful and what was not. For generations, whole societies have been taught that bodily pleasure is sinful, a teaching that has permeated our minds and souls. Our culture is a place where deep below our daily values lies the belief that our bodies are dirty and we must deny our bodily sensations, desires and pleasures so as to liberate the spirit, and that sex is sinful and the opposite of all that is sacred. Shame of our bodies and sexuality blocks many from sharing what can be blissful and transcendent.

As a result, treats that reward the eater with a wonderful taste are described as "sinfully delicious." When we indulge ourselves then we are enjoying "guilty pleasures." The well-established Puritan work ethic espouses a "work then play" order to activities, which imprisons us because in our culture, where many services are 24/7, work is never done so we cannot play. Play is for children, not for adults. In too many instances, adults have to be anesthetized by the influence of alcohol to relax enough to play. Pleasure, fun and sex are often viewed as non-productive activities. A side-effect of believing we are sinners is that many feel undeserving of pleasure or fun. Sex is also a form of play, in which playfulness can make the difference between mechanical actions and lovemaking, but, not experiencing ourselves as virtuous, we are robbed of the ability to relax enough to have fun.

Pleasure is as much a part of life as is pain. Acceptance of both as necessary parts of life is healthy, so long as our pursuit or avoidance of both is not in the extreme. Loving life requires that both conditions be embraced. Sex is another healthy, necessary part of life. Most couples do not engage in sex to reproduce (or be productive), as the church might like, but instead are sexual to reinforce their bonds of love, to practice merging into and celebrating life. Unfortunately, for those who feel guilty, to do so is not pleasurable.

> Criticism is to love what acid is to metal.

3-11. Curing the Sexless Marriage

Too many couples watch as days, weeks, months, and years pass without them having connected sexually. Lovemaking slowly becomes a thing of distant memory. Each partner knows it's not ok, but somehow it is just easier not to discuss it. Not a problem you say? Perhaps so, and if two consenting adult partners agree not to have sex, it should be ok. But the lack of sex in a marriage is usually a sign that something is wrong.

When cooking, there are certain foods that after being cooked, are best left to sit for a time before being re-heated and then eaten. In my house, we say, "The ingredients must marry overnight." This means that the food's ingredients must merge, mingle, and join to make the food fully delightful. People, too, must "marry" in this way. For a marriage to be a good one the partners must emotionally merge. A healthy sex life is the outward expression of this merging having taken place, but sex is also an activity that promotes this merging and is a symbolic on a physical level.

It is a sign when two people are married, or in a long-term love relationship, and are not actively sexual for weeks and months. These people are not merging. An essential part and purpose of being in a relationship is missing. As time passes without the bonding that sex provides, partners grow disconnected; they suffer. Their relationship becomes increasingly vulnerable to troubles, such as bitterness, conflict, affairs, and divorce.

If a love relationship has deteriorated to the point where it is sexless, then one or both partners need to grow emotionally. Emotions are experienced in the present but are a sum of our past. They powerfully influence our choices, our current experiences, and our behaviors. Negative emotions pull at us to be less than the best we can be. The weaker we are emotionally, the more we give in to negative emotions, which cause us to choose actions that are often not in our best interests. In the same vein, the stronger we are emotionally, the more we choose to act in ways that are loving to others and to ourselves.

Differences between partners are a source of friction. Developing the strength to negotiate differences in a loving way allows us to remain open to our partner in spite of the differences and the rigors of negotiating them. It is love that cures so many relationship problems, including sexlessness. Love is a choice, which when present, creates many new possibilities, including a satisfying sex life. It all starts at home, by loving ourselves. Those who grow emotionally stronger, will increase their capacity to love, and will experience a resurrection of what is hopefully, a sweet and pleasure-filled sex life.

3-12. Failure to Rise

In that awful moment, he is flooded with dread. Instead of being capable of fulfilling, he shrinks to limp, faded glory. Sometimes eyes meet with questions and with fear, but more often eye contact is avoided. It's just too uncomfortable. The answers sought are unavailable, so he offers equally limp excuses. It is an awkward drama when he cannot perform. Erectile dysfunction may have physical or emotional causes. This article focuses upon erection loss when its source is emotional, an event most men will experience at some point in their sexual lives.

The lingering memory after this kind of experience haunts men. They recall the embarrassment and feelings of inadequacy whenever they detect even a hint of a sexual opportunity. Without the confidence required for good sexual performance, some men choose to avoid the closeness of affection because it is a precursor to sex. Even men with formerly high sexual desire suddenly have none. Their partners may not understand why he is suddenly so distant. A single man with a history of failed erections may avoid dating. In fear, he mistakenly believes that every potential partner will want him to pass the sex test on the first date, one in which he will certainly crash and burn.

Because most men have a minimal awareness of their emotions, they may be unable to identify the negative emotions responsible for a sudden loss of arousal and erection. Confusion reigns at that moment, the first time his penis isn't doing what he wishes; men often can't figure out why. Facing a partner's questions is the second loss of control.

A female partner, when together with her male partner who is not performing, is thrown into a predicament for which there is no easy scripted response. She may feel it necessary to mask her disappointment, yet in doing so, she will be insincere, despite her wish to kindly reassure him. A less secure woman may believe his loss of erection is a statement about his feelings for her; that she is not desirable enough, or that her sexual skills are lacking. None of these are likely to be true. Each assumption heightens discomfort while fueling disconnection between partners. If the sexual opportunity is not salvaged, its memory may be the proverbial elephant in the corner; obvious, awkward, and unaddressed.

Anxiety, stress, and pressure are the most usual suspects; they kill arousal. Anger and emotional disconnection between partners do this too. As men age, they are increasingly vulnerable to aging's deleterious effects on sexual performance, though young men are not immune. If anxiety is a common emotional feature of a man's personality, he is even more susceptible to suffering erection loss when the pressure of performance is on. Good health protects men's erections, while poor health makes erections less resilient if it does not destroy sexual functioning completely. Medications, such as blood pressure pills, can often eliminate erections. Pro-erection medications are helpful to make an erection more confident and can also be a useful ally to destroy a negative, emotionally based cycle of performance anxiety.

Once it has happened, erection loss is an event that tends to re-occur. The experience of failure to perform is strongly anxiety-provoking, turning each subsequent sexual opportunity into a fear-producing event. Thus the climate is perfect for re-occurrence.

When there is not so much pressure upon a penis to produce results, it is better able to perform. Once successes are achieved, couples can practice and develop the skill of repair, regaining arousal even after it has been lost. When sexual partners can talk about their relationship, feelings, and sexual play, they are enabled to engineer low-stress, low-expectation sex, the right environment for erections to last. With moments of closeness, acceptance, and connection in a team effort, partners can slow, and ultimately defeat, the negative cycle of fear and failure.

3-13. Battling Desire Discrepancy

In terms of time allotment, sex is not a huge part of how a couple spends their time. It is barely a sliver on the pie chart, but when sex is a problem it negatively affects a disproportionately large part of the relationship. The saying is: "Sex is 10% of relationship; but when it's a problem, it becomes 90% of the relationship." Such is the case when partners differ in the amount of importance each places on sex.

Consider the fictitious married couple Rupert and Bertha, for whom the issue of sex had become a battleground. They both recalled how early in their relationship sex was the source of pleasure and how the frequency of their sexual exploits put some rabbits to shame. Rupert, who highly valued sex, lamented that "those were the days." He pointed out that because he initially experienced Bertha as a highly sexual woman, he considered himself a very lucky man for having struck sexual gold. As is the case for many men, Rupert felt deeply loved and connected with Bertha through their sexual play. During the recent past, as the frequency and passion of their lovemaking dwindled, he had grown distant and resentful. He had expressed feeling ripped-off. He and Bertha have been arguing often about sex. Due to their infrequent sexual encounters, he had questioned Bertha's love, since it was through their lovemaking that her love for him was confirmed.

Bertha, too, claimed she enjoys sex, but has never placed as high a priority on it as did Rupert. At the beginning of their relationship, she took great satisfaction in helping Rupert feel pleasure. The fact that he desired her really turned her on. Sex was not something she ever really did for herself. As the relationship aged, she found that she wasn't in the mood to be sexual nearly as often as she had been in the beginning. It wasn't that she felt less eager to please Rupert, but their lives had become more routine; she was more aware of his sometimes-annoying human eccentricities and did not enjoy the timing of Rupert's desire for a sexual encounter, which often seemed ill-timed to her moods. She also noticed that he was making less effort to get her in the mood by being what she considered romantic, through cuddling and gestures of his love. When he expressed a desire for sex, she didn't particularly like telling him “no,” and, over time, increasingly avoided those situations that gave Rupert the opportunity to initiate. When she did say no, he would act hurt and angry. She had grown to resent the pressure she felt to share herself with him sexually. True, she did feel guilty sometimes, but it seemed to be the easier choice. Sex had disappeared from their marriage, as had their emotional connection.

Over time, the spouses found that they were growing

apart. Each attempt at real communication repeatedly deteriorated into sarcastic allegations traded back and forth, which never arrived at a resolution or change. Both spouses felt powerless to alter the downward spiral of their marriage. Without third-party help, their marriage would have ended. They came to learn that the differences in their sexual needs could threaten their marriage if not openly discussed; that sex must be an active component and that their emotional connection functions as essential nourishment to keep their sex life active.

This is an all-too-common tale of a discrepancy of sexual desire, a small problem that can have devastating effects on marriage over the long haul. Sex is a vital part of a healthy love relationship. When it is not the source of satisfaction for both partners it is just a matter of time before the relationship loses its luster.

3-14. She Targets Sex

"If I never had sex again for the rest of my life, it'd be fine with me!" As a sex therapist, I have heard this phrase expressed in my office by dozens of frustrated, discouraged wives. It strikes terror into the heart of passionate husbands, while also confusing them. Without a doubt, this signals relationship difficulties in which sex is not a satisfying experience. Beyond that, what are the circumstances which cause a woman to reject her sexuality? Sex is a valuable part of being human. Would it be much different if she expressed hatred for her hands, hatred for eating, or hatred for life? It suggests an inner emotional conflict and a need for healing. When we reject any part of ourselves, our potential for wholeness is destroyed.

Women are vulnerable to splitting off their sexuality, thereby experiencing it as separate from themselves. Factors that contribute to this choice are the many pressure-inducing, media-delivered messages women receive about their bodies, about their beauty, about what sexiness is, and about desirability. If inwardly a woman does not feel good about herself, she may then regard with suspicion her partner's sexual desire for her. She may feel that he desires sex, but not her; that he values her body or sex parts, but not her as a whole person. The differences in the way men express sexual desire versus the way women want sex to develop only helps to promote this kind of disconnection.

Long-term relationships are difficult on so many levels. Negotiating a healthy sex life is among couples' thornier challenges, made even harder by the reality that for most couples, the male partner has a higher sex drive than the female. Many female partners avoid guilty feelings by making themselves sexually available, especially during times when they do not have much sexual interest. A loving wife who shares herself regularly to satisfy her husband's sexual needs bumps into trouble when her sexual generosity is not matched by the fulfillment of her needs for respect, connection, friendship and romance. At times like these, resentment builds. To a woman it can feel like sex is the problem, resulting in hate for sex. While it may seem so, sex is not really the source of the difficulties.

Because sex is at the intersection of all aspects of being human, sexual issues magnify any relationship or personal problems. If a woman feels insecure, or struggles with acceptance of her body, or has poor self-esteem, the odds are high that these may contribute to a discomfort with sex. It is more useful to identify the real problem, located within herself, her partner, or their relationship, instead of blaming sexuality.

Relationship difficulties contribute to making sex a battleground. Partners' success at controlling strong impulses greatly determines whether or not intimacy develops and is maintained within a love relationship. The following fictional people have trouble controlling their emotional impulses arising from low self-esteem, fear, anger and anxiety. While driving, when frustrated by other, stupid drivers, Burt hits the gas pedal hard, driving fast and aggressively. When his family is in the car, they fear for their lives. Despite his wife's complaints, Burt does nothing to change. Sally promised her husband she would rein in her spending, but since he mentioned this problem, she has hidden both her spending and her purchases from him. Relaxing doesn't come easily for John, so he looks forward to a couple of beers on the weekend. Routinely, two beers become three and this eventually leads to him consuming the entire twelve-pack. Once intoxicated, his personality grows mean and insulting, typically hurting his wife. If a man shows Jackie attention, even if her boyfriend is nearby, she fails to control her need to feel desirable by flirting without regard for her boyfriend's feelings.

Behavior patterns strongly influenced by these impulses constitute many of our routine daily actions, and therefore collectively represent a powerful force made up of many small choices. If negative, they harm loving connections like the proverbial "death by a thousand paper cuts." A disappearing sex life is often the first sign that damage is being done.

The failure to control our anxious impulses damages love relationships. Fear and anxiety get expressed in frequent, repetitive behaviors, each of which is like a spine on a cactus, stopping others from getting too close. No one wants to get close to a spiny cactus and risk getting stabbed. Bad behaviors will never make a good relationship or promote intimacy. Developing healthier coping methods to calm anxiety and discomfort is necessary if a close, healthy and passionate relationship is to be maintained. Practice controlling these destructive impulses! Love is our highest effort and paradoxically our most difficult task.

3-15. Opposite Paths to Arousal

Their sheets get twisted often enough, but their bedroom fun falls short of the satisfaction she knows is possible. Frustrated, she feels clueless about where to begin to make their pleasure better. Her husband also wants their intimate encounters to be steamier. He has begun to worry that, judging by her lack of excitement, his wife just isn't that into him. Without being armed with answers, neither dares to open the subject up to discussion.

Such is the situation between many lovers. Without being able to identify the nature of the problem, a solution is hopelessly elusive. They have the wood but don't know how to start the fire. This couple's trouble is a misunderstanding of the different, and opposite paths to arousal taken by males and females, a disconnect that is easy to correct.

Someone said: "Women are like crockpots and men are like microwave ovens." Both get hot and eventually cook, but the length of time it takes each to get to that place of steamy readiness is vastly different. If partners fail to respect this difference, their sexual experiences are at risk of falling flat. Younger men rapidly reach a boil in 30 seconds to two minutes. Older healthy men take a bit longer. Women heat up far more slowly, climbing gradually to high excitement in 15 to 40 minutes. For everybody, when negative emotions are present, getting aroused takes longer.

If the male partner is leading the sexual play, he will desire to begin intercourse far sooner than his female partner. Ready or not, many female partners defer to their male partner's timetable, intending to please. The disappointment and frustration that poor sexual experiences create will linger, and may contaminate future opportunities for pleasure and connection. Techniques or toys cannot circumnavigate such an obstacle.

Most men desire their genitals to be stimulated early and directly; no dilly-dallying about. Finding this deeply satisfying, men assume that women prefer this as well, so they will go right for their female partners' most sensitive parts, believing this to be the best approach. In reaction, women may feel misunderstood, rushed or even devalued.

Unlike men, most women are slow to become aroused, a fact men may have difficulty appreciating because their own experience is so different. Women's path to arousal requires attention to their entire bodies, with their erogenous zones being stimulated later. Brief teasing forays into her erogenous zones can expand as her arousal increases. Women give what they want to receive. They touch their male partners all over while avoiding early attention to men's sexy parts, an approach that frustrates men. Without correction, partners precipitously fall out of sync.

The path to mutual satisfaction, including high arousal and

high pleasure, must involve respect for the differences between partners. Males and females naturally give to the other what they want to receive themselves, an ineffective attempt to teach by example in which each fails to learn about the others' needs. It is much better to learn directly what the other likes and needs, and then follow through by providing it.

The sexual differences between men and women become insurmountable if communication is blocked. Discomfort or embarrassment with sex causes this. Within many loving encounters, silence is a symptom of the resulting loneliness and disconnection. In this intimate arena, a discussion about partners' feelings and needs can seem like a risky intrusion. Here communication is crucial; well-worded positive communication has the power to transform a sexual challenge into an adventure by allowing partners to teach each other about the mysterious, magical differences. When partners can say with comfort, "I'm not ready yet," "Please touch me here like this," or "This would feel good," then satisfaction is within reach without the risk of too-painful disappointment. When partner differences are respected, together, great heights of excitement may be scaled.

3-16. The Two Sides of Sexual Anxiety

Of the many obstacles couples face while creating a fulfilling and satisfying sexual life, anxiety is a large one. Sex is regarded as a physical experience, but in sex, our emotions play an even larger role than our bodies. Among our many emotions, anxiety features large on our emotional stage. It has been said that all negative emotions are related to fear. Anxiety is fear's close but smaller sibling.

Our success in life depends on how we manage fear. And for many people, the closeness and vulnerability that are essential for sex produces a fear that for many lovers represents a large and heavy door separating them from sexual pleasure. When facing a large change in one's life, people speak about simultaneously feeling scared and excited. These two emotions represent the dual nature of anxiety in sex as well. Lovers are often split between these two feelings, where each individual's sexual response is imprinted with one of these two forms of anxiety.

We live in a culture of anxiety, where anxiety disorders and dysfunctional reactions to the unhealthy environment are common. Anxiety problems cause people to shut down emotionally and physically. Sex is an arena in which this is likely to occur. A person feeling anxious about any aspect of sexual activity, such as fearing closeness, poor sexual performance, the partner's criticism, or the body looking unattractive, reacts to this fear by becoming sexually disabled due to emotional causes. Anxiety interferes with the ability to physically or emotionally function, causing the person to reflexively retreat inwardly.

These partners feel more comfortable with a sexual environment that feels safe and not challenging. Routine sex in which the partner knows which activity will happen when, what is expected, when and how stimulation will be given or received, and an exact recipe for orgasmic success results in a sense of safety, and ultimately an ability to relax. Assured privacy, emotional safety, and a sense of acceptance are high on this partner's list of requirements to make sex a pleasant experience.

Then there is the second side of anxiety; one that is about excitement. For the second kind of partner, safety, and routine lead to boredom. Instead of creating a shutting-down reaction, anxiety creates excitement. Trying new sexual activities and taking risks produces anxiety, which feels nourishing and alive, leading to a heightened level of sexual excitement. The eroticism for this partner probably includes a thirst for breaking through barriers and challenging authority. He or she thrives on adventurousness and possesses a thirst for new sexual experiences, which provide a sense of sexual freedom. Such a person may suggest being sexual in a risky location where the possibility of being discovered is real. He or she may require the sex life to include a wide assortment of positions for intercourse because novelty adds to the excitement.

When partners join, if each partner represents one pole in this dual nature of anxiety, the sexual relationship is primed for tension and conflict. The partner who requires safety must push his or her limits and accept that new experiences can also mean growth. The partner who craves excitement must also recognize that patience and love mean taking it slow, because sex is nothing if it is not paired with love.

{ Relax!

Good enough *really is good* enough. }

3-17. Coping with the Porn Factor

The issue of porn represents a divisive challenge to many couples. This problem is even sharper when the lovemaking has stopped and disconnection rules the relationship. Is porn a problem? In reaction to the use of porn, many couples experience conflict, partners are hurt, and trust is damaged. But is this porn's fault? It is similar to the age-old dilemma about guns; whether the problem lies with guns or the people who use the guns.

In most relationships where porn has contributed to an erupted crisis, the male partner (yes, most of the time, it is the male partner) has been discovered secretly looking at porn. The greatest amount of hurt is generated not so much by the porn as by the trust-damaging, secretive nature of his self-pleasuring. Good relationships are good due to openness and sharing between strong partners. Secrets and deception harm relationships. Porn can only truly be a problem if partners are not open with each other about their sexuality and freely talk about it.

So what's gone wrong? Most of the time, porn has filled a void already created by some kind of disconnection between partners. This is not porn's fault; porn use is just a symptom of an emotional and sexual disconnect. Female partners may feel betrayed by the male partner looking sexually at other women and fear that he will be more attracted to them. In actuality, if the male partner is in some way sexually dissatisfied or emotionally disconnected, pornographic material and masturbation function as a substitute which help him ***not*** to seek other real women...so in a way it may protect a disconnected relationship from dissolution and betrayal.

Studies have revealed that men who look at sexual images of women generally do not have feelings of disrespect for them, but on the contrary, tend to have positive, respectful feelings about women. I am not defending men who look at porn. If a relationship becomes disconnected, rather than turning to porn for sexual satisfaction, it is a better, stronger choice for men to openly discuss the problems with their female partner, who, hopefully, is responsive and receptive.

There are various scenarios which tend to lead to porn usage. A man is likely to hide it for the same reasons most couples have difficulty talking about sex; it is a source of shame, embarrassment and discomfort. After all, as an activity, masturbation is more taboo than sex itself. So unless a relationship contains openness about sex, such sexual behaviors will commonly be hidden. Some men have looked at porn habitually since their teen years and have not broken the habit. Some use it as erotic fantasy material to heighten their excitement so as to reduce stress; some of these men become compulsive in their need for sexual stimulation. Others use porn as a substitute when the sexual relationship is not satisfying, insufficiently active or completely inactive. Anxiety-ridden men who are not strong enough to risk intimacy use porn as an aid to achieve sexual satisfaction while avoiding closeness with their female partner.

When sex cannot be talked about openly, cloudiness is cast over the sunshine of potential sexual satisfaction. When men look at sexual images of women, they deliberately choose images containing women who appear to them sexually enthusiastic. Part of the fantasy is the imagined acceptance by the fantasy woman of the male viewer and his eroticism. The following factors are some of those which prevent sex lives from being relaxing, playful and fun: low sexual frequency, unenthusiastic partners, inhibited partners, unfulfilled eroticism and poor communication during sex.

The greatest protection from porn-related threats is provided by successful efforts at making sex satisfying, open and enthusiastic. For women who are challenged with beauty or body-insecurities, while you may feel threatened by the fantasy women with porn bodies, your ability to give or receive love and be a great sexual partner does not depend upon the shape of your body. Use your strength to put aside your insecurities and make the discovery of his porn usage an opportunity to learn about his eroticism. It may function as a step towards building a stronger, more intimate and more erotic love relationship.

Neither good nor bad, porn is a reality of our internet age. It is unlikely to disappear any time soon. Depending upon porn for arousal does not represent the healthiest sexuality; though porn can play a healthy role in singles' and couples' sex lives. Protecting a relationship from the destructive effects of porn use requires building a strong, active, erotic sex life through openness and emotional connection. The same elements contribute to emotional security.

3-18. Orgasm, Complicated

During their sexual experiences, for most couples, orgasm is prized. And yet, because men and women both experience and achieve orgasm differently, the entire issue is open to conflict. Men and women value this peak experience differently.

A sweet woman recently complained that her male partner usually insists that if she has not yet had an orgasm, she have one at the end of their lovemaking. She is troubled by this because she does not really care whether or not she has an orgasm, but when feeling pressured to have an orgasm by her lover, this robs her of the generated good feeling right at the end of their loving togetherness.

The issue raised by this woman is not unusual and is voiced by many. The issue of orgasm highlights the differences between men and women. For most men, it is a vital part of each sexual experience, without which an experience feels dissatisfying and incomplete. Some men go so far as to say that if they have a sexual experience without the release of orgasm, they are likely to experience subsequent discomfort in the form of "blue balls." For them, having an orgasm is a measuring stick as to whether or not an experience is "good enough." Women function very differently.

For most women, orgasm is not the determining factor of the satisfaction of a sexual experience, but instead, the degree of emotional closeness between a woman and her lover is the salient indicator. Most women do not orgasm regularly, and rarely from intercourse, unlike their male counterparts. Generally speaking, women have neither developed that expectation nor hold it as physically vital. Men value orgasm and ejaculation so highly that many men cannot conceive of women's truth that orgasm is not vitally important.

For decades the importance of their female partners' sexual satisfaction has been impressed upon men. Some shudder at the thought of being labeled a bad lover. In their struggle to learn about and understand women, many men fail to appreciate the importance of women's emotional experience; it plays a less important role in the man's world. Hence many men are poorly equipped to feel an emotional connection the way women do.

In men's misguided attempts to satisfy, the above-mentioned two factors collide; of blindly valuing orgasm and of wanting to be a good lover for their female partner. Men hold the mistaken belief that, similarly to themselves, if their female partner does not reach orgasm, then they have failed to satisfy her, and risk being viewed as a bad lover. Even when a female partner clearly expresses that orgasm is not important, many men, because of their own inner value systems, simply do not believe this.

One final issue contributes to his insistence that she have

an orgasm: many male lovers gain deep satisfaction from witnessing their female partner having the high excitement, hopefully dramatically expressed, of orgasm. Witnessing this spectacle, a man feels strong and in control. The surrender that must accompany orgasm, to men, is a sign that his woman is completely open to him. He is provided reassurance of her love.

Negotiating differences is difficult, and may often seem impossible. The openness that comes from learning specifically about how your partner functions and how he or she feels is superior to following myths or preconceived notions. That is what makes sex such a special experience; when understanding and sensitivity are not included, the feelings can be diminished. Protect these moments by being open to learning about each other.

SEXUAL PLAY

4-1. Digging the Dirt

Behind closed doors, and maybe even elsewhere, when people play sexually, some like to talk dirty. Others are turned off by dirty-talking partners. What is this dirty talk, and why do many people like it, while others do not? It can be controversial, the source of conflict between sexual partners. Some say, "Please! Say something dirty!" While the other replies, "No! That's disgusting!"

Dirty talk lives in the paradoxical sexual world where what is good can be bad, what is bad can be good, and what is dirty can be fun! But only for some. When it comes to sex play, partners do not always agree about what kind of sex is fun and what kind "crosses the line" into discomfort. For those partners, discomfort means being turned off.

What is at work in those who get excited by hearing dirty words from the lips of their loved ones? It is about the particulars of his or her eroticism. A universal aspect of eroticism is novelty. When something is new, it is exciting. This phenomenon is not unique to eroticism; this is why the car industry rolls out a new version of the old model every year to arouse consumer excitement yet again.

Long-term committed relationships struggle to cope with the lack of novelty, the same partner, the same habits, the same body, etc. Dirty talk is one method of inspiring novelty by encouraging new and uncharacteristic behaviors in a partner, especially when the kinds of dirty talk deviate from his or her normally-held values.

Another feature of eroticism is sparked by the breaking of rules, limitations and boundaries. The most potent kick of excitement comes from violating societal rules and values. Dirty talk accomplishes this by asking the partner to express sentiments, ideas and arousals that touch or break widely held moral and sexual values. This is exemplified by the male asking his female partner to “talk like a slut.” Another similar situation is when a woman wants her male partner to talk and act aggressively, or even as a rapist. The requested scenarios may be shocking, but in reality, dirty talk can be intensely exciting and coincidentally safe, good clean fun.

Where dirty talk bumps into trouble is when sexual partners have different levels of comfort with this kind of activity or the requested subject matter. If a female partner has strongly-held moral values, she might feel that she is betraying herself by stepping out of her comfort zone and filling the role of a slut. Women's newly possessed societal permission to own power may cause many women to be uncomfortable pretending to relinquish such hard-won power by adopting a subordinate role. A male partner, if not secure in his own goodness and power, may feel uncomfortable filling a role in which his power is used destructively, even if it is just acting. The line of comfort and discomfort delineates where a partner will set a limit and say no to dirty talk.

Violating boundaries can produce an erotic charge in many. This was often instilled in the teen years of experimentation during sexual development, when sex play had to be hidden and thus for many was only able to occur away from parents' supervising eyes in the confines of a car's back seat or other secret areas. Breaking rules, taking risks and being the "bad boy or bad girl," may all spur on excitement due to the freedom of entering into territory which is beyond conventionally accepted behaviors. Because sex challenges our boundaries, our discomfort is rendered a poor test for what to include or exclude from our sex lives.

4-2. Playing with Power

Sex and power are strongly linked and interact on many levels between romantic partners. The use of power can be split into two broad categories: the power to control others and the power to love others. Power to control is implemented through direct force, examples of which include authority, fear, or obstruction. The power of love also influences, but without domination. Instead, it offers nourishment, growth, connection, and freedom. The second power values you and your needs. The first does not.

Our personal power is granted from birth. True power is our ability to make our own lives satisfying rather than to control or manipulate others. Free will offers us the opportunity to oppose others and life if we so choose. If love partners battle for power, love will be blocked, resulting in emotional disconnection, tension and a withered sex life. Conversely, if partners share power and control, love will flow, opening the gates for emotional safety and goodwill, optimal conditions for a good sex life. Power imbalances in a relationship are bad for sex; it is no coincidence that a partner with too little relationship power is much more likely to have low or no sexual desire.

The opposite is true within the sexual arena, given that emotional safety has been established outside, as here, power imbalances are grist for the mill, with the potential to generate high arousal, intense excitement and highly erotic play. Beyond mechanical and unimaginative sex, much of sex play is rooted in experimenting with power. Even in the most basic of sexual experiences, power is demonstrated by who is on top versus who is on the bottom.

Life experiences with power, especially from childhood,

when powerlessness was acute, have a direct impact on emotional and sexual development. As children, many experienced harm through the misuse of power in unbalanced, poorly controlled ways. Most of us, at one time or another in our childhoods, had to cope with the simultaneous lack of safety and powerlessness, causing us either intentional or unintentional emotional wounds. Reacting inflexibly to power, with either defensive aggression or passive retreat, is the developmental result. These challenging life experiences show up in our sexuality in the form of erotic interest in power or powerlessness.

Significant themes in our human drama are the quest to obtain personal power, the experience of finding power unobtainable and feeling unsafe because of powerlessness. All this is manifested in sexual play where partners request and deliberately create scenarios that call for large differences of power assigned to each sexual role. This fosters intense excitement. Bondage, domination and submission, use of pain, or role play between people where there is a power imbalance are obvious examples. Playing with power during sex is an attempt to relate to, heal from, and grow from much earlier experiences with issues of power, but more often, powerlessness. Power dynamics spark an erotic charge because the possibility of healing and the potential for deeper completeness is near. Within sexual play, the kinds of power used do not signify that partners outside the bedroom possess these same kinds or amounts of power.

For most of us, having no power is undesirable. It is associated with weakness and vulnerability. Yet during sexual play, powerlessness has a hidden benefit, so long as safety is assured. By being taken, wanted and chosen, a less powerful partner's desirability is confirmed. Desirability is another large theme within sexuality and love relationships. Female partners have a propensity for obtaining desirability. Male partners lean towards possessing power. These are not rigid roles.

Playing with power during sex is a vital piece of what makes sex relevant and exciting in our lives. Most partners gravitate more towards either power or powerlessness. When partners possess the flexibility to experiment with both dominant and submissive sexual roles, their sex life has the greatest potential for fun, excitement and growth.

> A partner's highest obligation is to protect the partner from being hurt or negatively affected by him or her.

4-3. The Multi-players

The topic of sexuality would be done a disservice by staying safely within the comfort zone of my readers. Sexuality does not fit neatly into the general perception of what is good or bad, right or wrong. Moral or immoral judgements do not alter the reality that many people have sex with several partners simultaneously. In acknowledging it, I neither promote nor condemn such behavior, but risk condemnation for publicly writing about it. Because these kinds of sexual activities are considered immoral by the prevailing social environment, group sex tends to be covert and not often publicly shared.

Group lovers gather in several ways: there are the swingers, those who prefer orgies, the "wife swappers" and, less frequently, the husband swappers as well. Other group lovers may aptly be called polyamorous. Some participate in highly-organized, well-regulated group sexual activities, while others enjoy smaller, more relaxed, multiple-partner gatherings of just three or four people. In many cases, these unions developed without conscious intention, but were facilitated by spontaneous circumstances and situations where inhibitions were lowered by drugs and/or alcohol.

Those who are considered polyamorous attempt to form stable, loving, long-term relationships with more than one partner and for more than just a sexual intent. These individuals may enjoy sexual pleasure in dyads or in the group relationship. This is a different pattern from the swingers who gather specifically for group sexual activities, but without any continuous emotional attachment. Other swingers enjoy playing with particular couples or several other couples separately or simultaneously, which sometimes may be called wife swapping, a name which is most appropriate if the male partners are the motivating force behind the union of couples. There are many couples who desire to include a third partner in their sexual play. Depending upon the desires of the partners, a couple may choose a male or female partner as the third participant.

These sexual combinations are fluid and changeable. They may contribute to an individual's or couple's sexuality occasionally, intermittently, or on a time-limited basis. While multiple-partner sex does not accurately describe most people's sexuality, it is a significant and perennial sexual subset and therefore worthy of discussion if an understanding of sexuality is to be achieved.

For those who participate with multiple partners, great pleasure and joy can be experienced, but there is always the risk of potential problems. Among the dangers are attachments between primary romantic partners being tested by the attention and affection shared with others. Many committed couples' security and integrity are threatened by feelings of uncertainty and jealousy when one partner or the other has a particular fondness or excitement for someone outside the couple. Insecurities are easily raised; relationship triangles are prone to instability. Exposure to sexually transmitted diseases multiplies with the number of sexual partners.

The curiosity about bodies and sex, the attraction to others beyond a single partner, the need for connection and merging, as well as the unlimited and indiscriminate nature of sexual energy all motivate some to seek out multiple-partner sex. Further, adventurous lovers desire to increase the intensity of their sexual excitement by violating taboos of limitation, an attribute that is high in multiple-partner experiences. Participants enjoy feelings of intense intimacy when a group setting is safe and loving combined with the joy of unbridled freedom that complete openness offers, a sensation shared by nudists.

Sex with multiple partners is not a good choice for the majority of people, but it is and always has been a variation of sexuality. From a sexual standpoint, it is neither right nor wrong, neither good nor bad, but simply one way among many that some people choose to love and be sexual.

4-4. Bound to Have Fun

Excitement is the name of the game. To feel alive, we seek out many ways to be excited. This is certainly true in good sexual experiences. Yet to produce excitement, there is usually some degree of risk. Horror films are popular for this reason; they allow us to observe frightening, even life-threatening scenarios, with little risk of harm. Sexually, bondage is analogous.

People express their sexuality in many forms. Sex acts are judged as "kinky" when they cross the line into our discomfort zone. Sex that does not cross such a line is called "vanilla sex" by some; these are plain experiences in which little risk is taken. Without a doubt, some kinds of sexual expression are more "mainstream" than others. The risk of accepting danger and vulnerability while simultaneously testing the trust between partners is characteristic of bondage. I neither encourage nor discourage any particular kind of sexual experimentation; this article simply explores the ways people are sexual, and why.

Being tied up and rendered powerless while held captive to the whims of a partner is intensely exciting to some. Such an emotional experience provokes old emotions going back to infancy and childhood when we were totally helpless; a tied-up partner experiences this same vulnerability. For the in-control partner, it is deeply exciting for the other to be completely open in submission.

This sexual game is not appealing to all. The dark connotations of being bound, dominated, and punished do not inspire warm associations. The close approximation to real past hurts causes this kind of play to come too painfully close to reality to make it interesting for many. Why is this fun? The participants revel in the intense excitement and sensations of inner emotions not otherwise accessible. The darker places within, filled with rejected parts of the self, called the "shadow" by Dr. Carl Jung, are common to all of us. Feeling these emotions is an experience most avoid, but in the drama of bondage, these feelings are celebrated, and through acknowledgement, it provides not only excitement but also emotional freedom. Venturing into risky territory deepens the intimate connection of bondage partners.

All of us grew up being powerless children, without the capacity to make choices for ourselves. Negotiating this challenging environment had a long-lasting impact on our emotional and sexual development, especially regarding elements of power, desirability and living with limits. These are human challenges that are not indicative of dysfunction or past abuse. The emotions arising from early life experiences form the material that becomes erotic sexual play and causes bondage to be the sexual expression of choice for some lovers.

In the sexual drama, the powerless partner becomes an object of desire and attention. When bound, this partner receives all the attention. His or her value is demonstrated by the other's intense need to possess, abduct, or hold him or her captive. The dominant partner enjoys owning the power, and with it the opportunity to orchestrate the activity. His or her value is confirmed by the other's willingness to display openness and submission by placing his or her life in the powerful partner's hands.

Bondage play enhances the trust and intimacy of consenting partners. Like two people who endure an arduous ordeal together develop a deep bond, bondage partners, by reveling in their deep feelings and vulnerabilities, build a stronger connection. It is forged by complete trust which is tested by their actual drama.

Sexual exploration and experimentation furnish an opportunity for partners to invite previously repressed emotions to reach the conscious light of day. Fantasy is healthy but fantasizing about unsafe situations can be risky. Playing at being unsafe is vastly different than actually being unsafe! Play is about fun and excitement, not real hurtfulness. A safe word agreed upon before the beginning of their play establishes a signal so that both partners know when a request to stop is serious and is not play. This is necessary because sexual excitement knows no bounds.

4-5. A Threesome? Oh my! Why?

Linda (a fictional character), who has been married to Paul for six years, is uncertain how to deal with a situation that has arisen. Her husband repeatedly expresses a desire for her to invite her best friend to join them in sex. Linda has never had a thought about being sexual with another woman, or of including more people, other than her husband, in their sexual life. She wants to please him and admits that when he brings it up, she feels a combination of fear and arousal. Despite not encouraging Paul's desire, he often reminds her of wanting his fantasy to be acted out in real life.

People express their sexuality in numerous ways. For many, the pursuit of more intense sex and greater sexual adventure leads to the desire to include more people in their sexual experiences than just their relationship partner. Some people crave sexual variety in both sexual acts and partners. It is not uncommon for the eager and curious partner to request that the couple invite another into their sex-play. Rarer is the couple that actually makes real what for most remains unpicked fruit from the tree of fantasies, a realm where everything and anything goes including activities that never actually get acted out. In a fantasy, everything is safe, controlled, and summoned from the uncreated imagination for optimal erotic pleasure. Fantasies do not typically translate well into reality; the real experience compares poorly with the perfect drama dreamed up by the imagination.

For those who are more daring and adventurous, including a third person in sex-play is the source of tantalizing eroticism where the possibilities of excitement and pleasure far surpass the more common one-on-one sexual interlude. A threesome may be about doing something taboo, in which traditional sexual, moral, and religious rules are violated. Having sexual contact with a stranger, or a person other than the spouse, can intensify a sexual thrill many-fold. A threesome is just one sexual variation that includes more than one partner. Other multi-partner sexual arrangements include polyamorous relationships, partner swapping, voyeurism of watching others being sexual, multi-couple sex, swing parties, and orgies.

Few topics polarize people on a moral basis as often as sex. Are three-way sexual encounters right or wrong? This is not a particularly useful question since the answer is highly subjective. Three-way sexual encounters exist. They are wrong for people with conservative sexual values. It is not unusual for many members of a society to view numerous sexual practices as immoral, yet, when viewed without judgement, these sexual variations exist, always have and always will. Some people do choose to express their sexuality in these ways and experience them as highly pleasurable.

There are two distinct moral camps regarding how sex should be regarded and the proper reasons for choosing to engage in it. The first, and the most common perspective among most organized religions, is that sex is an activity through which to express love, to feel loved, and to deepen a bond of love between two people, usually a man and a woman. The second camp holds that sex is a wonderful and highly enjoyable activity which is about celebrating pleasure and expressing the freedom to live out all the enjoyable sexual permutations without limit. The two views are opposite in that one is about making a bond while the other is about celebrating the freedom from bonds. The primary values of each group, love versus freedom, are deep and virtuous.

Sex is common. Despite its taboo nature and the idea that sex holds an unhealthy place in our culture, most adults have a lot of sex, but not in a multiple partner modality. Many people may have participated in a three-way sexual experience at one time, but for most a threesome is not part of their regular sexual vocabulary. Instead, a threesome for many couples may function as an unusual, but exciting variation which happens due to the urging of an insistent fantasy of one of the partners. Among those who engage in three-way sex, are your regular neighborhood folks, Joe, Josephine and John, who are not necessarily any more, sexy, kinky, or wild than most of us.

But the dangers involved in multiple partner sexual experiences are many. From a relational point of view, three people form a triangle. Socially, triangles tend to be unstable in that it is far easier for two people of the three to be engaged while the third is left out. This tends to foster emotional friction or hurt feelings such as jealousy and insecurity. A three-way sexual experience can reopen old wounds as well as reactivate unresolved traumas in devastating ways. While the erotic allure of a three-way may be strong, it can de-stabilize a two-way love relationship. Questions about why a partner desired a three-way experience may linger long after in the form of damaged trust if partners are not careful. The more people involved in any sexual experience, the greater the risk of sexually transmitted diseases, pregnancy and emotionally complicated situations.

For those inclined towards sexual adventurousness and experimentation, the benefits of a three-way encounter are clear and enticing: heightened arousal and eroticism, a greater potential for pleasure, freedom of new experiences with new partners, more hands, feet, tongues, genitals, and orgasms, a potentially greater sense of sharing, and pushing the emotional envelope, and growing in a new way.

Want to give it a try? This writer neither encourages nor discourages the experience. Should you be tempted, let the following be your guide. A three-way sexual encounter should never be set-up without your partner's knowledge or consent. A partner pressured into a three-way experience is not likely to enjoy or value it, thus decreasing the potential for pleasure. No person should engage in this kind of sexual play if it is not aligned with his or her moral values. Before participating, ask yourselves if you are ready to live with the potential consequences. A situation where emotional safety is present creates an environment with the best possible outcome. First ask yourselves: "What is my motivation for wanting this?" A relationship needs to be strong and the partners secure in each other before a sexual experience of this kind can be positive.

4-6. Real or Fake?

Probably one hundred percent of men believe that their female partners don't fake orgasms, but in recent studies, approximately fifty percent of women admitted to having faked at least one. Do you remember the famous scene in the movie When Harry Met Sally? Meg Ryan's character was debating with Billy Crystal's about whether or not a male partner can tell when a woman fakes an orgasm. Her command performance, a loud fake orgasm in the middle of a bustling cafe, suggested that men cannot tell the difference if an orgasm is real or fake.

Since most people think a female orgasm should look dramatic and loud like Meg Ryan's, a male partner's ability to judge the difference between real and fake orgasms is limited, because many women actually orgasm quietly. The difference between reality and expectation causes uncertainty in which lovers have difficulty creating satisfaction.

Is faking an orgasm a problem? It can be. It is deceitful and signals a breakdown in communication. Without sincerity, the satisfaction of an intimate connection is limited. Yet a fake orgasm is a seemingly painless solution to a difficult problem, like a little white lie. On the surface, faking an orgasm can be motivated by kindness, to help a sexual experience end gracefully while saving face. It may spare a couple some awkward moments of discomfort. At first, the situation appears comical, but under the surface, some harsher truths are hidden.

The reality of sex is that it is complex and highly political. Partners' sexual choices are driven by both realistic and unrealistic expectations. Self-esteem is on the line in each sexual encounter, making sex a highly charged cauldron of pressure. When good outcomes seem unobtainable, something's got to give...and that is often a believable faked orgasm.

If sex were less burdened with expectations, a woman may feel freer to say she hasn't had an orgasm or doesn't desire one. This would be a vast improvement. Unexpressed expectations create pressure for a sexual drama to proceed along with a pre-defined plot, otherwise hurt feelings ruin a well-choreographed experience. A faked orgasm is a symptom that a problem exists.

Why would women do such a thing? Each woman's reasons vary. Most women don't orgasm during intercourse but believe they should, so faking an orgasm helps them to live up to their own "shoulds" about sexual performance. Other women make this choice to soothe their partner's sexual insecurities; many men worry that their female partner's failure to reach orgasm signifies their own lack of sexual skills, a misplaced burden that some female partners carry. Some women, if ready for sex to end, may fake an orgasm to gracefully conclude it. A faked orgasm also frees a woman from having to ask her partner for the stimulation she may really need to reach orgasm, a conversation many women prefer to avoid, especially if she fears the request would upset her partner.

Is it a victimless crime? The partner may never know how real a woman's orgasm is unless she herself reveals it. Openness is a relationship ideal and faking an orgasm violates it. If sex is troubled by emotional disconnection, a faked orgasm does nothing to address the problem, but only prolongs it. In an emotionally safe relationship, a more vulnerable but sincere approach may include having an honest discussion about sex, expectations and sexual limitations. Gaining more sexual information may be an important step. It takes a strong person to embark on such a journey. The results may lead to learning and increased sexual confidence that benefits the relationship and heightens the mutual satisfaction of sex.

4-7. Play Nice! Take Turns

In infancy, even before our first play date, each of us was taught from early on to share. Equality and sharing are fundamental concepts introduced to us in kindergarten. If we mastered the lesson well, our adult relationships and marriage benefit. In adulthood we say, "Turnabout is fair play." Mutuality and reciprocity are values deeply rooted even within our system of government, although not always well-enacted.

Yet some of our most deeply-rooted values do not translate into consistent behaviors. Take sexuality as an example. Within the sex lives of many couples, giving and receiving of pleasure is not performed with equality, mutuality or reciprocity, a tendency that not only expresses our individuality but also reveals an imbalance. The struggle to be balanced is fought within each one of us on a daily basis as we constantly adjust growth and change. Built into our being is a propensity to be more of a giver or receiver, a tendency that gets expressed when we make love. In each love relationship, there is a lover and a beloved.

Certain aspects of who a person becomes are inborn, a tendency to be a giver or receiver may be such a trait, or it may be a characteristic that is less deep within us and may be available for change. The elements of control play a large part in sexual dramas. Possessing or refusing control may be included in what a person experiences as erotic, but it may just be an echo of past hurts. A rigid need to be in control not only suggests inflexibility but also insecurity in which a loss of control feels unsafe. Being passive, without any willingness to possess control also points to an unhealthy past in which control was never offered, and thus never developed. In both positions, a person is stuck with the switch in an on or off position, interfering with their ability to share with mutuality.

Just as a wheel that is out of shape grows even more out of shape the more it is used, in our sex lives, any fixed tendency only becomes more fixed and ultimately becomes a problem if it is part of a rut. Growth is beneficial to each one of us, enabling us to become stronger in every area of our lives; that includes our sex lives. One kind of sexual calisthenics is to reach beyond the comfort zone by sexually taking charge if you are not such a take-charge kind of person, or to surrender and give up control if you are naturally an in-control kind of partner. By reaching into foreign territory we exercise parts of ourselves that are easily neglected. This is a method of balancing that moves each one of us in the direction of becoming more whole and healthy. Muscles that are used routinely become strong, but we also risk them becoming tired or overdeveloped, and then out of balance with less developed muscles. Changing the routine allows you to become more skilled in areas of less skill, and more comfortable in areas of less comfort.

We are not equals. An apple and an orange are not equal; they are just different. So it is with a man and a woman. It is not wise to ignore the differences while trying to force equality. The way partners sexually share is different as well. The differences will extend to the amount of sharing and the manner of sharing, but what most needs to be equal is the amount of satisfaction on the part of both partners. In sex, as in every other part of our life, we can maximize the benefit to ourselves if we live in the experience fully, by granting it our attention, focus, concentration and, at the same time, relaxation. The new, more equal sharing may rejuvenate what has become a lifeless routine, and as a wheel, it may help us to be more round.

4-8. More Than Just Lip Service

The pleasures of oral sex

Most sexual encounters are like a multi-act drama in which each act features a central pleasuring activity. Oral sex is the source of exquisite pleasure; a popular method to give and receive the gift of sexual attention. While common in the sexual repertoire of many, oral sex is equally avoided by many others. Sex is an intimate act, so much so that the word "intimacy" is commonly used to mean sex. Kissing, however, is rated as more intimate than many acts of giving sexual pleasure. Among sexual acts, oral sex is at the top of the list regarding what is considered most intimate.

Genitals are our "private" body parts. They possess a quality of being tremendously personal, whether or not the owner attaches to them pride or shame. Having oral contact with these intensely private parts is highly personal and highly erotic. Granting to another such close access to our private parts is exciting due to the risk of openness and vulnerability. So many people have ambivalence about their sex parts, because of the association of strong shame, a sense of dirty-ness, the embarrassment of vulnerability, but also a vital curiosity, which links our body to the magic of reproduction and the seduction of sexual pleasure. Whether you are God-fearing or not, it is difficult to prove that our genitals were created with any less attention or love than any other part of our bodies. Is it a mistake that the greatest bundle of pleasure-producing nerve endings are located so close to a place of elimination?

Oral sex is special, close personal contact with the lover's genitals, a body part that potently symbolizes the lover's masculinity or femininity. Our mouths and tongues are organs also exquisitely supplied with nerve endings. For the skilled lover, the tongue functions like a highly calibrated tool capable of excelling at stimulating sensitive nerve endings like no other. Intimately serving your lover by giving the gift of oral pleasure is certain to win gratitude and appreciation. It deepens the bond between lovers because of its intimate nature, but also because of the hint of dirtiness that exists within most minds, raising its erotic appeal.

But for some oral sex is emphatically distasteful and controversial. Too many lovers complain about their sexual partners, "If I get oral sex, then it must be the end of a decade!" Others express frustration; "My partner has no skill at oral pleasure." For the many people who associate genitals with dirtiness, oral sex resides beyond the line of acceptability. It is the sensitive lover who fully recognizes the place of hygiene in sexual and intimate matters. Hygiene is a gift of love that invites greater closeness and permits fuller pleasure. A good lover is a strong person who pushes beyond personal limitations to succeed at loving the partner so deeply that he or she feels divine.

Above all else, oral sex is about giving; it is about loving in a deep way which, by its very enactment, proclaims acceptance of the partner's worthiness as a man or a woman. The skill it takes to offer the full-bodied pleasure of oral sex must not be overlooked. Ask your partner what makes the difference between a mere sexual act and otherworldly pleasure.

MEN & WOMEN

5-1. A Man's Expectations

Within the relationship between a man and his closest friend, there often arise some difficulties. I am not writing about the relationship with his romantic partner, instead I am writing about the relationship with his penis, which defies female understanding because there is no female equivalent. For most men, his penis is his best friend and his special tool, which defines his emotional and masculine identity. It is his sexual power and masculine obligation.

Just after conception, we all begin life as female, becoming male means an added chromosome and increased testosterone. For our entire lives as men, we depend upon our penises to uphold and reinforce this one all-important distinction...that we are not women! The possession of a penis, how it well works and how often it is used, determines a man's emotional and masculine success. For men, this is a big deal! From a practical perspective, a penis is nothing more than a seed-planting tool, but from a man's perspective, it is a marvel of engineering, worthy of fondling, holding, and displaying so long as it works. If a penis doesn't work, a man will feel deep shame, inadequacy and emasculation. The penis defines the male gender.

In the relationship between a man and his penile friend,

there may develop some tension due to unrealistic expectations. Good sexual performance is ever threatened by lack of ejaculatory control, lack of an erection when needed, or the incomplete joy and satisfaction of his female partner. Men tend to have the expectation that their penises should work perfectly under all circumstances, on demand, with machine-like precision without fail, to completely fulfill the call of duty. The failure to live up to this ideal displays weakness, which undermines the strength and power of the masculine ideal. Each man would love to have greater control over his penis' responses.

This, for you women trying to understand your man, is the masculine ideal, and is without regard to your needs or expectations. This unrealistic ideal gets men and their penises into trouble. Missing from most men's calculations when it comes to expectations of sexual performance are the strong influences of emotions, relationship factors, energy level, health issues, and pre-occupations. While aging, all of these factors have an increasing impact on a man and his penis. As much as each man wishes for complete mechanical perfection, his penis teaches him as he ages that he cannot be a machine and that in some good ways, he is more like a woman than he would like to admit.

A man must learn that he cannot ignore his emotions; that closeness, sharing and openness with his partner are essential for really good sex; that patience is a virtue, and that good sex is best attained when control and power are shared. In doing so a man may avoid the dire consequences of failed sexual performance, which even Viagra will not completely correct. The instances when his penis has failed to perform up to his expectations represent a man's moments of greatest masculine fragility, but also the potential for masculine triumph if he adapts by enjoying a close and pleasuring encounter without reliance on his primary tool. From a penis' perspective, aging means softening erections, erections that fade more quickly, and slower response times, all of which to a man suggest loss of virility. If the acceptance of aging occurs gracefully by lowering his expectations, a man is less likely to find himself ensnared in the demoralizing cycle of performance anxiety.

A warning to the female partner: reacting with harshness or ridicule to your male partner's performance problems is committing sexual suicide. Nothing but loving patience and support will be beneficial. An older male partner has greater potential to be a more patient, creative, attentive, and sensitive lover who values slow, sensuous lovemaking and who has greater availability for an emotional connection. Such are changes which many female partners may welcome. The upside here is that sex has the potential to become more full and connecting, even if it is less Olympian.

> Making effort is not the same as producing results.

5-2. Women Don't Like Sex: Part 1

Within the cultural conversation and collective belief system is the reputation of women for not liking sex. Complaints come mostly from men in long-term committed relationships. They say, "I have tried everything, and despite my efforts, my wife/girlfriend/fiancée has no interest in sex. Having been repeated often enough throughout history, this scenario has solidified into a culturally held myth that is sadly expressed in the joke often shared between men, "How do you stop a woman from having sex? The answer: Marry her."

How true is it? No one blanket statement describes all women. Many women love sex, yet others would rather visit the dentist. Men, in their quest to succeed sexually with their female partners, are disadvantaged by their masculine approach unless it also seeks to understand their partner's feminine perspective. Sex is a necessary cog in the machinery of health, emotional balance, relationship satisfaction and even spiritual development. Women who are turned off to sex miss out on a vital, God-given gift. They would do well to make the effort to understand and remove the obstacles to sexual pleasure. The following is a short list of conditions that interfere with a woman being open to and enthusiastically embracing an active, passionate sex life.

Women who seem to dislike sex populate a choir who sing a song of complaints, most of which prove that it is not sex that they do not like. The majority of these women cite a bevy of unmet needs, describing the emotional closeness, safety, trust, respect, understanding, and experience of feeling loved, that are missing within their partnerships. For women, these needs function as prerequisites for sex. Unlike their male partners, who seek to build a connection via a sexual pathway, most women must first connect emotionally, and require that connection to be complete before sex becomes internally consistent with what they feel is in their own best interest. Unless the setting of a relationship is strong and positive, most female partners have little sexual desire. Men struggle to grasp the concept that the female partner's emotional experience is her reality and cannot be defined by him, even if to him it doesn't make sense. For most women, sex and emotional closeness *must* go together.

Living in a strong, well-connected and positive relationship is a challenge that sadly eludes many couples. The older the relationship, the greater the possibility that life's rigors and partner friction have caused an accumulation of deeply-layered negative emotion. The men in these longer relationships are the most vocal in complaining that their female partners have no interest in bedroom playfulness because these are also the relationships most locked into emotional disconnection. Couples that battle and have been unable to transform power-struggles into a loving connection are also likely to be inhabited by women who live in an emotionally unsafe environment unfriendly to their interest in sex. In such couples, the male partner will develop the impression that women don't like sex, but in reality, the conditions allowing women to have sexual interest are not being fulfilled.

It is true, however, that some women remain uninterested in sex. But most of these women are also saddled with difficulties that are distinct from a dislike of sex. Between thirty and fifty percent of women have experienced abuse at some time in their history. Unhealed emotional wounds block many women from feeling emotionally safe enough to risk the closeness, openness and vulnerability that sex requires. Other women suffer the blight visited upon most of the female population, of shame and hatred of their bodies, which interferes with the freedom to be sexual, and is a condition rarely shared or understood by male partners. Hormone fluctuations, especially during menopause, are also factors that limit sexual interest for some women.

To the outside world, and particularly to men, it may appear that women do not like sex, but the reality is that it is not specifically sex most women do not like. Instead, the absence of vital relationship ingredients renders sex an unattractive option for these women.

5-3. Women Don't Like Sex: Part II

It is not true that women do not like sex, but it is true that most women first need to feel loved within the context of a healthy relationship before being open to an active and passionate sex life. True, but only part of the story; there is more.

The pattern is clear: in long-term relationships, especially where the male partner has a significant desire for sex, the female partner loses sexual desire and thereafter remains less interested. This trend is the source of painful tension and frustration within many couples. Because of the complexity of this phenomenon, only a few of the elements may be discussed here. However, there is a force women must battle to embrace and comfortably express their sexuality. Many women lose in this battle. Women and their sexuality are potently influential in the quality and stability of our love relationships and culture.

Up until twenty or thirty years ago, women owned significantly less power, independence, influence, and status than they do today. A tremendous shift has occurred. This shift, however, does not mean that all women feel more powerful, but it does mean that greater societal permission exists for a woman to define herself and obtain power and influence if she wishes. Yet echoes from the past remain, in which women lived in submission to greater male-owned power, even if this power did not cause men to always feel powerful. Many effects of this past climate, which was unfriendly toward women's needs, continue to linger today.

Sex is an activity that is strongly linked and aligned with our personal power. True power is the freedom to be who we are in complete self-acceptance. That means affirming all parts of our humanness, including our sexuality. Yet for women, remnants of the past powerlessness lie deep within the recesses of the subconscious and still influence women's thoughts and emotions. Many women have not yet broken free from the chains of past feminine powerlessness, a cyclical dynamic which repeats itself in love relationships between men and women as it did years ago on a much larger scale between the collective masculine and feminine.

Sex, which at its best is an exchange of love, easily falls into a battle over power. Deep down many women fear that sharing their desire for sex results in giving away their power in the relationship: a notion that has its source in the belief that "men only want one thing," a remnant of the old power structure in which women had low value. The fear is that when a man gets what he desires, he will then have no need for her and she loses all her power to keep the man. Thus a woman retains power so long as she holds out sexually. But truly she has no power if she has no love…a conundrum that only reveals itself in the final failure and misery of a poor relationship.

Other links in the old rusty chains of powerlessness include the notion that a woman who is interested in sex is non-virtuous, a slut; that our bodies are sinful and only our spirits are sacred; that to be a moral, good woman, sexual desires must be rejected; and lastly, that a good woman is submissive and exists only to serve others, especially her male partner. Each of these is a distortion of a truth, which has been manipulatively used to dominate the feminine and has no place in healthy, passionate relationships today.

This entire pattern of female behavior may make it appear, on the surface, as if they do not like sex, but this is not true. It is powerlessness women don't like; the two have become confusingly entangled. Underneath the struggle to be powerful, women are intensely passionate and sexual. What does it take for a woman to break out of this collective pattern? She must assert her individuality and risk owning her power...be herself, but also have the right to be proud of her body and to have sexual pleasure...accept that her sexuality is a potent, healthy force for herself and not something intended only for the pleasure of her male partner. This is also the process of emotional and spiritual maturation and owning greater responsibility for her life, love and sexual satisfaction. Sex should be a celebration of life in all its glory and sensuousness. It is no less an integral and essential part of a woman's vitality than it is a man's.

> Each gender views the other as childish in areas of its own strengths.

5-4. The Male Zipper Problem

Almost daily, a new sex scandal fills the headlines. Revealed with such regularity, these shocking developments deepen the general cynicism of a society that is already wary of incessant bad news about wars, terrorism and recession.

The short list of some high profile sex scandals:

- Former President Bill Clinton,
- Former Governor Arnold Schwarzenegger,
- International Monetary Fund Chief Executive Dominique Strauss-Kahn,
- Superstar Athlete Tiger Woods
- Former NY Governor Eliot Spritzer
- Former NY State Representative Anthony Weiner
- Former House Speaker Newt Gingrich
- Former Italian Prime Minister Silvio Berlusconi
- Former Presidential Candidate John Edwards
- Former Presidential Candidate Gary Hart
- Former President Donald Trump

Most shocking is that the revelation of sexual improprieties by our male leaders, whose behavior ought to set an example, damages the trustworthiness of men in leadership. What is happening to cause this repetitive pattern of men's moral and sexual breakdown? Why can't men keep it zipped? What were they thinking!!?

Sex is a powerful force; so powerful that many men fail to control it. Professional and personal disasters can result. But most men are not out of control sexually. Common to these famous powerful men is a pattern of obvious flaws, but less sensationalized are the countless similar incidents that occur among the not-so-famous. Uncontrolled sexual impulses cause great harm, shame and embarrassment when extra-marital affairs, sexual addiction, immoral choices, impulse control problems, and deceit are revealed. When sex causes harm to another or oneself, it has crossed the line into unhealthiness. Due to the embarrassing nature of sex, the deceit and free-falling morals of men who are caught make for scandalous news. At the other, quieter, end of the sexual disorder spectrum are inhibited partners who deprive their significant others of closeness and sexual satisfaction. They are equally unhealthy, but in a way that is not newsworthy.

It is simplistic and dismissive to defend these men by saying that they are biologically designed to impregnate as many women as they can for the continuation of our species. Others say, "It has always been this way; men always cheat." After all, “boys will be boys.” It is like saying that children instinctually don't wish to grow up. This perspective ignores the maturation exemplified by growth, inner-strength discipline, self-control, and personal responsibility. When considering a deeper, spiritual perspective, men's primary life-task is to transform sexual energy into loving energy. Succeeding at this earns a man reciprocated love and societal respect. Growing up means accepting responsibility and realizing that we cannot have everything we want.

What is wrong with men? They account for most of the U.S. prison population. Men are far more likely to be violent than women. Significantly fewer women abandon their children than do men; you rarely hear of a female equivalent of “deadbeat dad.” Of all the high officials embroiled in recent sex scandals, all are men. Are men just a troubled gender? It is a big problem.

The question begs to be asked and answered: how could such intelligent men behave so stupidly? The answer is that their choices were not made with their intellect, but with their troubled emotions. For these scandalous men, their intelligence was off-line because they were overcome with painful emotions and responded to an urgent need to soothe them.

Partially responsible is the way modern societies like ours socialize boys into men. Obviously, it is not done well. We produce men who are not strong, and as a by-product, produce injured, angry women. Our cultural trend is towards males and females residing at extreme poles of masculinity and femininity, which encourages males to reject all that may hint at femininity. While growing from boys to men, puberty is the phase in which sexuality develops. Simultaneously, boys shift into man-mode by repressing their feelings, especially those which reveal weakness. Males do this skillfully to differentiate themselves from females, who have societal permission to feel and express emotion.

As sexuality explodes and feelings are repressed, the two connect and combine. Thus many men, especially those who are less emotionally aware, are unable to differentiate sexual urges from emotions. Most of the repressed feelings are deeply painful ones from childhood, a time of powerlessness. They are blocked from understanding and healing. Positive feelings are not repressed because they do not contribute to powerlessness.

By tacit masculine agreement, the expression of all feelings is disallowed except anger and sexual desire, the two emotions that look and feel powerful. For men, disconnection from their feelings results in two major problems, both arising from a lack of inner emotional awareness. The first is that impulse control is reduced without awareness of intensifying emotion. The second is the reduced ability to verbally communicate needs, an action that can help to head off escalating inner tension. Out of this formula comes a gender that is at risk of combining out-of-control power with poor judgement.

By rejecting their feelings, men suffer high costs but also benefit. Men achieve, make, build and compete. Hundreds of thousands of buildings, bridges, tunnels and roads have been built almost exclusively by men. Male pride is realized by not letting anything, especially feelings, prevent success. Allowing feelings to surface displays weakness. Men are taught to persevere despite the pain and discomfort...get the job done. Men who display weakness do not earn the respect of other men. Among the costs associated with this is that sexuality becomes the narrow channel through which men may own and express their emotions so as to feel powerful. Unfortunately, the relationship between sex and love is damaged by this arrangement. Power prevails.

Mixed messages about men and sex are prevalent. Young men are lauded for their sexual exploits. Men who sexually partner with many women are envied by their male brothers and viewed as especially virile by females and males alike. What do we expect from men? This phenomenon changes once a man ages and marries; the standard remains, but is only partially rejected. An older man who is successful at bedding many women is still envied as a "successful" male by other men, yet his failure to control his sexual impulses attracts a diluted but valid concern about values and morals. Among women who strongly value fidelity and commitment, the sexually uncontrolled man earns the less respected reputation of being a "player."

With a blurred distinction between emotions and sex drive, if a man becomes highly stressed, he is likely to seek a sexual solution, whether or not sex is the source of his malaise or the potential solution for the problem. Sex is the quickest path to comfort. Being found attractive by a female is intensely validating for men; the hunt, chase and possession of a woman bolster his self-esteem. An additional danger is that the relief provided by sex and orgasm can quickly become compulsive, a cycle in which a man has subjectively lost the ability to stop the behavior of seeking sex. Some call this sexual addiction, others sexual compulsion.

The masculine primary value is power, which is distinct from the primary feminine value of beauty. Ultimately men experience the power derived from their positions as dissatisfying. It is illusory because the power that comes from position or money does not heal inner powerlessness, the true quest for every man. Being sexual can offer a temporary feeling of potency and powerfulness. Sex, and a woman's attention, will not provide lasting inner power, which truly only comes from self-mastery. Real power is the ability to control all of one's sexual, angry or aggressive impulses, and channel that into loving purposes.

Possessing power, as do those men who hold high offices, only intensifies the stresses which may trigger a sexual scandal. Power is a doubly treacherous element in a man's life; first, possessing great power comes with high pressure and public visibility and second, power provides ample opportunity to have contact with women who are attracted to power. This double trouble is the undoing of many men.

What kind of man desires great power? A driven man who will place great pressure on himself to achieve. It is a well-known pattern that emotions and emotional defenses, which make up what we call a personality, are motivated by the need for protection from harm. Emotional defenses have a tendency to seek the opposite of the identified vulnerability. Thus a man who feels powerless within defends himself by cloaking himself in power. He compensates. Men who seek power are often strongly driven to prove their worth in order to mollify their own painful self-doubts.

Sex has an anti-depressive effect on the brain. By reducing anxiety and offering a general sense of well-being, sex is a great stress reliever. Many men utilize sex for just this purpose. Those burdened with inadequacies seek ways to soothe their pain. The more stressful our society becomes, the more men will seek stress reduction in both sexual and non-sexual ways. Equally destructive are the pain relief offered by alcohol or drugs. The healthier, but less popular approach for these men is to emotionally open up by facing their inner demons. While this is a lasting solution, it demands that a man experience his pain, something that most immediate-gratification-seeking men run from fast.

As our society's code of etiquette and morality deteriorates, men enjoy greater freedom to behave badly, thereby obtaining fleeting emotional benefits, like a drug addict. The anonymity of large populations, aided by the internet, makes hiding bad behavior easy. Greater opportunity, increased stress, reducing the demands for personal responsibility, and unlocked moral strictures creates a perfect storm for sexual misconduct.

A man who does not control his sexuality carries shame about his lack of control. Extra-marital dalliances are conducted covertly. If not truly shameful, there would be no need for secrecy. Deep down, the man knows that his sexual acting out does not come from a place of inner strength or virtue. What he really seeks is the power to feel good about himself and to be free of emotional pain. Using sex to solve an emotional problem will repeatedly fail, as will seeking an external solution to an internal problem. But it will give short-term immediate relief.

Marriage is challenging by nature. The marriages of famous, powerful people are at even greater risk than their less famous counterparts. For many men, their marriages and wives are the source of stress and unhappiness. Female partners hold no culpability here; this is the nature of marriage. By his wife, a man is known for his true, human frailties, not the idealized image he offers for public consumption. His weaknesses have a corrosive effect on his partner's respect. It is no surprise that powerlessness is something many a man experiences in marriage.

For a man struggling with self-worth, gaining the public's adulation, as performers, athletes, celebrities and politicians do, provides the large-scale validation which feels to be the proper prescription to soothe what ails him. Many men do not experience their wives as fans but as critics, especially in relationships where a man's failings have already hurt or alienated her. Familiarity breeds contempt, and in a married man, it breeds a growing sense of failure. This reality contributes to a man's motivation to look outside his marriage for sexual soothing, and is a strong contributing factor in divorce among the famous.

All of the above is part of an explanation but not part of an excuse for men's sexual misadventures. Being more aware of their painful feelings can protect men, and their families, from unzipping at the wrong time. Men's highest mandate must be to protect others, especially their partners and children, from being harmed by the destructive potential of their sexual actions. Men who act in sexually destructive ways have broken a male code of honor, which sadly has seriously eroded along with the decline of etiquette and civility in recent decades. By keeping his sex drive under control, a man demonstrates a triumph of masculine power and earns love and respect. Failure to do so produces shame. The strong man reconnects sex and love, so that his sexuality is a nurturing and constructive force.

Men who behave badly are in great pain, but the choices

they make, unfortunately, prevent us from being compassionate. Instead they earn our scorn. Men have an obligation to protect our society from their potential to be hurtful. Getting help before damage is caused is responsible, while continuing to behave badly and just hoping not to get caught is reckless. In pursuit of relief, such men are very selfish and blinded by their pain to the trail of destruction they leave behind.

5-5. The Erotic Nature of Men

In their friendly conversation, he jokingly described himself as a "leg man." His occasional golf partner laughed in understanding and followed with, "I'm more of a breast man, myself." The two laughed at their mutual admiration of and incessant hunger for feminine sexual attention. It was not, however, the kind of conversation two women would have, or would enjoy overhearing. Male eroticism is a distinct facet of being male, which women have trouble appreciating. To a women this would sound like objectification, a demeaning, disrespectful reduction of a person to her physical parts, without any regard for her personhood or well-being.

It is vital for a man to know intimately his female partner's need for emotional satisfaction and love, similarly it is also vital for a female partner to know, understand and appreciate her male partner's eroticism. Learning about his turn-ons may be challenging because male eroticism tends to be disturbing to the feminine. Non-judgementally, a female partner will be rewarded for understanding the flavor, interest and specificity of his excitement.

If this powerful force of eroticism, the man's deep desire to heal, grow and love himself more fully, is not met with understanding, then toxicity will develop out of his feelings of not being fully accepted and loved. Eroticism is such a deep, vital part of the self that if it remains unexpressed, invalidated and rejected, it will seek to get expression in unhealthy, illicit ways that may be destructive to a love relationship. The other route is that the erotic energy is buried so that shame, depression and frustration all may reduce the emotional healthiness of a man.

In their eroticism, men are often caught between their deeper desires and their female partners, who respond to this distinct male eroticism with discomfort, judgement and rejection. In their urgent need to find expression, men then seek out satisfaction secretly in isolation, through viewing online porn or, more actively, with sex workers or affair partners.

Many female partners are uncomfortable with their male partners looking at pornography. A lot of women experience the use of pornography as approximating cheating and betrayal. Men make a distinction between porn usage where no physical contact occurs versus unfaithfulness with a woman present. A female partner with conservative values or one with insecurities may object to porn because of their values or because they feel threatened. In either case, an upset female partner will miss the opportunity presented by his porn usage to learn about his eroticism. A man chooses specific pornography from the panoply available to satisfy his very unique erotic needs. From a male partner's perspective, he may believe his pornography usage is actually protecting his female partner and the love relationship from his "dirty" eroticism or his sexual dissatisfaction.

Male eroticism is often distrusted, having negative associations of being lusty and animalistic. Such feelings proceed more positive qualities, earning men negative appellations: "He's such a pig," or "What a dog!" Intense for men and uncomfortable for their female partners, couples do not always deal well with this eroticism, and fail to integrate its raw energy. Feminine influence is on the rise, and male eroticism is under attack. In his strong sexual desire and at-times extreme fantasies, a man, unconsciously or not, is relating to Eros, the god of love. Each man, internally, lives out this primitive energy to connect with life and merge physically, a drive so urgent that many men struggle to contain it while staying within social and moral boundaries. Erotic energy is not limited by moral or ethical considerations.

The male erotic nature is expressed in the individual man

by very specific desires, which may not be "mainstream." As a combination of the love energy and the man's unique emotional make-up, his eroticism manifests in very specific sexual interests. Men's eroticism tends towards fetish-like interests, as contrasted with female eroticism which is much more relationally based (body-part, specific sex-act focused). To learn more about it, take a look online at pornography, a medium that is overwhelmingly made by men, for men, to satisfy their erotic needs. Judgement needs to be suspended if learning is to occur, an effort that is not easy with a hot-button topic such as pornography. It is an expression and representation of male eroticism. Pornography is profit driven and created specifically to attract enough men to be profitable. Pornographers would not produce sexual material that attracts only a small audience. Perusing the online erotic offerings demonstrates that these images, videos and online experiences, such as live video chat, are tailored to suit very specific sexual tastes. Therefore, many variations of sexual interests are represented online.

Many men are excited by women's breasts. The men with a strong erotic interest in breasts will seek out the websites that specifically cater to this particular erotic interest or fetish, by offering a collection of images and videos featuring women with their breasts prominently displayed. Other categories include an almost infinite variety of female physical characteristics, such as long hair, brunettes, blondes, hairy women and those who are tall or possess large behinds. There are categories which address ethnic considerations, such as sexy Asian women or African American women. Some men are particularly turned on by women's feet, thus there are pornographic websites devoted to the eroticism of feet. Online pornography devoted to larger-sized women serve those men who are particularly excited by sexy heavy women. The variety is very detailed and categorized, as are men's sexual interests. Other erotic categories are formed by specific sex acts or intercourse positions. Some men are aroused by multiple women giving and receiving sexual pleasure. Still others are about older women or "amateurs." There are more categories devoted to sex acts performed by certain kinds of people, such as an African American man having intercourse with a blonde woman.

Darker aspects of eroticism exist as well, and may be uncomfortable topics for consideration. These are troublesome turn-ons that may cross the line of moral, ethical or legal limitations and are not the sole domain of men. Our personal histories include many kinds of injuries; attempts to heal the associated wounds may permeate into eroticism in disturbing forms: an erotic fascination of sex with children, voyeurism, sexual violence, rape, sexual slavery, sex with corpses, and bestiality, to name just a few.

A vast majority of these negative erotic interests never see the light of day; they remain never-shared shame-based secrets that are activated only in private and personal fantasies. Because sexual energy is not defined by limits, erotic interests that are unhealthy and harmful are equally present online. The prevalence of online pornography represents the variety of men's erotic needs, who go in search of erotic satisfaction with online porn usually as a substitute because they cannot or dare not share it with their partners.

In the shadows of male sexuality and eroticism is the "world's oldest profession," prostitution. The potent need men possess for sexual expression supports a sex business in every world culture. Many cultures hide it by relegating it to a location that is hidden from everyday eyes. The shame of the real truth about human sexuality dictates such choices and actively blocks healing by keeping such things hidden in the shadows. The presence of prostitutes, now often referred to as "sex workers," underscores the power and persistence of male sexual desire.

Literature and films have documented the sometimes intimate and loving connection a man and a prostitute can form. Men tend to more easily share their darker, shame-based erotic interests with a prostitute than they may with a wife or long-term female intimate partner. A deep bond can form between these men and the women they share their eroticism with because a man will feel accepted for his authentic self by a prostitute who witnesses him at his most shame-based and still accepts him.

Men struggle with the split nature of their sexuality and eroticism. There is the good, which is comprised of sex that is used to express love and to strengthen the loving bond with an intimate partner. There is self-focused sexual expression that takes the form of masturbation which may be shame-based and is more about self-care, regulation and self-soothing. And then there is the bad, which is the often-repressed pain that takes the form of erotic darkness, desires that men feel ashamed of, so they keep them hidden. Long-term female partners live in the good sector.

Male partners typically "protect" their female partners by splitting off their "bad" eroticism in a process that has been termed the Madonna/whore complex. The romantic partner gets allied with his good side and even elevated to a level of purity. She will receive only his good and best. Unfortunately, women in relationships with men who feel mostly bad about themselves receive little, because the women are experienced as better than they are, and the men believe that they themselves have little good to give. At the extreme, should his sexuality be a source of shame, a man will not be sexual with his romantic partner, fearing that sex will defile and contaminate her. His sexuality still needs expression so he finds a partner who he feels is commensurate with the "dirtiness" of his erotic needs, someone viewed as lowly, like a whore who is dirty, with whom he can comfortably share his dark desires. He brings his dark desires to his dark maiden.

Men do not choose their unique erotic nature. As unique as a fingerprint, their erotic constellation is a product of their early life environment, their experiences and their childhood reaction to it. Our eroticism dwells in a deep inner place and to share requires intense vulnerability. For many men, their eroticism is the source of deep shame and embarrassment. Relationships, which ideally include complete acceptance between partners, are often limited in their potential to achieve this ideal because of the male partner's eroticism. While often unexpressed, men experience sharp isolation by not taking the risk of sharing their complete selves. Too many men anticipate that their eroticism will be dismissed, criticized, belittled, ridiculed, attacked, judged or rejected if shared with their female partners. The hurt registered from such a wounding is too painful to risk again, thus many men simply take their sexuality away from "together" experiences.

A female partner who is open to her male partner's eroticism is rare. Learning about it, understanding it, and accepting it may be different than participating in it. If a very specific sex act is a turn-on for a man, it is not required for his female partner to take part. Accepting all of him is different than agreeing, but it also requires that judgement be suspended. At times, if his turn-ons are shared, strong limits may have to be enforced if the turn-on is not interesting to the partner. Once expressed, the erotic desire will want further expression.

Eroticism was named for Eros, the god of love. Women do not immediately view the male form of erotic expression as loving. Many sources of erotic interests are from pain and wounding, not nourishing love. Making your relationship a safe place where all facets of both of you can be explored provides the greatest environment in which a couple have the best chance of living up to their joint potential, the ideal of love. If not attended to, they risk a build-up of emotional toxicity, and the relationship becomes vulnerable. Learning about your man's eroticism is a deeply effective way to make him feel loved.

In current times, as women are increasingly empowered and more likely to influence the political and social conversation, male eroticism is under attack. It is viewed more and more as objectionable, immoral and inappropriate. The concern is that, if not encouraged to see the light of consciousness, male eroticism in all its forms will be repressed into the unconsciousness even further. Danger exists should further repression occur. The already dark state of much male eroticism gets expressed destructively in even more dangerous forms if it is rejected.

5-6. The Animalistic Side of Men

Writing about sex is difficult because any sexual topic is only true for a minority of people. For every sexual truth, there are many exceptions. This article will tease out two broad aspects of male sexuality, which I will call the Need and the Love. This article focuses mostly on the first aspect, the Need, because it causes the most trouble.

Both within men, and within the broader social discussion, uncertainty exists regarding what is good and what is bad about men and their sexuality. Men themselves are confused about these two sexual sides; they express ambivalence particularly about their Need, an instinctual, animalistic part of their sexuality. Men's Need may be appropriately named "the call of the wild," or "the duty to impregnate." It is not sensitive to feelings, does not consider relationship or morals, but only wants satisfaction. It is more concerned with frequency of sex than quality. On the one hand, having great sexual desire is a sign of masculine strength, health and virility, but on the other hand it introduces into society and relationships elements that are not regarded highly. It is not good, it is not bad, but is instead a force of nature, much like a storm or a flood which cares little for who it affects.

The Need, in my unscientific estimate, is part of the lives of sixty percent of men. It is an incessant, urgent sexual desire. The myth about male sexuality describes men who are constantly horny, dog-like, and whose strong sexual desire easily overrides their impulse control while contributing to poor judgement. This is not true for most men, but if combined with character weakness, chronic dissatisfaction or strong negative emotion, high sexual desire may compromise a man's strength to maintain his untarnished admirable qualities.

A strong incessant hunger, few men complain about their Need in public. It constitutes constant suffering. The Need functions like a magnet which is attracted to metal but has no mind about which piece of metal it is drawn towards. Many men struggle with this because their love for their partner and society's commandment of masculine faithfulness are in direct conflict with their Need which cares little about such limitations. For men with strong desire, satiation can only last momentarily. Prostitution, which has the moniker of the world's oldest profession, exists to fulfill the Need of male sexuality, as does pornography. The ever-presence of these sexual relief valves are a testimony to the strength of men's sexual Need. Society reluctantly accepts them.

Inwardly, men experience satisfaction of their sexual desire as a Need not a want; it does not feel to them like a choice. Instead, it feels like a constant, chronic hunger for food. It is a pain but satisfying it can be a joy. Commonly, romantic partners are hurt by the reality that the Need a man experiences is neither personal, loving nor convenient. Its insistent nature may make sexuality a difficult negotiating point between romantic partners and an issue around which many domestic conflicts revolve.

Many men voice guilt about pressuring their partners to be sexually available and admit to feeling uncomfortable with their irritability when their partner is sexually unavailable. A secondary cause for discomfort is that their sexual Need means that they possess a vulnerability; men do not like this.

The second side of male sexuality may be appropriately called "The Love." This part values relationships. For some men, this aspect opens only once the Need is satisfied, otherwise the Love is blocked by a wall of frustration. Eroticism, passion, and playfulness are all included in the Love. A loving connection with the partner, himself and the life that sustains him also characterize the Love. There is a focus on mutual openness and acceptance. It is less about "getting the job done" and more about having intensely exciting shared sexual experiences. Especially true in emotionally-aware men, the Love values variation of play, allowing greater openness and the sharing of a man's playful side. The possibility of this is greater within an emotionally safe relationship.

For female partners, who most value emotional connection, the sexual activity requested to fulfill a man's Need usually does not create satisfying, emotionally connected sexual experiences. Many female partners complain that to be available for their male partner with the frequency he desires results in their sexual experiences falling into a routine, obligatory and chore-like condition. They may also complain, "How come we can't cuddle without it *always* leading to sex?" Affection and cuddling are loving expressions that a man is better able to offer if his need is fulfilled. Men: be aware that if your partner makes an effort to fulfill your Need, expressing gratitude is essential. Partners who battle over the frequency of sexual activity will find that making the transition to the Love side of a man's sexuality will be nearly impossible. For complete satisfaction, most men ultimately need fulfillment of both the Need and the Love. Loving another is among life's most challenging tasks. A man's Need is a force of nature, which tends not to be receptive to negotiation, and thus represents a formidable challenge for romantic couples.

5-7. #MeTwo: Considering Men

Where gender differences intersect it's easy to miss the point.

Men and women are different. What is difficult to determine is just how different we are. At a time when the #MeToo movement has raised this in the national conversation like never before, the differences between women and men are at risk of being confused with woundedness, anger and power. Sex and sexuality are at the cutting edge of the gender differences, a place where differences show up in exposed ways.

Being male and writing about this topic risks sparking the dry tinder of rage. I am not an apologist for men who brought their power and sexuality hurtfully and inappropriately into relationships with women where it didn't and shouldn't belong. Such actions are not to be tolerated. A little hurtfulness is too much hurtfulness. Women have rightfully demanded safety, respect, equality, and having their concerns taken seriously. The #MeToo movement well articulates the need for these changes. Yet the vein of rage that runs through our society about this issue is a fuse which gets successively lit by the parade of revelations of inappropriate sexual acts where men violated women. The issue of gender differences and relations is complex, with multiple layers, nuances and subtleties.

A real risk exists of overshooting the balance point by the spreading of an emotional fire. Judgement and blame are not part of a successful effort to heal injured women, understand damaged men and improve our society. A paradox is that, while women have felt powerless and victimized, most men, too, inwardly feel powerless, even though it is men who hold most external power while behaving badly. Male sexual expression, welcome or unwelcome, can often be linked to an attempt to be rid of feelings of powerlessness and shame; an attempt to feel better.

Time and again stories erupt about another woman harassed, abused and violated by a man. The violence, sexual and otherwise must stop. In the mental health field, conventional wisdom has held that roughly one in three women have been abused but, given that many incidents go unreported, the number is probably closer to fifty percent and maybe even higher. Males are abused at a lower rate, roughly twenty to thirty percent. A majority of men are good, loving and peaceful, but there are enough troubled men that the problem is alarming. Women deserve better and must be safe. The conversation about how women need solidarity and empowerment is a good one. However, why have the succession of stories about mistreatment of women by men not raised a discussion about what is wrong with men in our society? When our high school students are being shot and killed in mass shootings, always by a deviant male, we talk about a gun problem. But when our women are sexually harassed and assaulted, a discussion ensues about the need for female power. Why don't we talk about a "man problem?"

Men struggle with porn addiction in epidemic numbers; this is more accurately known as sexual compulsivity, not because they are morally corrupt but because men are quite troubled and hurting. Engaging in online sexual activity is a desperate attempt to fulfill their obsessive need to be worthy and lovable, made desperate by deep-seated shame. A substantial male audience floods the U.S. porn industry with a revenue stream estimated at over $10 billion dollars annually. This is certainly not the symptom or tendency of a healthy, empowered group. The female equivalent attempt to soothe internal shame is the compulsive struggle many women have with negative body image, unhealthy relationships with food and compulsive shopping. Women, too, seek sex in unhealthy ways to soothe the fear of being unlovable, but they do so in ways that are less aggressive, thus rarely making headlines.

Male problems of coping with and containing sexual urges are super-charged by shame and low self-worth. While a strong sex drive is seen as a natural male flaw to begrudgingly accept, female challenges of self-worth are a new rallying cry for courageous empowerment. There is no equivalent movement in the male world. This is not a suggestion that men should ride the wave of female empowerment, but instead a recommendation that men ignite their own transformative wave. To overcome their current malaise, men need support from women, while men also must support women's wellbeing.

A largely unidentified factor of this problem is that male sexuality and the male value system show up generally as shameful and rejection-worthy in the female world. Men and boys internalize this. The message that men are corrupt is received subtly or blatantly from many of the important women during each boy's development, a trend accelerating due to advertisers who identify this as an opportunity to reach the female audience by making men look foolish and inept. The more women are harmed by men, the more women are fearful of and angry at men, and in turn, boys receive a stronger negative image of men.

Morality is much kinder to female sexuality than it is to its male counterpart. Male fantasy literature and pornography are tolerated but chronically teeter on the moral edge of banishment, while the female equivalent, the multi-billion dollar industries of romance novels and female-oriented love stories provoke no such moral debate. Female movies of empowerment typically include a demonized male abuser or rapist; such movies are not a target of moral judgement, yet function in the female world the same way porn functions in the male world. Both are satisfying because they soothe inner pain and shame. Fantasy literature simultaneously expresses consumers' inner experiences while also influencing outer-world relationships.

I am neither promoting pornography nor attaching any valuation, good or bad, to it. Male sexuality gets expressed erotically by breaking the whole into parts. It is exemplified by the common male tendency to erotically charge a very specific sex act or a particular female body part. In all areas of their lives, men break the whole into parts, a process that feels to women like a reduction, disrespect, and objectification. Men possess certain qualities that women will never favor. Yet in the tendency of masculinity to do this is, men are also not immune from its painful effects; it just seems to men more normal. Institutions that are run by men trap many men within similar cages of powerlessness to those about which women complain. Many accomplishments and advancements are the positive result of this male tendency, but when combined with male shame and inner self-hate it gets expressed in abusive and misogynistic ways that are repulsive and frightening to women.

Aspects of the male world are quite cruel. The military, a male-oriented organization, displays the breaking of the whole into parts in the form of a rigid, highly structured, specialized and hierarchical arrangement. On the surface, the military seems to support the successful taming of men's painful shame and controlling of their sexual impulses by instilling pride and honor. Women are increasingly entering a military where incidents of sexual assault and harassment have increased exponentially. An annual estimate shows over 22,000 sexual assaults and over 100,000 incidents of sexual harassment. The violence suggests that the apparent success of this male method to effectively sublimate sexual and powerlessness-based energies is only illusory.

Historically, male violence and destructiveness has been viewed dismissively as "boys will be boys." Perhaps men get a pass because of testosterone; "that's just how men are." Yet many men become doctors, educators, civil rights leaders and loving fathers who demonstrate a capacity to channel their energies morally and constructively. Why is it then, that in our prisons over ninety percent of prisoners are male and of single parent families, over eighty percent headed by a single woman? What is happening to our men? Perhaps if we really believe our men can do better, we would view the current crisis of female sexual abuse as a "man problem" for which a solution needs to be found. The current #MeToo movement is a discussion that needs to include ways that our society can raise emotionally healthy men.

In the shifting social and gender changes, men are being lost in the dust of female advancement. They are confused as their influence and relevance fades. Women ask, "Do we really need men?" Men used to have more external power, but as a group we have insensitively misused it by subjugating women. Men were wrong and should demonstrate sorrow by making a correction that really has not yet begun. Women have an opportunity to do better. However, in their hurt and anger, women are at risk of doing the same in reverse, by demonizing men instead of humanizing them. Understanding their painful pathology is the way. Anger, no matter how justified, is an ineffective tool for healing. Less emotionally aware, men have not matured as a collective. Men collude with the negative message that men and their sexuality are immoral and shameful by tacitly accepting the label of being hurtful animalistic beings who cannot tame their morally blind rage and lust.

Men tend to prefer denial over conscious healing. The "man code," a deep pattern of behavior and language which causes men to resolutely avoid any situation which may result in them looking or feeling weak, stops them from entering the territory of conscious acknowledgment. Men are desperate to live up to what they believe is a real man, the ideal of being strong in every way. They feel shame when they don't measure up. One way men defend against their failure is the formation of narcissistic tendencies, an emotional veil to cover up inner pain and vulnerability, one without empathy for others. Men collectively have not taken any steps to rid male sexual expression of unregulated impulse control problems, which only can be achieved with a balanced, strong and healthy sense of self. Men's failures to be emotionally healthy can never be an excuse for misplaced or hurtful sexual actions towards women; excuses are unacceptable. Emotional unhealthiness is the underlying problem fueling this dark pattern.

Sex and power are tightly entwined. Power and

powerlessness are major themes in all sexual eroticism, male and female. Each individual's quest for power is nothing more than an outward expression of an internal need for worth. Power is to sex what MSG is to food; it enhances and amplifies it. The pain of worthlessness fuels an obsessive quest for being valuable, a state sought primarily through love and sex, yet a state that, if sought externally will never be internally satisfying.

With the changing distribution of power, women have greater access to such positions. Men experience greater competition for power, an unwelcome change. Some men view women's entry into formerly male territories as unwelcome, and resent the interlopers. Once in a position of power, women wield it differently than do men, and in ways that feel disrespectful to men. Men who feel threatened with great inner shame and weaker impulse control react violently at times.

A deeper dive into the emotional obstacles to male pride and mental health is vital to understand the workings behind problematic male behavior. Men mistakenly look upon women and their love as a lifeline when drowning in a sea of shame. For a woman to be sexually available to him confirms his desirability, positive masculinity and value. But women cannot and do not want to be their man's substitute for strength and confidence. Porn for men is their totally safe substitute in which they will not be exposed to judgement or rejection. Men who doubt their own worthiness cannot bear the acute pain of rejection; it too openly reveals their worst fears about themselves; that they are weak.

A tendency among men is to look upon women and their sexual attention as a form of emotional food and nourishment...not unlike how their mothers' bodies were literally food when they were newborns. The more fulfilling those early developmental days were in a man's life, the more able he will be when looking at a woman to see her as a human being instead of as "food." To men who are chronically hungry, women are a non-personal source for nourishment. Boys who grow up emotionally malnourished become men who seek to gain external power and success to give the appearance of being worthy, but internally they will feel an insatiable hunger for power and love. This can go on throughout life. External improvements have little or no effect on their internal insufficiencies. The state of malnourishment is fixed. Men whose shame is deeply pathological, even sociopathic, may attempt to steal "nourishment" by use of coercion and immoral force, because deep down they do not believe they deserve it and therefore they must get it surreptitiously. Men are enraged about this reality.

It is a painful realization for a man's female intimate partner, that she ceases to become a satisfying source of nourishment once his shame has been revealed to her and he feels her knowledge of his shortcomings has reduced her pride in and respect for him. He then looks to other women for feeding, either through porn or infidelity. In broken families, over eighty percent of single-family households are headed by women. Most have been left by inwardly powerless men who chose seeking sexual nourishment elsewhere over the needs of their children. We can easily judge these men as morally blind, but it is more constructive to look upon their tremendous pain and inner shame as a deeper source for solutions to this complicated problem.

Many women, consciously or not, judge their male partners by comparing them to a fantasy "white knight," unrealistically expecting their men to live up to high levels of character, perfect morals, and strength. She hopes he will save her from all the troubles of life, an ideal at which men always fail. Some women, upon realizing that their man is imperfectly human, develop a contemptuous attitude towards him. This is not unlike, and even equal to, the impossible and destructive ideals of beauty and sexiness by which men measure and rate women.

The personality flaw that can cause a man to thirst for power is the same one that weakens him from controlling his sexual impulses. Many of our politicians and executives, men who have obtained power, are prone to this flaw. Adding to this combustible cocktail is the fact that women are attracted to men with power. Powerful men interpret eager and available women as permission to enjoy unlimited, unfettered sexual freedom.

The scale must be balanced to view the relationship between the genders with an undistorted perspective. This relationship is at times more of a battle than a love affair. In the battle, women are not passive spectators, but equal competitors. The manner in which each wages war is different.

Beauty, sexiness, and the female body all are powerful. It is an obvious truth to men. Most women are unaware of how men experience their feminine attributes. Yet many women use this power, consciously and unconsciously, overtly and subtly without fully knowing or appreciating their effects upon men. Sometimes the use of beauty shows up as non-physical violence in the man's world. At times women use men's sexuality as a vulnerability to be exploited. Simultaneously, most men recognize the indirect threat every woman poses, the damage that can be done by an accusation alone of sexual inappropriateness, harassment, abuse, or rape. Most men are acutely aware and fearful of the great amount of destruction to careers, marriages, financial well-being, jobs, etc. by accusation alone. All without the due process of the law. It is not uncommon for women to falsely make claims or to threaten to do so, thereby inflicting non-physical violence on men to gain an advantage.

In violence towards women, there are some innocent victims, but there are also some less innocent victims. Admittedly, no amount of prior guilt justifies violation or violence. The perpetrator alone must bear responsibility for this. The truth cannot be denied, however, that some women have used the power of accusation alone to effectively do harm to men, which causes women with legitimate accusations to be doubted. Women who have been abused are harmed a second time by a system that has grown insensitive. In some cases, situations between the genders operate like this: the man brings the dynamite, the woman shortens the fuse then lights it, the man's dynamite explodes, the woman screams about how bad he is for allowing it to explode. Without feeling fair, it is true in this drama that the explosion crosses a line that must never be crossed. Men need to possess enough strength, character and leadership that they can always avoid crossing the line. They must instead solve problems constructively. It is a lot to ask of men and does not feel fair. Fair or not, men must do better.

Power starts so small. The ability to have a voice, and to know and believe in oneself enough that one can acknowledge that voice, is real power. Real power is also expressed by compassionately listening, understanding and deeply respecting another's individuality and autonomy. The voice within the sexual dialogue, whether it is a national discussion or a quiet dialogue between potential romantic partners needs to grasp that power. It is ultimately the power to love others, life and ourselves. Not just to say yes or no, but to say, "I know myself and I am valuable." We are getting closer to a solution when both men and women feel valuable.

The genders are inextricably linked. When we get stuck in a cyclic debate about which gender is superior, the most valuable point is missed. Woundedness in one leads to a weakening of the other. If the pendulum of power swings between them and each one thirsts for dominance, both lose the most essential and vital part of humanness. Each wounded woman who mothers a son passes her pain onto him in the form of shame and powerlessness; the son will struggle to possess positive self-esteem and healthy sexuality. Each damaged man who fathers a daughter dooms her to grow up as a wounded woman; the daughter will struggle to feel worthy and lovable. To be healthy, each gender is dependent upon the health of the other. To transition to a situation where men are healthier and stronger, women's love, support and understanding are necessary.

Without arriving at the core issues, the debate about sexual harassment, violation and degradation will just be like a rapidly swinging pendulum which blasts through the point of balance, damaging the potential for men and women to be healthy beings and healthy sexual beings. To protect women, the "man problem" of male suffering and unhealthiness needs to be understood.

Women should feel proud of their swelling empowerment. Yet in the long run, without enlightenment, empowerment will just be a destructive imbalance. The only real power is the power to love. Loving the differences between men and women is a challenging example. Instilling institutionalized support for both love and complete individual responsibility in our communities is a simplified roadmap. Men and women, we are in this boat together. If one of us jumps up and down too strongly on one side, the boat tips and both of us fall. We are different, we both struggle, yet we deserve an equal amount of value, love, healing and respect.

5-8. Sexual Desire and Men

Women often bemoan their burden of monthly menstrual cycles, pregnancy, the labor and the pain of giving birth, saying, "Men are so lucky to not have to go through this." Women's suffering is real and worthy of compassion. Yet the suffering men experience due to their sexual and reproductive capacities is real, but not fully understood by women, probably because men rarely talk or complain about it. Men rarely share about being burdened by incessant sexual desire. The suffering that men endure from constant urgings far outweigh the pleasures they have during brief sexual interludes.

My non-scientific estimate is that high-desired men constitute between 50 and 75% of all men, with a higher percentage among those who are younger. Sexual desire is a physical experience for men, which is turned on at puberty and cannot be turned off. Sexual desire slowly diminishes for a majority of men as they age.

Heterosexual men experience the intense desire to be sexual with women they don't like, women they shouldn't like, and women who are unavailable. Men experience sexual desire for other women when they are married and even at times when there is no real sexual opportunity. For many men, the sexual desire just will not go away. The physically-based desire of men is an intense, purely instinctual driving force, which lives outside of all moral, ethical, and civil considerations. Men will rarely share about their suffering, but instead are more likely to joke about it with other men, especially when referring to the too-influential beauty and physical charms of women. Only a small fraction of the sexual desire men feel is ever transformed into action, most of it men try to ignore.

Do men like being this way? The simple answer is "no." A majority of men do not give it much thought and have simply grown accustomed to the intrusive urgings and impulses. They consider it part of being normal. But at its deepest level, desire is suffering. Needing sexual satisfaction makes men vulnerable to a force which is beyond their control, and most men do not like being out of control. Otherwise good and loving men are accused of rubbernecking and gawking at other women. At the sight of an attractive woman, without choosing to, men grow weak at the knees and lose their intellectual functioning while their lustful desires are intensely aroused. Men's physical urgings often cause them to behave in ways that are not loving and are outside of both their values and interests. Sexual desire often gets men into trouble.

Due to their chronic desires, men are not easy partners for women, who may be hurt by men's sexually motivated behaviors. While not as vital as breathing or eating, from the male perspective, sex is a need. High-desired men view sex as non-negotiable; much the way food is a non-negotiable need for survival. Sexually unfulfilled men grow irritable and can be mean. Do men want to be this way? No they don't.

A girlfriend or wife may notice a significant and positive personality shift in her male partner after he is sexually satisfied, in part because of his temporary relief from the inner longing of sexual desire. A man's sexual desire is an opportunity for his female partner to express compassion by fulfilling his need and earn his gratitude for which in return he should offer kindness, loving acts, patience and generosity.

5-9. For Men, There is No "One-Size-Fits-All."

Ask any man who is in a relationship with a woman, and he will tell you that figuring her out is nearly impossible. Oscar Wilde said, "Women are not to be understood, they are to be loved." So while attempting to please her, the strategy that most men use simply doesn't work. Men are eager to find "the single answer," the one-size-fits-all. And this happens on a daily basis, when trying to make her feel loved, and when trying to please her in bed. The daily disease is applying one answer all the time hoping to get the job done.

Women are more like the weather than they are like the sun. The sun rises each morning and sets each evening; it can be predicted. Whether skies are cloudy or blue, the sun will come up and the sun will set. But women are less like that. Women are like the moon with its many phases. Women embody the constant changes of life. Men are more like the sun, which is even and steady and not influenced by the drama of the world. From a male standpoint, women are infinite and ever-changing. The saying we have where I live in New England is that if you don't like the weather, wait a minute. Women are like that. The weather has constant variations and many moods, each with its own distinct beauty. But if we make plans needing the weather to be one way, you can be sure that it will be another.

For men, women's variations demand that we stay present. There is no single prescription, or single answer, or canned laughter, that will work every time. Women teach us to be real, to be alive and in the moment. So for you, man, be prepared for the reality that as soon as you settle on a theory, your theory will be proven wrong. As soon as you say, "she is like this," she will probably be different.

Many men are fond of predictability. In so much they do, they figure out the one way that something will work, so as to get it done most efficiently. There is that elusive "right answer," that will provide us the security of always being the same. But with our female partners there is no such answer. She will always baffle us.

And it is like this too when it comes to sex. As soon as we settle on a way to please her, we find that one day to the next it doesn't get the job done. So as soon as we get settled on clouds, the sun shines; once we are prepared for the sun, that's when the storm arrives. And in her very nerve endings, her mood is reflected.

Learn from her and her flexibility. It means do not settle on any one outcome. Accept that you must live in the moment without expectation and without prediction, be ready for the gift that she gives you today. The answer is that there is no answer. Because if we decide that one color in the rainbow was best, when the other color shows up, we will be disappointed.

OUR BODIES

6-1. Anatomically Unfair

In the most essential sexual act, men and women are unequal and different. Expectations about how intercourse should go differs from reality, interfering with the satisfaction of lovers. Many partners expect that intercourse should lead to orgasm, that all-important blast of bliss. Most men believe that during intercourse, if they are physically adequate and sufficiently skilled, their female partner will reach orgasm. Most female partners, too, believe that this is how it should go. When sex differs from expectations, problems are not far off.

The myth that women orgasm during intercourse persists despite the reality suggesting that this is largely untrue. The statistics show that roughly 30% of women orgasm during intercourse but most of these women most do not climax consistently. The expectations that women "should," pollutes a potentially joyful act with tension.

With men there is little problem or question; almost all men reach orgasm during intercourse. Responsible for such a large difference in response between men and women, is that during intercourse, a man's penis is directly stimulated. The female organ analogous to a man's penis is the clitoris, similarly loaded with pleasure-giving nerve endings but located outside of a woman’s vagina. The clitoris is not directly involved in intercourse. In a strange choice of nature, the experience of intercourse is far different for women than for men. A woman's vagina, which is fully involved in intercourse, has far fewer nerve endings than does her clitoris. Most women are orgasmic, just not from intercourse, or intercourse alone.

To illustrate the point more clearly, let's reverse the genders. If a man's lower belly were to be stroked, few men would reach orgasm. Most men would react by saying, "It's not going to happen, because touching my belly won't produce that result." Exactly, and that is true for women as well. Yet the erroneous myth of female orgasm persists. Women, who seek to enjoy an orgasm when alone in private, overwhelmingly stimulate their clitoris for pleasure, arousal and orgasm. Far fewer mimic intercourse by involving their vaginas in the experience.

But what about the 30% of women who do have orgasms during intercourse? Such women are successful by being deeply relaxed, achieving high arousal and experiencing intercourse as highly erotic. Their successful strategy is less body-based and more mental, emotional and occurring through the proper flow of sexual energy. Some people are able to orgasm without any physical stimulation at all, solely by thinking erotic thoughts.

To reach orgasm despite their anatomical disadvantage some women choose to stimulate their clitoris during intercourse. Other women are too embarrassed to attempt it. But this work-around comes with some risk, since some male partners feel threatened by a female partner's self-stimulation. He may interpret her actions as suggesting that he is "not enough for her." Women who believe that orgasms should occur during intercourse, but are unsuccessful, may struggle with feelings of sexual inadequacy. If her partner also subscribes to this erroneous belief, a woman is susceptible to concluding that "something is wrong with me." Couples who try hard to force an orgasm in their quest to correct the problem complain that "she takes too long."

The long-held ideal of simultaneous orgasms causes more disappointment and pressure than it does satisfaction. As the "Holy Grail" of sexual experiences, simultaneous orgasm is a bar set too high and risks becoming a case of perfection that prevents good enough.

Yet if a woman does desire to become orgasmic during

intercourse, she may develop this ability. Some women are successful at learning to relax, focus and redirect the flow of sexual energy within their body to increase their capacity for pleasure and orgasm both during intercourse and beyond. However, it may be simpler to let go of the myth that women need to orgasm during intercourse, and instead seek to more fully enjoy the relaxed pleasure that is more easily obtained.

6-2. Politics of the Little Blue Pill

With the introduction of Viagra in the late 90's, many men who could not otherwise sexually perform were granted a new lease on their sex lives. Since then, Cialis and Levitra have joined Viagra as options men may turn to when their penises don't respond as they or their partners wish. The opportunity for impotent men to once again celebrate potency upset a delicate balance many couples had emotionally engineered to cope with sex and sexual needs. Floating in on the tide of new-found sexual performance is the complexity created in a sphere of human interaction that benefits from simplicity.

Pro-erection medicines offer great help but do so in a part of our lives that is shrouded in misinformation and secrecy. The result is that these medicines are frequently used incorrectly, with unrealistic expectations and disappointing results. Contrary to widespread erroneous beliefs, Viagra and the others do not alter low sexual desire, strengthen ejaculatory control, fix relationship disconnection or solve the emotional problems that hamper good sexual performance. Yet for some men, the pill's placebo effect can temporarily seem to suggest otherwise. Despite the medicine's narrow purpose, men and their doctors continue to prescribe them without sensitivity to the actual cause of erection problems, which is often broadly emotional and relationship based.

In addition to being misapplied, many hold tightly to unrealistic expectations that these medications are guaranteed to be effective. While very helpful when properly used, uncomfortable side effects may outweigh the benefits for many men, the most common of which are headaches. They eliminate the pleasure of a successful sexual encounter by swapping one problem with another. And what of those erections that last more than four hours? The side effect is not as common as the jokes made about it. The men who have difficulty performing due to strong anxiety or other negative emotions may obtain little relief from using medication. Very powerful emotions can easily override the medicine's help. As a group, men have practiced avoiding their emotions for a lifetime. When facing an emotionally based problem, men routinely opt for an action that makes them feel more in control rather than facing their irrational feelings. Upon learning that the true source of their erection loss is emotionally-based, many men perceive this as the worst-case scenario. Most men would prefer the problem to be concrete and physical...something they could get their hands around with a simple and direct fix, such as a pill.

Ideally, sex is a simple and natural act. Viagra and its siblings inject complexity into the natural rhythm that couples develop. Even if reassured multiple times, female partners tend to fear that the real cause of her male partner's failed erection is his lack of attraction for her. Aging women are even more likely to hold this insecure assumption. Knowing and fearing this, many men obtain the erection prescription secretly.

Because men are generally acutely uncomfortable talking about their sexual failures, so pro-erection pills are often obtained covertly, especially in those relationships most in need of greater openness. Messy situations can develop when a female partner unexpectedly discovers that a pill is responsible for her partner's arousal. She will ask, "How long have you been doing this?" She will wonder how many of their historical encounters were truly motivated by his love and attraction for her, and for how many times he needed help because she isn't enough? And if he hid this from her, she may ask, "How many other things has he lied about?" Deceit, and the insult to trust, is a wound that is hard to heal. Should he take the pill guessing that they will be sexual while risking the waste of an expensive pill? If he asks her, the spontaneity is lost, and he has reminded her of his embarrassing dysfunction. But what if she learns that he has taken the pill? Will she be insulted that he expected a sexual experience without considering her choice? Pro-erection medications upset the natural order and instead of being easy and spontaneous, sexual situations become artificial and complex.

There is no simple fix, yet emotionally based problems call for emotionally based solutions. If used properly, Viagra, Cialis and Levitra can be of great help. Their placebo effect may help a man escape from the thorny cycle of performance anxiety. Yet a sexual problem should be a couples' problem and not an individual problem. Being open about difficulties and solutions while inviting dialogue offers an opportunity for partners to get even closer while facing the adversity of dysfunction. If treated this way, the highest and best values may guide partners to good, loving solutions.

6-3. Time to Take Out the Garbage

You live in your house, but you are not your house. You live in your body, but you are not your body. After all, when someone dies, their lifeless body remains empty without them in it. Our being and our bodies are different. This concept is vital to achieving emotional health and good loving, as is the concept of where in our body we place the center of our being.

Pain is a normal and inescapable part of life. Still, most people do their best to avoid pain. One way it is accomplished is by burying the emotional pain deep down within the body; a practice called repression or internalization. Doing so seems to successfully make the pain go away. But it doesn't truly go away. The pain is just temporarily out of awareness. Internalizing emotional pain is effective as a temporary solution, but it is unsustainable.

Internalizing painful emotions is using the body as an emotional garbage can. Its limited capacity is no different than a real garbage can; it can only hold so much. If a garbage can is continually filled until it reaches capacity and you keep adding to it, the garbage will overflow and make an ugly mess. The high toxicity of painful emotions becomes apparent months or years later when there is no longer choice about feeling them because the "garbage can" is full.

The ugly mess is emotional dysregulation, demonstrated by emotional instability, depression, chronic anxiety, anger management issues, irritability, and negativity. The cost to physical well-being is high as well. An emotionally toxic body is vulnerable to disease, organ dysfunction, and physical deterioration. Headaches, digestive troubles and sleep problems are common when toxicity is high.

Living in toxic waste is obviously uncomfortable. The habitual internalization of negative emotion gradually makes a body uninhabitable. Sharply painful experiences like trauma significantly accelerate this process. To further avoid discomfort, many people shift the center of their being as far away from the pain as possible, often to their head. It is like filling a house with trash and gradually relocating the center of living to the attic so as to not see or be reminded of the trash. The head is a place of thinking, not feeling. When there is no feeling, pain will not be felt.

A life lived out of the head is a bit like listening to music with speakers that have no bass. The sound quality is high-pitched and thin. When a person's experience is dominated by thinking, the connection has been broken between the individual and his or her emotions, and things will easily fluctuate out of control. The unstable emotions interfere with being effective, content, and a successful romantic partner.

To bring the emotions back into a healthy balance, an internal body-based focus is necessary along with an acceptance of the rejected feelings. As a body is emptied of toxic emotion, the center of being may be comfortably relocated back into the center where it belongs. By focusing non-judgemental attention on the physical experience, with a willingness to feel the full range of sensations, a connection to old repressed emotions is reestablished. Choosing to scan the body for related sensations further facilitates the healing process. Meditation is a practice that is used for the effective maintenance of healthy emotional balance once it has been achieved. It is not nearly as difficult as it sounds. As calmness, emotional balance and emotional regulation are restored, a person grows far more capable of loving him or herself, a romantic partner, and others.

6-4. The Body of Love

Talked about, joked about, the source of fascination and unease, physical intimacy provokes strong reactions. Of the mind, body and spirit, loving the body is the most challenging and controversial. Occurring behind closed doors, the general quality of couples' physical love and satisfaction is difficult to ascertain. Bedroom problems are far more frequent than is generally acknowledged. Most problems, and there can be many, remain secret due to embarrassment. Partners suffer in silent frustration and disappointment. When a relationship or marriage fails, a dissatisfying physical relationship is often a contributing factor, though is usually not the publicly shared cause.

Each one of us is complicated. When two people join together in love, the complexity is more than doubled. For intimate success, multiple systems must all coordinate well. The physical endocrine, circulatory, cardiac, and pulmonary systems join with the non-physical emotional, cognitive, relational, and energetic systems. They must all work together seamlessly. Considering fluctuating levels of stress, economic conditions, relationship rigors, dysfunction, and aging, it's a wonder that satisfying experiences can be achieved at all. Just being in a relationship is difficult, but when a close connection has been bruised by conflict or tension, physical intimacy is quick to disappear. For some, it never returns. For too many couples, what ought to be the source of pleasure and connection becomes one of disappointment and disconnection when they trip over one of the myriad obstacles that can derail a love life.

Rarely is a person as close to another as during lovemaking. The vulnerability of closeness makes sharing physical pleasure emotionally challenging by awakening inhibitions. Feelings of shame, as well as concerns about body-worthiness block the openness and relaxation needed in pleasure. A history of strong religious impressions may produce an inner conflict between the sacredness and sinfulness of pleasure and physical love. The terror of old trauma may be reactivated. Concerns about dysfunction and adequate performance may weigh heavily. In our busy world, many adults have long ago buried the child-like spontaneity which allows physical loving to be play-like instead of work-like.

What constitutes a good and satisfying experience is highly subjective; what a partner finds erotically interesting may change over time. The sources of excitement for each one of us is as unique as our fingerprints. Unresolved differences regarding the preferred path to satisfaction show up as tension or conflict between partners. The most common difference is about the frequency with which lovemaking should occur. What starts as a minor bedroom problem will quickly infect and harm the entire relationship.

Physical love strengthens and deepens the bond between partners, whereas an absent or troubled intimate life actively erodes the bond. A strong bond maintains and protects fidelity. What happens outside the bedroom directly impacts what happens inside the bedroom. Loving in numerous non-physical ways throughout each day keeps a relationship warm, making the jump to “hot” that much easier. Partners who share a high degree of emotional intimacy are far more likely to enjoy satisfying physical intimacy.

Physical intimacy is not a large part of most love relationships. In terms of time spent lovemaking, it is probably less than two percent of waking hours. But its minor role is not representative of the high significance of giving and receiving physical pleasure. Like a clock with many parts, remove a tiny gear and despite the gear’s small size the whole clock stops. Confronted with numerous potential obstacles, couples rarely seek out help when physical intimacy is dissatisfying or troubled.

6-5. For the Love of the Female Body

For heterosexual men, women's bodies are the source of fascination and erotic nourishment, but the relationship between women and their bodies is more like a war zone. In my capacity as a sex therapist, I recall treating an eighteen-year-old female patient whose body would elicit drools from most men and envious contempt from most women. Despite her actual shape and proportions, she could only express criticism of and contempt for her body. She spoke harsh words about her thighs, attacked her behind, and when she mentioned her tummy, her face contorted into an expression of revulsion. If the sampling of women I have had the honor to treat is representative, this eighteen-year-old is not atypical of how many women feel, regardless of the attractiveness of their bodies.

It has seemed odd to me that many of the women's male partners do not share this negative perception. Most men say, "I like her body. It isn't perfect, but that doesn't matter to me as much as her ability to relax so that we can enjoy closeness and pleasure." Unfortunately, the negative relationship between a woman and her body has a direct and negative effect on the healthiness and quality of her sex life with her partner. Good lovemaking requires the ability to relax. A woman who dislikes her body cannot relax during sex.

Beauty is a primary feminine value; just as power is a primary masculine value. To possess beauty is to own a potent source of a kind of power, but because beauty has grown into an unhealthy societal obsession, many of us have been deluded into believing that unless we have high physical beauty, we have no value. This is not true. The media constantly pushes the beauty/sexy button knowing that it can elicit a spending response, but this unintentionally fuels women's shame and insecurity about their bodies.

Some men and women have received the gift of physical beauty, but, honestly speaking, most of us have not. Especially as we age into our middle or later years, if we have not given up on our need to have magazine looks, our vanity and our disappointment damages the beauty of what inner gifts we do possess. Perfection is an unrealistic goal.

Men and women manifest and experience struggles with self-esteem differently. With a primary value of strength, men see low self-esteem as a weakness. Many men will express struggles with themselves through a high desire for sex, wishing for each experience to pump up and validate their virility, as an expression of masculine strength. In a different way, women, whose primary value is beauty, will experience their lack of self-esteem by witnessing their bodies as distasteful and even disgusting. A woman's poor evaluation of her physical self may be contrary to how all others see her and this disconnect represents a distorted self-image.

It is wise for women to set a goal of physical, emotional, sexual and spiritual health rather than perfection in physique or beauty. This can be accomplished by making friends with your body, despite its limitations. Do you end your friendship when your friend develops an imperfection? Be just as forgiving with your body. If you harbor negative emotions, your body's health will be harmed. To feel badly about your body is to be less than your best; it is unkind to rob your partner of access to ***all*** of you. Do make the most of your physical assets, but don't let that be the source of obsession or self-hate. If you make it your friend, and if you can let go of negative emotions, your body is still capable of providing you and your lover with great pleasure; *that* is truly beautiful!

LOVE

7-1. Loving to Grow

Why do we enter relationships? Why do we need them? With all the drama, challenges and heartache, sometimes it just doesn't seem worth it. Every relationship ends, whether by death, divorce or break-up. Each lover is going to feel hurt. We can pretend that it is possible just to feel the bliss, without feeling the pain of love. In a perfect world, it would be so. By looking deeper within, we can uncover the truth about why we continually seek out and connect with romantic partners in spite of the pain and adversity it causes.

Our existence is composed of more than our conscious awareness. The dreams we have at night, which utilize an odd symbolic language, make little sense to our daytime minds. Our dreams provide a clue that there is something underneath, something more than what we experience when we are awake. Religions and spiritual traditions give this underlying something a variety of names and, beyond chasing away loneliness, our love relationships are in service to the evolution of this deeper part of us. Love is the active ingredient.

At our center, each one of us has a spark of life. By growing in our capacity to love, we nourish the spark. Our relationships require us to practice love and then live with the love we create. When it comes to relationships, the love we cultivate is the love we get to experience. Nourishing our spark is accomplished by relating through love and aspiring for personal and partner growth.

To obtain what is valuable typically requires a lot of effort; otherwise it wouldn't be valuable. A strong and positive love relationship is a case in point. For most couples, intense effort must be expended by each partner, digging deep within themselves, striving to be caring and non-hurtful. A desire to act in a loving way is often at odds with intense and painful feelings and self-centered wants. Growth nourishes our inner spark; it always comes with discomfort. By allowing ourselves to be pushed to our extreme, we look to our most deeply-held values instead of just what feels good on the surface.

If a partner will not put in this hard work, and refuses to grow by eliminating hurtfulness, weaknesses and selfishness, the essence of the relationship will die. In this way it is like a job; if we stop doing the work, we risk losing the job. A partner who refuses to grow puts the relationship at risk, because growth is necessary for the relationship to remain relevant. In a love relationship the importance of commitment to our partner is balanced with the importance of being true to ourself. Without growth, these two vital factors will be in painful conflict.

In troubled relationships, the growth process has gotten

stuck. Two continental tectonic plates pressing against each other build stress until eventually a tension-reducing earthquake is triggered. Similarly, between partners, tension builds up until conflicts erupt: the manifestation of a stuck growth process. Arguments are attempts to resolve stubborn obstacles which are preventing progress, but if unresolved, the painful effects may create a destructive "earthquake" crisis. Some partners refuse to change. Breakups are the broken promise of the relationship's potential for growth.

From an unconscious perspective, the partner we choose is a deliberate choice to complete very specific growth-oriented tasks, while our surface self usually wishes for a partner with whom to share pleasure, valuing that over the hard work of progress. Forming a love connection feels like something we do for our own satisfaction, therefore the growth required of us feels like it goes against our nature; it takes effort to grow into the stronger, more loving person we are destined to become. Our love relationships are truly a vehicle for our growth.

7-2. Loving Yourselves Promotes Passion

Older couples often say, "All that lovey-dovey stuff is for kids," as they look enviously at the younger couples who express their mutual love passionately. The passion in a relationship is a measure of both satisfaction and success. Yet it is difficult to maintain a long-term connection. For each partner to have loving regard for him or herself is a critical factor in being a successful loving partner. If you want the passion in your relationship to last...love yourselves!

Our society emphasizes two important life paths: career and relationship. To excel at our career, we are encouraged and forced by rule of law, to go to school for years, get training, and possibly even attend higher education. Much energy and effort go into ensuring our financial success. Careers are intellectually based while relationships are emotionally based, a basis which is less culturally valued. For the relationship path, no formal training is available, encouraged or provided.

Regardless, the expectation remains high that our relationships will be good. Such expectations are unreasonable.

If there was formal training, it would focus upon the strength and loving nature of the relationship each potential partner possesses with him or herself. No other factor gives us greater bang for our buck when it comes to forming and maintaining passionate relationships. The name for this is self-esteem. It is a measure of how much a person loves him or herself. Paradoxically, the more we feel good about ourselves, the less self-centered we grow, and the more capable of loving others we become.

Upon hearing this, many of us are tempted to reply quickly, "Of course I love myself." Yes, you probably do. Still, our potential to love ourselves is infinitely deep, and can always be further developed. Some of the many indicators of low self-esteem are: negative thinking, past hurts which remain unforgiven, accumulated resentment, low confidence, self-criticism, inability to set good limits with others or ourselves, judging ourselves or others, not speaking up about problems, making choices we later regret, character weaknesses, conflict avoidance, ignoring our needs, being anxious and fearful, and disliking our bodies. The list can continue, but I think you get my drift. Each of these limits our ability not only to love ourselves fully, but also to love our partner, other people, and life.

Having passion within our relationship or marriage is essential. Our relationship's satisfaction, health, longevity, and success depend upon it. Some couples express this through affection, some through kindness, others through an active sex life. To be a skilled lover, especially within the context of a long-term intimate relationship, positive self-esteem is of prime importance because sex is emotional in nature. Emotional strength provides a lover with the ability to relax while simultaneously allowing deep intimacy.

The more positive our relationship with ourselves is, the greater our capacity to love another will be. If the love for ourselves is not deep, then deep love will be invisible to us; it will be hidden behind the blind spot of our emotional limitations. You limit your own love. The relationship we have with ourselves filters how we experience others and our world. If it is a poor relationship, then the world and others will not seem loving.

7-3. Romantic Nourishment

The topic of sexuality can never be complete without a discussion of romance. Women, wives, and girlfriends, in unison, want more romance in their relationships. Many male partners express having little clue about what their female partners want and self-admittedly populate the ranks of the romantically challenged. What is romance and why is it so important to women? Men spend much effort to make their female partners happy, which isn't bad, but romance is more about adoring them.

For most female partners, romance is an essential ingredient in a completely satisfying love relationship. Receiving romantic gestures confirms her desirability and causes a woman to feel deeply loved. Nothing is a greater aphrodisiac for a woman than romantic love that fills her heart; it unlocks her passion. The merging oneness that passionate sex can achieve is the culmination of the romantic endeavor.

Sincere romantic behavior expresses a burning desire for the woman. At its most intense, it is greater than the partner's impulse control, so that he is completely moved to actions showing his eternal and undying love for her. Lost in overwhelming desire, the romantic lover will abandon self-concern and play the fool to impress and potentially obtain her affections. By such actions, the would-be lover expresses, "I cannot live without you!" It is a love for the indwelling goddess of which each woman is a manifestation.

What are those romantic gestures? The ones that show that she is valued; the unexpected giving of a gift; spontaneous compliments; gestures of affection without any sexual intent; providing unrequested help and support; arranging a candle-lit dinner where she is the focus of loving attention and genuine adoration. But also actions that show sensitivity to her feelings, which are known because she has been keenly observed. Being a strong partner who takes charge by showing her she is desired or protected from danger may cause her heart to flutter. All these may be experienced by a woman as romantic; they show her that she is special. These efforts will nourish her heart and function as an essential, special kind of food for her deeper well-being.

The challenges associated with long-term committed relationships produce an environment that is unfriendly to romance. Emotional complications render male partners romantically limited, but only within the relationship context, because if a male partner sees another beautiful woman with whom difficult emotions are unassociated, his romantic urges to court and flatter easily surface.

For many female partners whose need for romance is unmet, the fantasy genre of romance novels fill the void. The growth of the romance literature industry demonstrates how important romance is to women. Ninety-one percent of the romance novel readership is comprised of women, who spend roughly $1.36 billion (2010) annually in the U.S. on romance stories, according to the Romance Writers of America. Unlike other literature categories which have seen declining readership, romance novels continue to enjoy growth, and are the most sold fiction genre in the US. Women may find the comparison distasteful, but romance novels are to women what pornography is to men. Both provide fantasy fulfillment of a vital kind of loving connection, though each gender builds such a connection and makes meaning of this connection very differently.

Most couples have in their history a time when romance was excitingly alive. The passionate feelings that lead to romantic actions need to be actively protected for their survival. To learn about which actions are most romantic to your female partner, ask her, though a male partner who gleans her romantic preferences on his own will find a shorter path to her heart. She will probably be happy to talk about her feelings as long as her sharing leads to future romantic actions.

> Relationships: act how you feel like acting and your relationship will be like a train wreck.

7-4. I Love You, Please Change

Conventional wisdom says we should never try to change our partner. Yet partners always try. It is natural. Each one of us seeks the most satisfying relationship possible. We want the strongest, most successful, most attractive and the most loving partner. Over time, all relationships have a way of revealing partner limitations and weaknesses. Irritating behaviors and habits are on the initial wish list for change, but the truth is that each of us could be a better partner and person with some growth.

Change and growth are not the same in relationships. Change happens effortlessly, but not always in a positive direction. Growth, on the other hand, takes time, but usually produces beneficial and lasting results. How each partner attempts to encourage growth in the other can make a difference between relationship success or failure. The characteristics which make up the list of desired improvements point to the emotional place where partners need growth. If personal growth was easily accomplished, all relationships would be satisfying.

Conventional wisdom encourages accepting rather than changing our partner. The double-edged sword of acceptance reveals the challenge of relationships. By accepting our partner the way he or she is, our own need for satisfaction remains unfulfilled, but acceptance is the path of growth. An attempt to change our partner is likely to make them feel rejected because a painful underlying truth is revealed: he or she is not good enough as is. That hurts. Injury neither feels loving nor promotes positive change. On the contrary, it makes one partner resistant to the others' influence. The more a partner feels loved, the more open to the other's suggestions he or she will become.

Resistance to change tends to provoke reactions leading to a cycle of hurtfulness between partners. Refusal to change may provoke outright disrespect and contempt. Where attempts to encourage change have failed, many partners turn to criticism—a bitter way of expressing the desire for change and mounting resentment. Hurtful actions such as criticism have a disproportionately large and negative impact on the quality of a love relationship, compared to the positive impact of loving efforts.

People cling most tightly to qualities and behaviors which protect their pain and vulnerability. Deliberate change or growth often only occurs when there exists no other choice – unfortunately after much damage and pain have been caused. Too often, partners' efforts to create change, such as the common use of criticism, are negative and hurtful. They send a negative message which communicates to the other, "You are not good enough. You are failing." For some, a critical tendency is a negative legacy from their family of origin. For others, criticism is a response to the real-life suffering that most relationships provoke, such as a partner who is limited and flawed and who often fails to love well.

Criticism is to love what acid is to metal, and each criticism is like a small dagger thrown at our partner. Over time, negative communication corrodes love and connection. If left unchecked, it causes an accumulation of hurt in which all good feelings are drowned. Rather than encouraging success, criticism douses the flame of motivation with negativity and tears the partner down.

Expressed in tone of voice and attitude, nonverbal criticism cuts just as sharply. Sarcasm is one variant. Many frustrated partners criticize chronically and indirectly, suggesting, "You are unreasonable and stupid; what is wrong with you?" No one likes to be judged. Each one of us possesses flaws which make us vulnerable to the pain of a negative evaluation.

Criticizing is an act of becoming a self-appointed judge, who hands down judgements from on high. Love is different; it comes from a position of acceptance. Love finds a partner worthy even if growth is needed.

Protecting our partner from hurt is part of a successful strategy to maintain a warm and passionate connection. Thus criticism, negativity and force will not do. With skill and care, growth can be encouraged constructively without falling into the trap of destructive criticism. Instead of proclaiming what your partner did wrong, ask or say what you want. A "request for change" is far more positive and less hurtful than criticism. Slow, persistent, loving assertiveness offers the best chance of generating positive results. Cultivate the loving practice of patience, as growth is a gradual and sometimes slow process. Generously applying love while seeking to gently influence our partner is the best combination.

7-5. The Avoidant Partner

Some people avoid intimacy. Strangely, these people still form intimate relationships and, in a pattern that defies logic, they engage in lovemaking during the relationship's initial months. What happens next can be the source of confusion, frustration and finally outright anger for the partner. After intimacy deepens, the avoidant partner loses interest in being sexual, in hugging, kissing, and perhaps even holding hands. Some avoidant partners will seem to actively limit physical proximity, such as sitting far apart on a couch where contact may be possible. Most avoidant partners do not possess conscious intent to cause hurt but chronically reject the other without awareness. Even if asked directly, the avoidant partner will deny any avoidance because it is not a part of his or her conscious awareness. Avoidance of intimacy falls along a spectrum from mild to extreme.

Those in relationships with an avoidant partner commonly take the avoidance personally; it feels like rejection. They may question whether the avoidant partner is angry with them, or if they are no longer found attractive. Reactionary efforts such as going to the gym to get fit or experimenting with a new hairstyle to increase appeal are unlikely to alter the avoidant partner's low level of engagement and will fail to increase the amount of emotional or physical closeness in the relationship. A female partner may suspect that an avoidant male partner is gay or having an affair due to the prevailing myth that all men want lots of sex. The negative effect that deprivation of warmth has on the other partner can be significant, ranging from anger to low self-esteem and even depression. The lack of closeness and sex may raise the importance of sex to an extreme make-it-or break-it status, where threats such as, "Have sex with me or we're through!" are not unusual; even if sex has never before been that important.

The sting of rejection is sharp if it is discovered that an avoidant partner has been taking his or her sexuality away by having self-pleasure in private, or has been having an affair. Yet it is almost impossible for the hurt partner to embrace the reality that this is not a personal rejection. Avoidant partners are uncomfortable with closeness and real intimacy, which is what is really being avoided. Affairs are really far less intimate than long-term relationships, and masturbation involves no risk of emotional intimacy. Hurt partners' patience may be exhausted by such exclusionary sexual behaviors in conjunction with chronic emotional deprivation, and choose to end the relationship.

When confronted, an avoidant male partner is likely to say, "I am just not a sexual person;" words which contradict his or her active sexual behavior from the honeymoon phase of the relationship. If the avoidant partner is female, she is likely to say, "Sex is not that important, why are you so obsessed with it? I think you are a sex addict...you need to get help." It is normal when deprived of affection and sex to desire these forms of nourishment to increase, just as someone starved of food cannot get thoughts of food out of their minds. This differs from an unhealthy obsession.

Avoidant partners have developed this pattern in reaction to a childhood history which typically included some form of abuse or lack of emotional nourishment, even though the avoidant individual is likely to describe their upbringing simply as normal. Some families do not recognize or value emotions or emotional expression. In such families, emotional needs go unmet. A general and recurrent disregard for a child's feelings can produce in them avoidant patterns as an adult. Work in therapy can help an avoidant individual outgrow these tendencies; however, their strong motivation to do so is a vital ingredient for successful growth and change. Why a partner was attracted to an avoidant individual may also be a useful direction for exploration.

> Falling in love
> is easy.
> Staying in love
> is not.

7-6. Enticing Love to Stay

Falling in love is easy but staying in love isn't. A life without sharing love is considered by most to be an incomplete life, but with the divorce rate hovering near the fifty percent mark, the truth is revealed that many of us are not very good at loving. Getting clear on love, which is an essential aspect of life and relationships, may help more partners keep their relationships positive, satisfying and long-lasting. Subtle and hard to pin down, I define love as efforts and actions which encourage the well-being, nourishment and growth of another or oneself while also protecting him or her from harm. Successfully sharing such efforts produces the warm feeling that people commonly confuse with love, and hope to preserve in their relationships.

Love is always pure and perfect while we are not. Love is like gold, which no matter how tarnished it appears, may always be returned to its pure state. Love always wants us to grow towards perfection...we will never be perfect, but our capacity to love or be loved may be. Many stay away from love because it first activates our wounds in order to heal them, a painful process. Love demands that we maintain a vulnerable state of openness, which feels unsafe and uncomfortable. Love represents an ideal that serves as a distant beacon guiding us in the right direction to grow toward completeness, a destination at which few will ever arrive.

Why is it so hard to love another? Because we struggle to love our wounded, imperfect selves. Most of us are conscious of perfection and find ourselves shamefully lacking. Unwittingly, loving another is the practice of looking in the mirror. Most find their reflection unflattering. Conflicts with the partner are akin to shadowboxing with oneself. Loving well our fallible partner, faults and all, is good practice to perfect our ability to love. Loving in a relationship is a balancing act of simultaneously nourishing ourselves and the partner. When one direction of loving dominates the other, trouble is sure to ensue. If our partner is hurtful or self-destructive and refuses to grow, then loving ourselves may mean ending the relationship out of self-love. In a relationship, if either partner refuses to grow, the essential spark of life and love will die.

Our relationships are love's practice grounds, the place where we stretch to get love right. But just like the kindergartener who is just getting familiar with the alphabet, being a poor reader and making mistakes are a normal and expected part of the learning process. As lovers work to get love right, mistakes cause inevitable hurts. Trying to love another is also difficult because the human love that we receive often feels insufficient and dissatisfying; we suffer from its incomplete nature. Most lovers hunger for the nourishment of complete love.

Some of the human weaknesses that block love and damage relationships include being closed due to fear, causing hurt due to poor impulse control, not loving oneself and, as a result, being unreceptive, and having low self-awareness which causes limited ability to share. Couples who have not yet succeeded at loving effectively fall prey to the swinging pendulum of hurts, an alternating rhythm of angry blame and recrimination. Some couples tend towards a cold and silent style of reacting to hurts, one which is equally ineffective at resolving problems. The partners who succeed have learned the secret of remaining emotionally open to each other while also possessing a willingness to adjust, quickly and compassionately fixing problems when hurts occur.

A lot is demanded of romantic partners for love to remain between them. Love can't stay when negativity, tension and conflict are present, in the same way that silence scatters when noise erupts. Partners who avoid the mistake of mutually punishing each other when love is not given effectively, and instead teach each the right way to love, are on the right road to enticing love to stay.

7-7. Anatomy of Commitment

When lost in a delicious fog of love, many lovers propose the commitment of marriage. Despite their intent to share life "until death do us part," more than half of those unions end unhappily far sooner than that. Is there confusion about the nature of commitment? The high frequency with which marriages fail and commitments are broken suggest that romantic partners have either unrealistic expectations of marriage, do not possess sufficient strength, or both. Today, the wedding altar is a place where fiancés commit with a wink and a nod, because every engaged partner knows that if he or she becomes unhappy, there is always divorce as an escape route.

A commitment is a promise. People make promises to obtain a benefit now by "promising" to provide something in the future. Whenever a promise is given, it is really made to oneself, an opportunity to prove strength of character and integrity. Our entire society and economy are based on the good faith of promises, which, if empty, will erode all the freedoms we value in our society.

Too many partners seem to forget that a commitment is a permanent promise to "love, honor and cherish," in which failure is not an option. By offering a complete commitment, great life benefits may be gained. Marriage is more about deep lessons for the soul than ego-based happiness. Many partners seem to want the benefits of a commitment without doing the work. Only if a lover is "all in," can a marriage bloom to its potential. Lovers who half-heartedly commit will almost certainly experience accumulating troubles. Partners make better relationship choices if escape is not an option, and also become ardent influencers to keep the other at his or her best. A strongly committed relationship offers safety from the risk of rejection; each partner has the security and confidence to open up completely by revealing all of him or herself.

Marrying is a bond of love that is similar to a chemical reaction. The commitment is the reaction's container and love is the catalyst. Once activated, the chemical reaction melds partner qualities. The fizzing and churning of the chemicals in emotional terms produces discomfort as the pain of old wounds is brought to conscious awareness to be healed. The worst of each partner surfaces during this process. If the healing is successful, each partner develops a deeper capacity to love. The discomfort and adversity associated with loving is a normal part of the growing process. Typically each partner blames the other for his or her pain, but truly, the discomfort belongs to oneself and is a by-product of one's limitations of loving.

On the surface, a commitment appears to be to and for the partner, but in reality, loving another and making a commitment of love is truly a commitment to one's own growth and well-being. It is a commitment to oneself. A lover who breaks the commitment is failing to cultivate the best in him or herself. The adversity that flows from a commitment of love is one's own; failing to resolve an issue means that personal limitations linger unresolved.

Committed partners are at risk for confusing their emotions with the deeper part of themselves. Emotional struggles are a normal part of the work of love and not a signal that a relationship or partner choice is wrong. At times intense negative emotions may signal that the growth process has gotten stuck. During the work of love, happiness, at times, is not experienced, but unhappiness does not indicate dysfunction. Rather than questioning the value of the marriage or the rightness of the partner, better to seek to fix the problems and search deep within to own and take responsibility for one's contribution to the problems.

The choice of partner involves deeply unconscious and wise parts of ourselves and ought not to be taken lightly. Marital partners are selected carefully and deliberately; the chosen partner possesses certain qualities and characteristics that are vital for one's own development. There can be no mistakes when it comes to partner choice and commitment; however a lover may underestimate the amount of work required and may not be prepared for it. The best partner in terms of facilitating our growth is not a partner with whom a relationship will be only easy and comfortable. Not even the weather gives us only sunshine. If turbulence exists within a marriage, it may actually mean that growth is happening. Love your spouse well, even if you do not believe he or she deserves it; fix the problems instead of ending the marriage...after all, you promised.

> Feeling hurt
> is no excuse
> for bad behavior.

7-8. What Did You Expect?

Loving another person may be among life's most difficult challenges. It is made more difficult by the unrealistic expectations so many romantic partners possess about love relationships. Some such expectations come from poor examples set by partners' parents about what love is and how it should be expressed. Other expectations are strongly influenced by the golden "honeymoon period" experienced with the onset of new love. Many romantic partners think, "If it was possible then, it must be possible now."

Most who have lived through a honeymoon period reminisce with a sense of loss about this sweet time because it failed to endure. Because the bliss makes such a strong impression and is so desirable, often it is held as template for how a relationship or a partner should be. Instead, the intense loving connection felt by so many lovers shortly after learning that their attraction and interest in the other was mutual was nature's way to entice the lovers to enter love's arena to begin love's work. The golden glow of love also served as a small sample of what may obtained later should the lovers complete the work of love...much the way a business gives away free product samples to get the customer to come back for more.

But if the partners unrealistically compare their relationship during the process to this initial enticement, of course they will find it miserably lacking. Without realizing that the honeymoon phase is only a sample, romantic partners bemoan the loss of the delicious love. Many conclude that their relationship is a failure and the partner was a poor choice. It's as if when building a house, the owner sees the beautiful house design before construction has begun, but shortly after building has started the owner says, "This doesn't look like the design, and there is no roof...I can't live in this...this is a failure." The builder would respond, "The construction has only just begun. It takes many months to build a nice house; it will not be finished immediately. Be patient; it will be beautiful after all the work is complete."

But within love relationships, partners become so disappointed that all is not complete that their reaction interferes with or even stops the process from moving towards completion. Unrealistically, too many believe that a relationship should just be good, instantaneously, without effort. Like building the house, which takes much time, effort, and care by skilled workers, for a love relationship to be good, requires these as well, including the developing of greater relationship skills. Without skilled carpenters plumbers and electricians the house will not be well-built; and in a relationship without good relationship skills, neither will the relationship be well-built.

Continuing the analogy, once the house is built, and the owner has moved in, living in a nice house protects the inhabitants from the weather, but it does not guarantee that their life will be happy and trouble-free. Houses do not protect one from the rigors and struggles of life. Relationships, too are this way. The expectation of many, even those in relationships, is that a good relationship should provide happiness and a life free from difficulties. Life is difficult. People are imperfect. When two imperfect people join together in a relationship, the amount of imperfection is doubled. Being in a relationship is even harder than being single. A relationship does not protect from life's challenges as many unrealistically believe; it compounds them.

Many believe that being in a relationship will solve problems. When applying to college, being accepted by the school may be cause for celebration, but it is only the first step of much hard work to come. Forming a love relationship is also this way; the work has just begun. Contrary to what most believe about loving another, once the work phase of a relationship is underway, difficulties surface as a reaction to getting closer to another.

The most common unrealistic expectation is a that a good relationship is trouble-free. In fact the reality is that if the partners work to deepen their love, problems can be a signal that progress is being made. Partners who believe that a good relationship is trouble-free have great difficulty working to resolve relationship adversity. An unwillingness to let go of misconceptions is a problem that blocks couples from solving others. Just like an office in-box; when the top document is addressed the next one is revealed.

It is not unusual for a partner to mistakenly expect the other to know his or her feelings, thoughts, wants and needs, without communicating them. Mind-reading is not among most partners' skill set. During the honeymoon phase, being of "one mind," partners complete each other's sentences and share the same thought at the same time, and this is a cherished relationship ideal; one that may even return later once the work of love is further progressed. Without relinquishing such an unrealistic expectation, partners will be unable to form that deeper, harmonious bond.

There is the idea that if partners are right for each other, the "chemistry" between partners will last forever. Some lovers then believe that the disappearance of chemistry is proof that the relationship and partner choice was a mistake. On the contrary, loss of chemistry is more an indication that the hard work of love is underway, a process that exposes the ugliness within before the beauty and potential shine. In reality, chemistry, connection, and closeness ebb and flow throughout a relationship.

There is the belief that once in a partnership, you will be safe, free and be given to...instead, the best will only be received by you once you are ready to give unselfishly, without expectation of return...but balanced by being strong and advocating for yourself.

Clinging to the hope that someday a relationship will grow beyond problems, many work tirelessly to improve the relationship. But very few relationships are without at least a couple of perpetual problems. There are those partner differences which will never be resolved. Partners may choose to hold tightly to their frustration and opposition with regard to a stubborn, unresolved difference, but even unresolved, these problems do not doom a relationship to "bad" status. The relationship will never be perfect, and instead must be accepted as good enough. Persistent issues challenge the partners to develop strength of patience and acceptance rather than demand change.

The notion that two lovers will be one is an enduring ideal that unrealistically sets lovers up for disappointment. During the honeymoon phase, love can appear to blend partners into a blissful union, but that cannot truly exist until love's work is complete. Part of doing love's work is loving oneself balanced with loving the partner. As an individual, neither partner is ever lost in the togetherness of a couple. On the contrary, the stronger both partners are individually, the stronger and deeper the bond between partners may grow.

Of the unrealistic expectations explored, many arise from mistakenly transferring Heaven-like experiences from the honeymoon phase into the work phase. No amount of wishful thinking will eliminate the challenging, human work required of us when we love another, and replace it with what feels like perfection. The work of love is to deepen and refine our capacity to love. Over time and if, as lovers, we cooperate with love's work, we may develop a more perfect love, one that does not eliminate imperfections but grows to accept them.

> Hold yourself to
> a high standard of love.
> You will suffer less
> this way.

7-9. Choosing Love Over Power

Sharp, angry words are used by some in relationships to dominate their partners. Expressed loudly, angry words can intimidate with fear while bolstering a position of power. Relationships in which partners have unequal amounts of power are locked into a qualitatively poor state in which love is blocked and partner growth is restricted. Power will not create a loving relationship. The way dominance is maintained may be more habitual than deliberate; subtle and mild, or rising to the level of overt abuse. Regardless, it is harmful, especially to the less powerful partner.

Unless anger is used to resolve a problem, it is being misused. Other power-maintaining tools in a dominant partner's arsenal include criticism, threats, humiliation, and unilateral action. Less powerful partners may also actively contribute to a power imbalance by refusing to own their rightful power. The need that dominant partners have to possess power is rooted in fear of unworthiness. Carl Jung, the famed Swiss psychiatrist said, "Where love rules, there is no will to power; where power predominates, their love is lacking. The one is the shadow of the other."

In some relationships, this unbalanced dynamic results in stable co-existence. In others the imbalance is expressed as chronic tension and angry flare-ups, symptoms of an active power struggle. Over time, if not corrected, a power differential grows more extreme. Without repair, relationship crisis will eventually follow. Unbalanced relationships are draining.

A couple ready to depart from this dissatisfying cycle will have to reconsider their power-related roles. Powerful and powerless roles must change equally for the relationship to successfully transition from power to love. The powerful partner, in exchange for a truly loving relationship, must relinquish habitual control-maintaining tactics that diminish the other. Practicing non-hurtful behavior while developing sensitivity to the other's well-being is essential, but difficult for a partner who may be blind to the negative impact that domination has on the other. He or she will have to practice discriminating between hurtful and nourishing behaviors.

Powerless partners are most often the agent for change, because powerlessness is uncomfortable, it is a position in which self-esteem gradually degrades. Living in constant fear that the powerful partner will become upset and unleash hurtful anger, less powerful partners grow weary of choosing peace over self-respect. Because possessing power feels good to the powerful partner, he or she is likely to resist giving up the advantages even though both partners suffer as a result. A dominant partner may only realize the benefits of trading power for love once the exchange has long been completed.

To avoid further intensifying the power battle during a relationship transition, positive love-based rules of engagement offer necessary guidance and structure. The rule that directs the less powerful partner's growth is: each person has the right to possess and exercise individual power to obtain well-being. Assertiveness, limit-setting and choice of participation are efforts that serve this purpose. He or she must take a stand by insisting upon nourishing and respectful treatment. Doing so risks upsetting the dominant partner. The price of change for the less powerful partner is giving up the ability to blame the other and letting go of victim-based righteousness. He or she must begin to own his or her power and use it assertively for self-determination. Such efforts will only be effective if delivered in a firm, but loving manner. By seeking change, the less powerful partner is engaged in the risky task of renegotiating the relationship's contract. Rebalancing a relationship is a beneficial growing development for both partners, but a successful transition is not guaranteed.

For the powerful partners' growth, the relevant rule of engagement is: a partner's highest obligation is to nourish the other while protecting him or her from harm caused by him/herself and others. Powerful partners must give up their power, which is only the power to dominate, not the power to love or be loved. Doing so necessitates developing compassion and sensitivity for the other's experience while eliminating behaviors that painfully negate the others' individuality. He or she succeeds by supporting their partner's strength and individuality while offering a connection rather than domination. Using control is a closed emotional state in which true relating cannot occur. The new position is one of openness to love.

The fears of battling for power or living within a cold stalemate are the vulnerabilities of love. Only if both power-imbalanced partners simultaneously succeed at implementing positive change will a relationship arrive at balance where power struggles fade and love may flow.

> Where love rules, there is no will to power; where power predominates, there love is lacking. One is the shadow of the other.
>
> *-Carl Jung*

7-10. On the Road to Loving

Our culture's love affair with cars and driving form a suitable analogy for many of the complexities of love relationships. Cars are everywhere. They can be associated with freedom, independence, power, and cooperation, but also safety concerns; associations that driving and loving another both possess. The concrete, physical nature of cars and driving help to make clear aspects of relationships that are subtle and invisible.

The iconic double yellow line dividing many roadways boldly but silently warns drivers "Do Not Cross!" The double yellow line is a well-accepted symbol for danger and limits for safety. Challenge the lines by crossing over, and you risk fatally crashing into oncoming traffic. The equivalent in a love relationship is completely invisible, hence easier to cross, but nonetheless important to observe and respect; these are the limits a lover accepts upon agreeing to participate in a romantic relationship. The lines are the partners' expectations of respect, love and safety, that are commonly spelled-out in marriage vows. Crossing the line is unfortunately all too common when a partner abandons moral and ethical considerations in favor of individual pleasure, relief or satisfaction. Where does the line exist in your relationship? In successful relationships both partners staunchly stay on the non-hurtful side of their relationship double-yellow line by refusing to cheat, lie, be disrespectful or behave insensitively. Those who do cross over tend to crash in the form of volatile drama and divorce; such are relationship fatalities.

Installed between the vehicles moving in opposite directions on busy, fast roadways are concrete barriers to prevent collisions with oncoming traffic. Without the barriers, direct contact between vehicles would undoubtedly result in death, and also multiple car pileups and enormous traffic jams. The barriers provide safety and protection. In love relationships, the need for safety is equally important. Boundaries between partners may be less visible than concrete barriers, but they are just as important for safety. Relationship boundaries and barriers are made from understanding, agreements, relationship rules, promises, and limits. If these are clear and well-executed by both partners, with a well-formed understanding of individual obligations and responsibilities, partners can drive forward safely in their relationship.

Two cars may collide only if they are near each other. The closer two cars are, the greater the risk that they will collide. This is true in love relationships as well; the closer two lovers are, the greater the likelihood each will cause the other hurt. Both on the road and in love, we are vulnerable to damage and injury, which is easily caused, hence much care is needed.

A driver's responsibility is to be in control of his or her vehicle at all times. Weighing thousands of pounds, a speeding car may easily maim or kill a vulnerable person. A partner, too, is vulnerable, especially in their heart. Once a person's heart has been given, its owner may be easily hurt. When in a relationship, each partner ought to be "in control" at all times so as to not harm the other. Partners who lack the ability to be in control form troubled relationships. During times of emotional intensity, strong impulses are the most dangerous. Without good brakes, the nicest car is useless. For a person to be a good partner, he or she needs strong "brakes" in the form of impulse control to prevent intense emotions from fueling hurtful behavior.

On the roadways, a successful trip is one without accidents. Even a minor fender-bender is expensive and inconvenient. Drivers must exercise great care and attention to prevent contact with other cars. In your relationship, "bumping" into your partner means causing him or her hurt or a negative impact. A bump need not be physical to cause emotional pain. Just as an insurance company may refuse to continue providing coverage if a driver has too many accidents, a partner may question continued commitment if he or she is hurt too often.

Driving in traffic, which is unpleasant and restrictive, is not dissimilar to the inevitable rocky patches in a romantic partnership where each struggles to feel positive. Like the interminable stop and go of traffic jams, partners get stuck in tough times and just can't seem to move forward. Just as gridlock forms in intersections where the traffic has backed up in multiple directions, romantic partners also create emotional gridlock when competing needs prevent both partners from shifting in a positive direction. The feeling of being stuck or "relationship grid-lock" builds tension, negativity and hopelessness.

Intersections are places of complexity. Usually well marked with lines, every car wishes to travel through the intersection, so they must take turns. If the drivers refuse to take turns, many cars will crash as drivers compete to use the space. This parallels the moments when partners argue. When both partners have an agenda and insist on pushing it without regard for the other, the partners compete for space, time, and attention. When both partners seek to be heard at the same time and simultaneously refuse to yield, they crash. This is an argument. It is just like when two cars try to use an intersection at the same time. Damage is caused. Taking turns to listen and talk is like respecting the green, yellow and red of the stop light, allowing for the safety of taking turns.

As you and your honey travel along the roadways of your lives, be safe, keep your hands on the wheel, eyes on the road, and put the pedal of your love to the metal.

7-11. Strength is Love's Vital Ally

When discussing romantic relationships, love gets all of the attention. Less associated with relationship success is strength. Each partner's strength is as essential as love for long-term relationship satisfaction and longevity. Some refer to this as maturity — but if that were true, we would be forced to conclude that many adults never mature. Without strength, love will not last. Strength is the ability to do the right thing or to make the necessary changes needed for both individual and relationship well-being, despite discomfort. Using strength is what generates a stable, good life.

The forces contained within a love relationship are powerful. Desires and passions can challenge romantic connections. Often, old childhood patterns that are unfriendly to intimacy assert themselves. When loving and being loved, potent emotions are awakened that are dangerous to closeness. Many of these emotions are painful; they inflame strife. Much the way a farmer must corral the horses so they don't trample the crops, romantic partners must use strength to contain intense feelings and passions to protect the other partner.

As a teammate, friend, and lover, our highest obligation is to protect our partner from being hurt or negatively affected by us. A dilemma is formed by the inner conflict between honoring feelings and doing what is right. In other parts of our lives this dilemma is far less ambiguous; we go to work daily even if we do not feel like it. Parents feed their children whether or not they are in the mood. Great strength is required to put emotions aside in order to fulfill obligations. Significant discretion is also required to choose whether the time is right to express or reject feelings.

As unpopular and unromantic as the idea may be, the strength side of loving is similar to a job. Responsibilities guide our actions, deadlines cause our stress, and professionalism dictates our behavior. The concept of being a "professional partner" may be rejected because it is unromantic, yet it may be effective so long as duty doesn't overshadow humanness. Strength provides a structure so that love, playfulness, relaxation, and pleasure have protected spaces in which to thrive. It takes two strong partners to make one strong love relationship.

Discipline is another important aspect of strength. Within a relationship, each of us fills a role that includes dependability, reliability, and trustworthiness. Discipline is not craved the way love is; it is the all-important work-side of being a romantic partner. Strength has to be used to maintain giving and loving, even when conditions are adverse. Following through on promises, doing an inconvenient favor, being supportive of the partner even when he or she is wrong, rejecting feelings of attraction for another, and loving despite being angry are all examples of positive outcomes born from preventing underlying feelings from harmfully influencing choices and actions.

If you always behave the way you feel, you will have a terrible relationship. Strength is the force protecting a loving bond from unruly feelings. Without it, partners would be unable to make the important changes necessary to fulfill the partner's needs, to protect the relationship from random desires and to fix the relationship if it becomes troubled. Habitually soothing pain with alcohol or drugs, undisciplined spending, and expressing anger explosively are additional examples of feelings run amok.

Strength is needed to tolerate confrontation, to be patient while feeling uncomfortable, and to do the right thing even when one doesn't feel like it. Strength forms a vessel that is absolutely necessary to hold love so that it will last. In the face of unchecked partner weaknesses, accumulated resentment will erode love.

Water is essential for life. However, to make it useful, a container is necessary to carry it to where it is needed. The container limits the water from spilling wastefully. Strength is love's container. For a relationship to endure, love must last. Love is the precious element giving relationships value, but without strength, it is as useful as water without a pail to carry it.

> Love is:
> action and effort which
> supports and nourishes
> another's well-being and growth
> while also protecting
> him or her from harm.

7-12. Love, But Not Like

We don't always like our spouse, his or her choices, behaviors or attitude. So sometimes the love we have for the partner comes into conflict with the emotions we feel. For married couples, the promise to forever love, honor, and cherish places feelings of dislike at odds with the commitment. How can we love our partner when we don't even like him or her?

It is to be expected that you will dislike your partner at some point. Such situations present a dilemma: live out of surface emotion, which feels bad, or live from deeper love and values, which is difficult. As human beings we are complex. Several emotions, values, and ideals may be experienced simultaneously; they may even be contradictory. But when we realize that love is not actually a feeling, but a choice that always benefits us, then arrives the clarity that there is no paradox or conflict at all.

When in dislike, the desire or preference for the partner to be different may trouble daily life. It is a truth that most of us want what we want when we want it. Our society highly values our desires and celebrates them by fulfilling them as quickly and easily as possible. Valuing these desires by investing in rather than disregarding them is the rule rather than the exception. We want to be taller, stronger, more beautiful, thinner, funnier, richer, more successful, etc. The list of preferences is very long. We want our partner to possess some of these improvements in order to to reflect our worth, to earn our admiration and to excite us.

Preferences and desires ultimately come from our inner sense of incompleteness. They arise from our wounds and reflect our deep pain, not the best parts of us. Each time we act to fulfill a desire, we are demonstrating through choice that we are incomplete by lacking the object of desire. We believe that upon fulfillment, we will be more complete. Perhaps you have had the experience that satisfying a desire leads to a temporary feeling of satisfaction which ultimately fades into the disappointment that completeness, and the freedom that is hoped to come from it, remains elusive.

The acceptance of life as it comes and accepting the partner the way they are is painfully difficult at times. "What is" often deviates drastically from what we want it to be. To rail against the partner and the world by trying to change what we don't like is exhausting and usually futile, producing little benefit and many costs. Instead, it is better to increase the capacity to tolerate the discomfort that comes from disliking aspects of the partner and relationship while remaining open and loving.

Every partner tries to change the other. Hopefully, it is done with the same loving, unselfish spirit with which every parent tries to change his or her child, sensitive to the partner's growth and potential. Gentle, loving and respectful influence in the face of unhealthy or self-destructive tendencies may be needed, but force provokes rebellion. When love is continually shared, the partner and his or her objectionable qualities are more easily influenced as they remain fluid instead of locked in the ice of resistance. Acting from love is always in your best interest and absolutely your best policy. Setting the best example is among the most powerful ways to influence. Doing so is hard, but not impossible and requires patience.

When facing something we don't like, instead of seeking to change the partner, we must look inside ourselves to uncover the reason why it affects us so greatly. We only have the power to change ourselves. This is often our only option, and our growth will be fueled every time we do so while using love as a benchmark. Dislikes are nothing other than our limits of loving ourselves.

Loving when you don't like is neither foreign to most people nor impossible; parents do it all the time with their children. When not liking your partner, loving him or her is the best way forward. Love makes the world go round; no one says that about like.

7-13. Love's Gymnasium

The quest for a deeply loving and satisfying love relationship is only slightly less strong than the instinct to survive. The pervasive need to couple with another is evidence of that. The urge to improve love relationships by deepening connection and resolving problems for most feels vital and continuous. Love relationships are a vehicle for individual growth, which if successful are marked by an increased capacity for love and compassion. Our relationships are love's gymnasium. Much like the way we use weights to strengthen our muscles, working at love relationships are the exercises to strengthen our love. The weights are just the method to achieve stronger muscles; the exercises are not really about the weights. In outward appearances, partners seek to resolve relationship problems to make their relationships better, but the deeper purpose is for partners' growth regarding love.

Couples develop the patterns they do because of a combination of partner strengths and limitations, but dysfunctional patterns that provoke pain and anger are caused by partner limitations. The work of love is to resolve and overcome such limitations. The pain and frustration partners experience when love is insufficient, blocked or withheld is significant and may rise to a high level of distress. Within a relationship, blocked love may have a large negative effect on partners' well-being and self-esteem. That the impact may be so large and negative proves the high importance of love. The painful truth is that not all relationship problems will be solved. Many a partner has neither the will nor the strength to tackle a particular issue. An unresolved problem indicates weakness or fear. The other partner in response may practice patience or acceptance so that his or her growth continues. The other's limitations are not an excuse for failure to love completely, that limitation is within you. Your capacity to love is about yourself, and not about the degree to which you believe that your partner is deserving of love.

The changes and areas of growth most requested by partners will prove to be the least popular and most difficult to achieve; this is the reason why the obstacle exists in the first place. Each and every change is the healing of a wound around which a defense has been wisely built for safety and self-protection in response to a past hurt. Partners are rarely eager to dissolve a wall of protection that has long provided emotional security and safety.

In no other place in our lives do these protective walls become more evident than in our love relationships, where partners dream of, hope for and expect complete love. Within an intimate relationship the demands for love and openness are high. Paradoxically, in no other place in most partners' lives is vulnerability equally as high. Full love means complete openness, which means complete vulnerability. Once a defensive wall has been dismantled, a wound has to be healed. Such is the process of self-discovery and personal growth. Desiring something, such as more fulfilling love, is a reaction to the experience of being incomplete; it feels as if the desired object will complete us. But once the object of desire is obtained, it will only lead to a deeper awareness of incompleteness, which once again fuels greater desire.

However, in the context of a love relationship, the problem or issue targeted for change rarely appears, on the surface, to be difficult, but usually proves to be an involved process. It is easy to say, "I would just like my partner to be more romantic," or "I wish my partner showed me more attention." On the surface a fix may appear to be a simple adjustment of attitude or behavior. Much like the proverbial tip of the iceberg, each problem is but a small hint of what may be the pain of significant wounds operating under the surface. Like getting at the contents of a tightly closed jar, the delicious contents are easily visible, but opening the lid may be a tough first task.

Most partners dream of a more fulfilling love. Each one of us can always love more deeply. Our capacity to love is unlimited. If you want to be loved more deeply, are you willing to increase your ability to love to obtain it? Because a love relationship is a system, change always has to be reciprocal for any change to be supported, maintained, and long-lasting.

The healing of your relationship is the process of love doing through you what love does… completing incompleteness, becoming stronger and more open to giving and receiving; like opening the curtains of a dark room and letting in the sunlight. It is the process of becoming completely open and vulnerable, a process that sounds good in theory, but raises fear like nothing else. Your love relationship is a vehicle for your growth...growth in your capacity to love, ever deeper, yourselves, your partner, other people, and life itself. The problems in your relationship are evidence that in order for you to be fully open, more work must be done.

> One hurtful action destroys the positive effect of a dozen loving gestures.

7-14. Careful Does It

Getting into a love relationship is a risky proposition. Closeness means getting hurt. Feeling fear when first facing a potential love relationship is a common reaction because when sharing love, hurts are inevitable. While many lovers have a tough exterior, once their heart is open to another, it is easily hurt. The baseline for succeeding in love requires partners to work as a team to reduce and eliminate hurts. The more important the partner becomes, the more easily we are hurt by him or her.

In the center of our hearts, each one of us is as tender as a newborn baby. When "in love," the tender center of our hearts are open. Being completely accepted is of monumental importance to experience the full extent of love. Because openness creates a high degree of vulnerability, many may never fully open to experience the fulfillment of love. Being loved is such a vital dream that to be rejected is just too painful; so painful that many people avoid taking the risk. The dilemma each lover faces is that to protect oneself means being safe from hurt but then closeness and connection becomes unobtainable. At our center, we long with every fiber of our being to be fully loved and accepted. To practice full acceptance of a partner is to reach towards the boundary of where human love becomes divine, like the way each plant reaches towards the sun.

How easily are we hurt? A sharp tone, a disapproving glance, or a cutting sarcastic word is enough to emotionally injure a person. A brief lapse of care can cause defensive closing down. A thoughtless remark hinting that the other isn't good or valuable enough can invite an angry counterattack. Personal weaknesses, character flaws, and tendencies towards the extreme are usually at the root of most repetitious hurts. Insufficient care and lack of awareness cause an accumulation of hurts the way snowflakes pile up in a blizzard. Because most romantic partners were raised in family environments in which power struggles and conflict were common, many lovers cannot conceive of a relationship without hurtfulness. If left unchecked, a steady flurry of unintentional hurts creates an emotionally toxic relationship environment.

When water is exposed to very cold air it begins to freeze immediately. The water doesn't wait to think about whether it wants to freeze or not. The same highly dynamic, natural cause and effect is manifested when partners close off their hearts in self-protection. Large hurts are obvious, but in most relationships, it is the accumulation of many tiny unintentional hurts that is responsible for disconnection. This is like relationship death by a thousand paper cuts. Laziness and insensitivity can produce this. Every romantic partner must grow and change; the way partners seek to influence each other to encourage this growth need not be hurtful.

Being in a relationship with a partner who regularly fails to listen well, or with a partner whose communication rarely leads to action is unpleasant. It is similar with a partner whose promises usually go unfulfilled. Occurring chronically these kinds of actions will cause a partner to gradually feel unimportant and unloved. He or she will eventually close off. What about a partner who often criticizes the other? Or a partner who does not emotionally open up when closeness is requested? These actions cause hurt, too. If such instances happen routinely, a relationship will gradually cool and grow disconnected in response, this is not a recipe for passion and closeness. A partner who makes important decisions without consulting the other is unintentionally sending the message that the partner is unimportant. If occurring repetitively, over time such actions have a cumulative and negative influence on the partner.

The success of loving another is not made with large, grand gestures, but instead it is all the little, common efforts which protect the other from harm. A soft tone, carefully chosen words, and deliberate, positive actions are effective at maintaining a loving connection. Most partners do not yet possess the sensitivity required to eliminate most relationship hurts. Cultivating it takes an intention that many lovers prefer to not develop; it is hard work.

We are easily hurt and most of the injuries are minor, each not worthy of a lot of attention. The deterioration of most relationships is imperceptibly slow, like when grass grows. The result is summed up in the often-expressed words, "I've fallen out of love." When it snows, no single snowflake is noteworthy, but when billions of them fall, the resulting blizzard now has a large effect. The accumulation of many minor hurts destroys a loving emotional connection. Partners succeed at loving when they ratchet up their sensitivity by becoming highly aware of how their words, actions and choices may have a positive, loving effect. By treating each other as precious, you two may build a safe and loving togetherness.

> Police yourself and your partner will not have to or want to.

7-15. Teaching You How to Love Me

Like a fingerprint, each one of us is unique and has preferred ways of being loved. When our partner fails to understand this by loving us ineffectively, a common reaction is to feel hurt, and express anger by either attacking or distancing. When both partners are involved in this kind of dance of hurtfulness, the result is a downward spiral of disconnection and unhappiness. Such a dynamic describes a common but unfortunate pattern of relating, an ever-tightening knot of emotional gridlock. Most partners try hard to succeed at loving, but when what they are doing is wrong, trying harder tightens the knot instead of loosening it.

Loving the other only when we believe he or she deserves to be loved is part of the problem, and is disastrous compared to a less conditional approach. The easiest thing to do is to love the way that comes most naturally to you, rather than your partner's preferred way. The resulting negative cycle can be difficult to repair. Anger is a poor teaching tool. Instead of teaching, anger hurts, intimidates and usually provokes a defensive "walls-up" reaction that harms connection. Additionally it motivates a partner to resist change. Successful relating can only happen if a partner feels loved. Teaching your partner how to love you right, instead of punishing him or her for their failures, is part of a successful recipe.

A widespread but incorrect assumption is that if our partner loves us, he or she will know how to love us. Greater confusion is added by the reality that many partners demonstrate effective loving in the early phase of togetherness, a sweetness which sadly disappears along with the relationship's deepening. As partners grow more connected, deeper and older emotional patterns surface. Partners face the task of "re-training" each other in the ways of loving within an evolving togetherness, an effort which can easily take many years.

The tendency of partners is to take personally the other's failure to love them properly, and interpret it as rejection. When both partners react to pain and disappointment, the relationship becomes embroiled in a destructive and accelerating negative dance. The way out of this conundrum is for one, but preferably both partners, to adopt a strong commitment to act towards the other in loving ways while teaching the other how to deliver love in the right way. Love is always part of the answer to a relationship problem, though loving efforts may not offer immediate results. A commitment to be loving under all circumstances is simple; it requires much strength, but offers an eroded relationship hope for a brighter future. Unconditional love is impossible to humanly achieve, but it is always a worthy endeavor.

Teach instead of being sensitive. It is more effective to inform your partner in a positive way that you wish to be treated differently than it is to be critical of your partner in his or her failure. The more specific you are on how you want to be loved, the better. Examples are: "Touching me more gently feels nicer," instead of "You're too rough!" and "Generosity makes you more attractive to me," instead of "I can't believe how cheap you are!" and "When you listen well and understand me, I feel closer," instead of "You never listen to me!" Along with voicing a suggestion, an affectionate touch can motivate the partner to try even harder.

Resist the seemingly natural tendency to act out of hurt when your partner fails to love you in satisfying ways. Punishment is a less successful method of teaching than offering loving help. Loving behavior models the right example while also causing the partner to be more open to change. You are an expert on yourself, and you are the best teacher from whom your partner can learn how to succeed. Teaching about love is not an easy task and will require a lot of patience. Lessons may have to be repeated dozens, even hundreds of times. Your teaching tools are your love, your strength, and your power to influence. However, do understand; a partner will never be forced to love. When using any kind of force to produce constructive results, it must be combined with love. Actions which hurt your partner slow progress greatly.

Someone who feels loved will be more open to their partner's influence than someone who does not. Permanent change arrives slowly. The goal is to gradually wear down your partner's resistance to loving you in the right way by applying incessant but loving persistence...like the Colorado River which eroded the beautiful Grand Canyon incessantly over millions of years. Be a loving force of nature that never gives up! Let your partner's failures motivate you to act more lovingly towards him or her, and surely over time your love will triumph. Teaching your partner to love will simultaneously accelerate your own growth and capacity to love.

7-16. Love is perfect

Love is perfect and we are not. Our humanness is at the center of our struggles within love relationships. We tend to love poorly and inconsistently. We rarely succeed at purely loving and fully accepting even ourselves. Also, we tend to love our partners intermittently and rather badly. The heights of unconditional love are so lofty that few come near them. The sun gives its light unconditionally every day to everybody without exception and without fail, while never asking for anything in return. Love relationships are highly complex; two imperfect people joined together. When coupled, their union possesses twice as many imperfections as each owns individually. The relationship is bound to be a test.

Love is a natural connecting force; it joins and bonds. When fully given, love nourishes, while chasing away all separateness. Love embraces and accepts, while including us in belonging. When we are fully loved, we feel valued and important. If we cooperate with love, it encourages us to let go of all selfishness. One definition of love within a relationship is supporting the partner's nourishment, well-being and growth while also protecting him or her from being harmed. Each one of us has the option to strive to grow beyond our highly conditional lives to love unconditionally.

Many relationships begin with intense excitement and transcendent feelings of bliss. Time and again this is referred to as the honeymoon phase. Rarely does the experience of bliss last more than a year, but usually less than six months. The good feeling is so profound that it becomes many partners' definition and expectation of love; they hope and expect that it will continue unabated throughout the relationship. Celebrated as the pinnacle of excitement, Hollywood and advertisers repeatedly use this blissful experience for their own purposes, while continually sustaining an illusion about real relationships. We are trained to unrealistically expect relationship perfection, a perpetual honeymoon bliss, which ultimately undermines a relationship as it can never be "good enough."

Hugely less glorious, but far more common, is what may appropriately be called the "work phase" of a relationship, the long period following the honeymoon phase in which partners do the hard-growing work of love. And it truly is hard, sometimes ugly, work. Hard work usually feels uncomfortable. Enduring change is painful, and growing in response to change is harder still. Most partners are not prepared for the magnitude and long duration of the challenge of the work phase. It is as if in our culture, all the attention and excitement has been devoted to the honeymoon phase, but the work phase, representing the majority of the relationship, has been denied. Because of unrealistic expectations, romantic partners resist growth and change, refusing to cooperate with love's process, while not having anticipated that growth is a necessary and normal part of successful relating. As a result, many romantic partners are deeply disappointed and disillusioned once firmly in the throes of the "unromantic" and painful work phase. Expressions of "I did not sign up for this," signal another impending broken union. The reality of the work phase is dismissed by the phrase, "unlucky in love." When it comes to love, it is not luck.

The "work" in the work phase is about improving and increasing the capacity to love ourselves, our romantic partners, family members and life itself. Because each one of us grows up inheriting our family's patterns and limitations, and because while growing up we sustain emotional bumps and bruises, healing and growing is required in order to be more capable of complete love. Growing is especially hard. Striving to unconditionally remain open while accepting of all life's experiences, even painful ones, is essential to realizing love's essence.

Few get to live a life of continuous stress-free vacation, with all our needs fulfilled, enjoying chronic pleasure. For most of us vacations occur occasionally, only small islands in a large sea of daily work. Love relationships are similar. The honeymoon phase is a special time that does not last. Truly, there is no love without pain. Realistic expectations include a readiness to complete the emotional tasks required of us in the work phase, which in the long run allows for more relationship "vacations."

7-17. Important, Special, and Cherished

In the big wide world, most of us are relatively unimportant. Within love relationships it is an entirely different matter. Not feeling important to our romantic partner causes pain and disappointment. Being important, special, and cherished is not only a common expectation within romantic relationships, but if not fulfilled, becomes a point of growing dissatisfaction that exposes the relationship to the risk of dissolution.

Economics tells us that when something becomes common and easily obtainable, its value drops. The same concept holds true between partners in long-term relationships; the partner, already obtained, becomes common; a factor that erodes specialness. Being taken for granted develops easily. Another factor is referred to in the well-worn phrase, "familiarity breeds contempt." Knowing the partner well means knowing his or her human limitations, frailties, insensitivities, and insecurities, no matter how painful this knowledge may be. Such qualities are not endearing. Success at maintaining a relationship at a positive level demands efforts that counteract such seemingly natural but erosive forces.

Shouldn't feeling good and special just come naturally? When experiencing newness, excitement and good feelings arise spontaneously. When any experience, person, place, or thing grows familiar, it loses the luster of novelty as it joins the ranks of the ordinary and the excitement wears off. Anything of value, whether it be a satisfying love relationship, building a successful business, or raising a healthy child, takes effort to achieve. Hard work, commitment and dedication will be needed, otherwise the value will not be achieved. Giving your best to that which you wish to create is essential for success.

A recipe for maintaining some of the excitement that comes when a love connection is new includes making consistent effort to show that the other is important, special and cherished, which results in the other feeling loved. As a young child, each of us needed this same kind of loving attention from our parents. If given, this high regard helped us to develop emotional security, positive self-esteem and resiliency. Unfortunately, many of us did not receive this kind of compassionate attention. Our love relationships are a second chance to give and receive this kind of loving attention. The words, "You are special and important" may not be necessary, but to show it in thoughtful and careful action is necessary. If the second chance is well taken, emotional, relational healing and deep positive bonding is possible. In every love relationship, partners emotionally "parent" each other. Rather than being a power struggle, this parenting is positive if it is loving and patient.

Couples run into problems when partner interactions provoke rejection, anxiety, disappointment, and fear of failure. Showing the other that he or she is important and treating them in a cherishing way can soothe such painful feelings. Showing the partner that they are important is done by giving their emotional well-being a high priority. Responding compassionately to a partner when they are in pain or discomfort communicates importance by demonstrating that "I am here for you." Showing that the partner is special is accomplished by consistently having his or her back at all times, meaning that support will be offered when needed. Additionally, actions that show that your partner is repeatedly chosen behaviorally communicate that "you alone are mine" and serve to cultivate specialness. Cherishing happens when we are highly responsive so as to keep the other safe by consistently showing up to protect him or her from discomfort, or difficult or potentially harmful situations.

The kind of close relationship that most partners seek and

dream about is only obtainable when partners are successful at creating a safe relationship bond that is sensitive to well-being. Coming from emotionally tough family environments, some partners may scoff at the level of sensitivity needed, viewing it as rewarding weakness, but such a perspective is a thinly veiled defensive expression of personal pain and vulnerability. Sensitivity is a strength that serves couples well while they demonstrate that the other is important, special, and cherished.

7-18. Falling out of Love

It is creeping into awareness, just a feeling here and there at first, and met with dread. It does not bloom fully until years into the relationship, once the ecstatic honeymoon phase has fully faded. The relationship takes daily effort now. Falling out of love is an experience that strikes terror into the hearts of partners in stable relationships. Is there any lover, partner or spouse who doesn't fear the words, "I love you, but I'm not in love with you?"

Grappling to make sense out of this upsetting emotional development, an out-of-love partner grieves the loss of loving feelings and may experiment with trying to get them back, only to slip deeper into this loveless hole. Announcing it to the partner may seem like an afterthought, though it marks the beginning of a new tortuous chapter. How can one stay together where no love feelings exist? This is not the way a good love relationship should feel.

The disappearance of love and passionate feelings seems mysterious. To an out-of-love partner a quick appraisal of the other will find plentiful qualities, characteristics and habits suitable to blame for love's abandonment. The obvious conclusion is that the other was simply the wrong choice as a partner: If my partner was more attentive, patient, sexy, or just not so annoying… This external search for causes feels natural and is the path of least resistance. Introspection is much harder as plumbing the emotional depths seems fruitless and our own defenses and years' worth of repression represent formidable barriers to a diligent search. With the emotional gates firmly shut, there may be nothing visible as a cause.

Negative emotions which constitute the "falling out of love" phenomenon show up consciously from two sources. The first source is the relationship and partner interactions, including things such as poorly negotiated differences and accumulated pain from hurts. Most out-of-love partners do not wish to give consideration to the larger and more significant second source: reawakened painful emotions from old wounds, traumas and the profound, often negative, impact of childhood development. The surface layers of the emotional personality have been eroded, uncovering unresolved hurts and the anger associated with events long past.

The convenient conclusion is that the partner and their imperfections are the cause; the easiest corrective action for an out-of-love partner is to get rid of the relationship and thereby get rid of the pain. The more he or she ruminates on internal dissatisfaction, the more intense the desire to get away from the other. For many, the quickest way to stop the emotional pain is to find a new lover who sparks the ecstasy of new love. Love is the best anti-depressant.

However, the lack of love we feel or experience is always about us. Blaming the other is easy, but our challenge is to meet every situation with love and acceptance. By rejecting the other, an out-of-love partner fails to practice the life lessons the relationship is trying to teach. If we have fallen out of love, we have blocked access to our true nature.

Our love relationships, if we allow them, will teach us to be emotional adults; they have the potential to expand our capacity for real love. The lessons can be uncomfortable; the medicine may be bitter, but character strengths are the hallmark of maturity. Love relationships cannot be ruled by emotion, otherwise they will be inconsistent and unstable. Until we switch to a perspective in which love is realized, not as a feeling, but instead as a choice expressed in action, we will be vulnerable to the uncomfortable emotions that convince us that our love is gone. Loving our partner only when we feel like it, or when the other seems to deserve it, is a narrow, incomplete perspective that almost guarantees relationship failure. The broader view is that love is our very essence, that if it seems gone, we must accept that we have blocked it. Owning such a responsibility is the beginning of the journey towards an unconditional kind of love.

7-19. Many Fish in the Sea... Sharks too

Searching for a romantic partner with whom to share love can be uncomfortable. Risks include being judged and potentially hurt or rejected by new potential partners. Singles are likely to come across many who are a poor fit, and most hopeful experiences end in disappointment. Among the potential partners are sociopaths who are deceptive and ultimately cause pain. We all want to be loved, yet there are those people who naturally use guile and deception to obtain selfish satisfaction, and who care little about the impact on others.

Hungering to share a togetherness makes each one of us vulnerable. Sociopaths sense vulnerability and skillfully use it as an opportunity to gain an advantage. In the bay, fishing boats depend on warning buoys to inform them when there are dangerous rocks just under the surface. In the dating scene, no such buoys exist. The wise who are looking for love do so slowly, and take great care.

A proportion of the population have some degree of mental illness, which can be largely invisible to the majority of people. It may be subtle and deliberately hidden, and of course when dating, no potential partner chooses to put all their weaknesses and character flaws on display. Each one of us puts our best foot forward in the hope of attracting another. The sociopath is no different. Like the shark that stalks its prey, these actions are not personal; it's just what they do. Sharks want to be loved, just like every other fish in the sea.

A sociopath is a person, most often male, who has poor mental health, often damaged by growing up in a harsh and harmful home environment. The term "sociopath" is a popular term; mental health professionals use the diagnostic label Antisocial Personality Disorder to describe this set of emotional problems. A sociopath's inability to empathize with another's experience, an essential trait to form a healthy love relationship, interferes with the development of relationship stability and emotional safety.

Sociopaths prioritize narcissistic fulfillment of personal needs and wishes, often at the expense of the partner's well-being. Being devoid of empathy or compassion, if the pursuit of satisfaction harms another, the sociopath cares little. After hurt has been caused, the sociopath tends to give a callous response, accepting no responsibility and shifting blame elsewhere. His or her conscience is a quiet inner voice that is often dismissed, a task accomplished more easily by them than by non-sociopaths. Possessing a poor sense of right and wrong, he or she may derive a twisted pleasure from possessing control and using it to keep another off-balance and uncomfortable. As their need for survival awakened, the sociopath learned early on how to be manipulative, how to sense others' vulnerability, and how to turn on the charm while easily attracting others. At its core, the personality of the sociopath is unstable, resulting in difficulty maintaining a job, making friendships last, and controlling impulses that can manifest in violent rages, hot-headedness and a fondness for risky behaviors. Instability is further manifested by a propensity towards promiscuity, infidelity and addictions.

Strength is attractive and sexy. Time and again women are attracted to the "bad boys," whose rebellious, defiant individualism appears as strength and at times leadership. A male who is strong and attractive, and who a woman cannot control is perceived unconsciously by her as a potential partner who has what it takes to provide her with safety and protect her from harm. Such a male registers high on the tummy-butterfly meter. But although the bad boys, of whom male sociopaths are card-carrying members, possess a charisma as well as the surface appearance of strength, they lack the depth of real strength of character and good mental health. For women, bad boys are wonderful fantasy partners, they are exciting and suitable for throw-caution-to-the-wind weekend romances, but they cannot deliver a healthy, positive and stable love relationship. Instead of being a partner who can protect from her harm, this person ends up being someone who causes harm, offering long-term pain, misery and disrespect.

Truly getting to know someone takes time. Romantic feelings and "chemistry" quicken the pace of joining together, but undermine a slow and safe approach to the development of closeness. To avoid falling for the deception of a sociopath, or any poor partner, assertively setting a slow pace is essential while gathering information to determine the mental health and goodness of fit of a potential partner. The intensely exciting passionate hookup is the friend of the poor partner. With any kind of falling, including falling in love, it is uncomfortably difficult to fall slowly. Love is so enticingly delicious, and this is not fully dulled by the possible pain of loss of control, broken heartedness, and grief. A romantic partner is the single most influential person in one's life, a poor partner can be the single most destructive.

Ask the right questions while taking a budding relationship very slowly. Does the potential partner have friends? Sociopaths have few friends. Is he or she financially stable with a solid work history? A criminal history? A history of drug or alcohol problems? Did the potential partner have a smooth or rough experience in school? Was his or her early family life supportive or harsh and unkind? An emotionally healthy potential partner will have little problem offering transparency about the past. Learning this information before the heart is fully invested is necessary because finding a new love is serious business. If the fit is not proved to be safe, the new-found relationship must be swiftly, decisively terminated.

> If you are
> going through hell,
> keep going.
>
> — *Winston Churchill*

7-20. Mothering Kind of Love

The loving bond between a mother and her child is unique. No other relationship is as pure and selfless as the one between a woman and the innocent infant she brought forth as gift into the world. Becoming a mother changes a woman deeply and has a profound impact on her romantic partner as well. Some female partners have difficulty distinguishing between mother's love and passionate love in long-term relationships, a fact that many male partners complain about.

"Stop mothering me," is a chorus sung in frustration by many male partners, a reaction to moments where their female partners give instructions with an all too familiar attitude. The dynamics of the relationship between mates are complicated, and made more complicated by struggles for power and control. The reaction of men to moments of mothering range from a momentary angry look to an explosion of rage. This kind of female expression wounds their men in a way that is completely lost on most girlfriends and wives.

How male partners hear it differs wildly from how a woman intends it. A mother-like expression often seeks to correct instead of connect. The words or tone are more commanding than requesting and get a male partner's back up, since he interprets it as she knowing better than he. Collectively these communications form a cocktail of sometimes not-so-subtle declarations that the female partner is in control. Domination and servitude are fine if both partners are satisfied with the arrangement, but love demands greater equality. Mothering tends to infantilize husbands and boyfriends, often non-verbally suggesting they are not capable.

Mothering communications, while often innocently intended, touch upon the wounds of childhood powerlessness for many men. These emotional injuries are often not completely healed, and motherly statements and actions take the man back to a time before he was a man, emotionally recalling a time when, as children they possessed far less power than their mother and were also completely dependent upon her. As a way of affirming their masculinity, men enjoy possession and displays of strength, including independence. Many men distance themselves as much as possible from all things child-like, which for them is associated with powerlessness and weakness.

Many female partners are thoroughly confused by what may seem to be a huge, irrational reaction to a few minor words. She just reminded him, "Be careful." What's the big deal? she thought. Coming out of nowhere, his angry response seems worthy of disregard, when what is really lurking in such a moment of disconnect is a power imbalance. If not corrected it will grow to be a big problem. As with most relationship difficulties, they build from behavior patterns that are frequently repeated.

When a male partner says angrily, "I need a lover, not a mother," the words may not find a home in his female partner's consciousness. The mothering dynamic is lost in her blind spot. Unlike males, females are born of a mother who later becomes her role model, for better or worse. Daughters develop emotionally in part by identifying with the role of mother, one that is reinforced once she begins her own family. As a result, this is a behavior pattern that it is almost impossible for wives and girlfriends not to fall into. The kind of love a mother gives her child is nourishing and celebrates the infant's complete dependence on her. An infant's need for the mother is profound. In an adult love relationship, emotional neediness is unhealthy evidence of codependency. In contrast to that is the passionate love that promotes desire and admiration between adults balanced by individual strength and autonomy.

For men, the mothering kind of love is associated with several kinds of "bossy" communications; contained within and between the words are an attempt to gain or assert power. Unlike the ideal loving mother, who just seeks to love and nourish, real-life mothers are understandably frustrated and maxed-out at times, and mothering words convey this uncomfortable reality. For an anxious and fearful female partner, the tendency to "mother" her mate may be turbo-charged. Couched within mothering-type language are assumptions of male incompetence that often violate his boundaries by giving unsolicited help and guidance. Male partners interpret such interactions as his female partner viewing him as stupid. Any lingering childishness in men emotionally inhibits their ability to challenge these kinds of assertions. Most go silent. Some explode.

A love relationship is a system between partners in which every patterned interaction is supported by both partners. The sarcastic verbal tournament, "You are not my mother," vs "I want a man for a partner, not another child," is evidence that our relationships are places where we try (and struggle) to grow up. As much as male partners loathe their women's mothering tendencies, they generally do not notice how they unwittingly support it. Men who fail to take full responsibility, or avoid taking initiative, invite mothering. A male partner who really wishes for all mothering to be gone from his relationship will gain this reward by maturely owning his power through the demonstration of full responsibility, and by asserting himself firmly without domination or hurtfulness. The mothering kind of love is an ineffective way to encourage partner maturity, which is better accomplished through passionate love.

7-21. Caring by Being Careful

Getting into a love relationship is a risky proposition. Closeness invites getting hurt. Feeling fear when first facing a potential love relationship is a common reaction because, when sharing love, hurts are inevitable, and while many lovers have tough exteriors, once they open their heart to another they can be easily hurt. The baseline for succeeding in love requires partners to work as a team to reduce and eliminate hurts. The more important the partner becomes, the more easily we are hurt by him or her.

In the center of our hearts, we are as tender as a newborn baby. When "in love," the tender center of our heart is open. Being completely accepted is of monumental importance to experiencing the full extent of love, but because openness creates a high degree of vulnerability and the high risk of hurt, many never fully open themselves to experiencing that fulfillment. Being loved is such vital dream that being rejected is just too painful; so painful that many people avoid taking the risk in the first place. The dilemma each lover faces is that self-protection means being safe from hurt, but also makes closeness and connection unobtainable; yet at our center, we long with every fiber of our being to be fully loved and accepted. To practice full acceptance of a partner is to reach towards the boundary of where human love becomes divine, the way every plant reaches towards the sun.

How easily can we be hurt? Just a sharp tone, a disapproving glance or a cutting sarcastic word is enough to emotionally injure. A minor lapse of care can cause defensive closing down. A thoughtless remark hinting that the other isn't good or valuable enough can invite an angry counterattack. Personal weaknesses and character flaws are usually at the root of most repetitious hurts, and insufficient care and lack of awareness causes an accumulation of hurts the way snowflakes pile up in a blizzard. Because most romantic partners were raised in family environments in which power struggles and conflict were common, many lovers cannot conceive of a relationship without hurtfulness. Unchecked, a steady flurry of unintentional hurts creates an emotionally toxic relationship environment.

When water is exposed to very cold air it begins to freeze immediately. The water doesn't wait to think about whether it wants to freeze or not. The same highly dynamic, natural cause and effect is manifest when partners close off their hearts in self-protection. Large hurts are obvious, but in most relationships, it is the accumulation of hundreds of tiny, unintentional hurts that results in gradual disconnection...relationship death by a thousand paper-cuts. Laziness and insensitivity can produce this. Every romantic partner must grow and change; the way partners seek to influence each other for growth need not be hurtful.

Being in a relationship with a partner who regularly fails to listen, or whose communication rarely leads to action is unpleasant. It is similar with a partner whose promises often go unfulfilled. Occurring chronically, these kinds of neglectful actions will cause the other to gradually feel unimportant and unloved, and eventually to close off. What about a partner who routinely criticizes? Or a partner who never emotionally opens up when closeness is invited? These actions cause unintentional hurt, too. If such instances happen routinely, a relationship will cool and grow disconnected over time in response, not a recipe for maintaining passion and closeness. Someone who makes decisions without consulting their partner is not unusual, and the message is unthinkingly sent that the partner is unimportant. If this occurs repeatedly, over time such actions have a cumulative and negative influence on the partner, since the pain from unintentional hurts is no less painful than that from intentional ones.

Successfully loving another is not accomplished with large, grand gestures, but instead it is all the little thoughtful efforts which protect the other from harm. The hurts run most relationships, but a soft tone, carefully chosen words and deliberate, positive actions are effective at maintaining a loving connection. Many partners do not possess the sensitivity required to eliminate most relationship hurts, and cultivating it takes an intent that many lovers prefer to not develop; it is hard work.

We are easily hurt and most of the injuries are minor, each little cut seems unworthy of much attention, so most are dismissed. The deterioration of most relationships is imperceptibly slow, like the pace of grass growing. The result is summed up in the often-expressed words, "I've fallen out of love." When it snows, no single snowflake is noteworthy, but when billions of them fall, the snow has a huge effect. The accumulation of many minor hurts destroys a loving connection. Partners succeed at loving when they ratchet up their sensitivity by becoming highly aware of how their words, actions and choices may have a positive, loving effect. By treating each other as precious, you two may build a safe and loving togetherness.

7-22. Love: Who is it for?

While attempting to create satisfying and enduring love relationships, love is of central consideration. More than half the commitments to life-long love end sooner than promised, suggesting that the concepts and practices we culturally hold about love are incorrect. The way we love is ineffective, and when we delve deeper into the nature of love, illusions fall away. So when we ask the question: "Who is love for?" the answer, ultimately, is you.

There is a widely held belief that love is a feeling. Not only is this incorrect, but the fallout this causes places our long-term relationships in jeopardy. My definition of love is efforts and actions which encourage and support growth, nourishment and well-being while also protecting the other or oneself from harm. So love is action that comes from a choice. When traveling through the normal and inevitable rigors in the life of romantic relationships, negative feelings commonly arise. If love is considered a positive feeling, the natural conclusion if it disappears will be that we no longer have love for the partner. Many a relationship crisis is hatched from this misunderstanding. If love could only be given when positive feelings for the partner were present, no relationship would ever improve once in trouble, and few relationships would stay positive. We must persistently love our partner, whether or not we have loving feelings, just as good parents do for their children. It is not unusual for a parent to be angry with their child, but they never stop loving them. Love is what we give to be our best, and it cannot be based upon our fluctuating emotions and moods. Unless we get love right, obtaining satisfying relationship results will be elusive.

Paradoxically, we need not have good feelings about our partner to love him or her. On any particular day we may not even like them, but we can still love them by making loving efforts. A significant cause of relationship failure is the repeated practice of withholding love when the partner is judged not to deserve it because he or she has behaved in a way that is objectionable. In reality, an "undeserving" partner and the coinciding at-risk relationship need love the most. A badly behaved partner is an opportunity to practice loving compassion, this is not done because your partner deserves it, but because to do so is the best thing for you.

When facing relationship adversity, anger and bitterness are usually provoked, but if we respond with loving actions, our growth results. By choosing loving actions we increase the chance that our relationship may improve, our partner will open to our influence, and we will be clearer about the role we play in the relationship drama.

Love is the energy we bring when we give our best to nourish and support, and in long-term relationships it RESULTS in loving feelings. Typically partners practice the opposite, only giving love if warm feelings are felt. Loving is a practice of focusing nourishing efforts on another, attempting to do so unconditionally. The process is purifying. When offered completely for another's well-being, it comes from deep within our center. Love's positive effects are magnified the more unconditional it is.

A majority of us grew up in a family environment in which love was incomplete, and this is instrumental in the development of a definition of love which is limited and distorted. For most, the emotional definition of love blends it with fear, dependency, attachment, domination, submission, and powerlessness. Love is not these things and the purer love is, the more effective it will be. The best efforts to love are those which value our own needs in loving consideration. Careful attention to giving, receiving and self-care allow love to stay, like water which cannot be possessed with a greedy grab, but will rest in a gentle, patient palm. The more we love, the greater our loving capacity will be.

Relationships are a closed system. During instances when we cause hurt to our partner, the result also negatively affects us. Like the flight of a boomerang, what we put out comes back at us. The emotional quality created between partners lingers within the relationship container. If a relationship is doing well, you benefit. Similarly if it does poorly, you are negatively affected. By loving your partner, you indirectly love yourself.

When you love, the gifts of pride, peace, and a good love

relationship are obtainable. In loving, grand gestures and heroics are not necessary. Love is your best practice of being you. Of course, when both partners simultaneously make such loving efforts, all negativity evaporates, and harmony and a loving connection prevail. Just giving love cleanses you of toxic emotion while nourishing those around you. Choosing to be loving is a gift to yourself. Who is the greatest beneficiary of your love? You.

7-23. Loving Our Partner, a Spiritual Discipline

A majority of people join with another to form a love relationship. Coupling up is just what we do. Of those who have become single due to breakup or divorce, many go on to search for a new partner with whom to form a loving bond and probably more people commit to love than do not. What is beneath this urge to practice love?

In our lives, love is of primary importance. Years ago, a song declared in its refrain, "Love makes the world go round." Many songs are about love or loss of love. A similar theme is expressed in almost every world religion and many spiritual traditions, loving the divine, loving life and gratitude for life. Is the consistency of these themes across popular music and spirituality a coincidence? No. Whenever and wherever we love, the deepest purpose is always the same. Music is considered a universal language, but an even more compelling element of universality is love, which exists among every people everywhere throughout time. Only the manner in which love may be expressed is unique in each time and place.

The strong pull of attraction to another often results in a loving bond, and early in a new relationship, the intensity of that attraction and connection is ecstatic. It leaves an impression that lasts throughout the relationship or life. When a deeper love is possible, it is hard to resist. Love is as essential as every breath we take, it is the most powerful drug that exists. An even more magical quality that love possesses is its unifying ability to transform separate people into a community, a nation, a world, and two people into one couple.

If love is so wonderful, then what about all the adversity romantic partners experience in maintaining a love relationship? The divorce rate is near fifty percent, and unmarried couples end their loving connections even more frequently. Relationships and marriage are hard, yet there is truth in the frequently expressed statement that you have to work hard to obtain something of truly great value.

Just as people work hard in the gym to get fit and strengthen their muscles through sweat, and maybe tears, our love relationships are the arena in which we practice so as to strengthen our love; not the love that is most often spoken about, but the love that is unconditional and perfect. It's not easy. Love is much bigger than getting fit. Love, or in other words the Divine, wants us, and the way to get more of us is through love.

In spiritual traditions, seekers, aspirants or monks practice discipline to rid their lives of anything which separates them from the Divine, to have an ever-closer relationship. It is an arduous grind, characterized by asceticism. Loving the Divine through longing and devotion prevents anything coming between themselves and the One they seek. For their hard work, and some grace, they are rewarded intimacy with the Divine.

For those of us who are not consciously following a spiritual tradition, the love we practice serves us similarly. By making effort to love more deeply, to love more kindly, more patiently and to stay with our loved one through adversity and dissatisfaction, we are perfecting our love which results in being ever near to love, which is none other than the One who is the love: the Divine. All along we didn't realize that by being attracted to our partner we were being called to travel the path of love towards a closer relationship with life. Our love relationships are the discipline and practice that grinds us and perfects us so that we get closer to pure love, closer to the Divine. It is hard work; no easier than the ascetic or monk, but nothing is easy that has real value.

Blame:
among the best ways
to not solve a problem.

7-24. When Love is Troubled

There are those difficult times when partners don't get along and emotional disconnection grows. Frustration and hopelessness build when, instead of greater closeness, the efforts of both partners produce only disappointment. During such times can the love and the relationship survive? Relationship experts and conventional wisdom instruct us that we shouldn't try to change our partner, but within real relationships, partners *always* try to change each other. Our relationships are nature's pathway through which partners are strongly encouraged to change and, preferably, grow. Most of us desire a strong partner. Universally a partner will seek to transform the other's weaknesses, the cause of diminished attraction, inconvenience, or pain. So what happens when the other steadfastly refuses to be influenced? Pressure builds between partners. It isn't pretty.

Living between a rock and a hard place is uncomfortable. Within the silent desperation of so many lovers' are deep cries for love, growth and strength. In that deepest place inside all of us, we are aware of a lover who is perfect. By comparison, our flesh and blood partner fails to match up. What is one to do? If tension grows unabated within a relationship, the emotional well-being of the partners will deteriorate.

Satisfied partners believe that what they get from a relationship should be equal to or more than what they put in, otherwise it doesn't feel like a good deal. Being loved, belonging in a partnership and being nourished by another are all soothing to one's self-esteem. If a relationship's environment is emotionally toxic, a partner's self-esteem will probably fall to unhealthy levels. Most lovers are strongly motivated to make their relationship habitable, passionate and vital. Repeated unsuccessful attempts at fixing it place him or her in a bind characterized by powerlessness and undesirable options. "Should I give more or should I end it? Can I produce the changes I desire?" These are difficult questions when years of togetherness, kids, a house, and finances are all on the line.

The bird of love needs two "wings of loving" to fly. The first wing is being true to oneself; this is where love starts. The second wing is giving of oneself so as to love the partner and build a connection of love. When placed in a bind by a troubled relationship, the partner will emotionally swing between these two opposing good values. He or she will act out of self-interest at some times, but act very differently when living out of the value of giving love. To others, the swinging between these poles can seem irrational, disturbing, and similar to the symptoms of bi-polar disorder. To the partner this emotional ebb and flow can feel internally like craziness but represents the internal struggle about which direction to go in order to get important relational needs met.

When attempting to be true to themselves the partner's actions will be influenced by an internal dialogue that goes something like this: "I am tired of feeling hurt and disappointed. I am sure that my partner can do better than this, and if he/she cannot, I am certain that there is another person who will love me in a way that will be satisfying. How is it that my partner cannot see that loving me in a way that is fulfilling is not an unreasonable request? It makes me so frustrated and infuriated."

Conversely when "giving of oneself", the partner's actions will be expressed in accordance with this kind of internal dialogue: "While I am aware of my own frustration and unhappiness, I'm certain that my partner does not intentionally disappoint me; he/she is essentially a good person. Perhaps if I just love him/her more fully and completely, then it will all work out. Perhaps I am not patient or giving enough and by improving myself so that my partner is more deeply loved, our relationship will improve. I'll try that and maybe our relationship will be more satisfying."

Actions generated by each of these sides will produce behaviors and emotions that are quite different. An unhappy or frustrated partner will switch between these two sides, causing them to appear inconsistent, unstable and highly confused.

Einstein said that a problem cannot be solved by the thinking produced on the same level at which the problem was originally generated. A problem can only be solved from a higher level. Within the troubled relationship, this means one or both partners may *grow* out of the problem, through strengthening of love and acceptance. If accomplished, the relationship survives and flourishes. Without growth, partners risk remaining together while stuck in an unhealthy relationship characterized by anger, resentment and depression. The last alternative is that the relationship ends.

> Focus on positive solutions instead of negative problems.

7-25. Simultaneity

Simultaneity. This is a word that I have recently made up to describe the perfect conditions within a couple to produce or reproduce that delicious feeling many couples had in the beginning of their relationship. It's simple and goes like this: when each partner is successfully loving the other, and the effort and success is mutual and simultaneous, a magic of passion and loving connection results. For this to occur, the loving effort of each partner must be effective at causing the other partner to feel loved, which means it must be sensitive to, and tailored specifically for the partner. If both partners do this at the same time, something really special happens, in the form of the kind of loving bond we all crave.

Think of two people dancing a traditional dance. The movements of each dancer are synchronized with the movements of the other. If the movements are well executed and synchronized with sensitivity to the other, the dance manifests the magic of beauty, in which emotion or a story may be told. But for this to happen, the dancers' movements needn't be precise.

In a love relationship, the efforts of the partners, too, need to be correct and appropriate to produce the best result, a building bond of love. As individual as a fingerprint, each one of us has a unique way of being loved. If our partner loves us in just this way, we are easily and fully nourished.

The trick to benefitting from the reality of simultaneity is that *both* partners need to be making effective efforts at the *same* time. If only one partner listens to the other and offers love in the way that meets the other's need, while the second partner is less giving and less effective at it, the cycle is prone to deterioration.

When partners first meet and find the attraction mutual, both partners are highly receptive, excited and motivated to give generously. At this stage, the experience of each new partner has the love flowing. Later in a relationship, after the friction of differences and the stress of daily life has had a chance to dampen the partners' enthusiasm, re-energizing this cycle of love takes more effort, but has a greater potential for each partner's growth.

Sex, too, may be accurately viewed as a cycle where simultaneous effort has the ability to energize a relationship and generate the flow of love between partners. Sex is one method of giving love that can help to repair a damaged relationship. However, it may be a smaller eddy in the river of love. Sexually, if partners are loving each other's bodies with the same effective attention to the other's pleasure and satisfaction, then connection, satisfaction and love may be generated.

The influences between partners are cyclical, thus it is very difficult to isolate the contribution of each partner. Within the relationship, when frustrated and troubled, partners may be unable to determine to what degree he or she contributes to relationship troubles. Which came first, the chicken or the egg? Typically each partner believes that the other is responsible for the majority of the relationship troubles.

> Care about people's approval and you will always be their prisoner.
>
> — *Lao Tzu*

7-26. Love's Expiration Date

"When did these problems begin?" is one of the questions I ask many couples at the start of couples' counseling. The average answer falls into the range of five to ten years; a long time to needlessly be in pain. If the couple has informed me that I am their last hope before contacting a divorce lawyer, I then ask, "Why did you wait so long to try to fix these problems?" For this, most patients have no good answer. There are those unfortunate brokenhearted souls for whom the work on their marriage is simply too late. For these people, the damage done by neglect, by lack of consideration, selfishness, or even meanness has completely drained the goodwill from their romantic connection. By nature, people are hesitant to invite a stranger into the most intimate relationship of their lives. In all too many cases, their hesitancy to seek help proves fatal, ending in divorce or breakup.

The test is quick. Ask yourselves these questions; "Is this the best my relationship can be?" and "Am I or is my partner capable of loving more deeply?"

Where is the invisible and hard-to-detect line that separates secure territory from that dark area in which lovers are no longer connected? It is invisible and is often crossed without a lover's knowledge. Further into that darkness exists a different line demarcating where the damage becomes permanent. Once that line is passed, the relationship grows increasingly vulnerable to affairs, conflicts, and emotional distance. Even little problems, if unaddressed for long periods of time, will cause toxic resentment to accumulate.

A lover's heart becomes fragile if denied the nourishment that loving acts provide. A car's battery, if drained too many times, can no longer be recharged. The heart is similar, if depleted of love; it, too, cannot be refilled. Some relationship problems are not easily fixed without a third party to provide guidance and objectivity. Relationship problems, if not fixed, will permanently contaminate togetherness. Please don't wait until it is too late. If there are problems in your relationship, the sooner you seek help, the sooner you can have a healthy and satisfying love. Otherwise, without you knowing it, love's expiration date may have passed.

> Know your partner
> better than you know
> your assumptions.

7-27. Does He or She Deserve Love?

We give love, in the manner that the other needs to receive it, because of the kind of person we are, because it honors us; it is really the method to gain the best relationship with ourselves. Being a loving person is not about others, but about being the best we can be. Giving love, therefore, is not about whether the partner deserves it or has earned it, but is about the measure of ourselves.

The efforts our partner receives from us largely depend upon how we are feeling. For instance, if we are angry or resentful, most likely we will withhold our best. Yet love is unconditional and not based upon circumstances. Emotions may function like antennas, which communicate to us when conditions are safe or right for openness and giving. Emotions inform us when it is right to be loving or more defended, or even punitive.

Yet it is these very same feelings that are strongly influenced by our past, especially when provoked by the intensity of a love relationship. If we could be fully in the present, free of past events, it would be much easier for our love to flow. When we are upset or unhappy due to partners' actions, our choices may reflect an attitude that the partner does not deserve our love at that time. So when does our partner deserve love?

During tense times, love is what is needed most to repair and improve the uncomfortable relationship situation. Isn't it true that a partner who feels loved is a partner who is most motivated to be loving towards us?

Consider the relationship between a parent and their child. There is no doubt that children can be challenging because they seem to intuitively know all the parents' "buttons." Parents become angry with their children, but the question of whether or not the parent has love for the child does not arise. Questions of whether or not the child deserves love also do not arise in the same way as they do with a partner.

The ideal is unconditional love, a situation that seems disappointingly elusive, especially in love relationships. Unconditional love normally seems to be present between a mother and her child. Pet owners fall deeply into despair after the death of their pet because that bond has an unconditional quality about it.

But within the love connection, the relationship provokes the surfacing of all our unfinished childhood business, injecting serious complications in the union. Without thought or hesitation, the moment our partner hurts us or has failed to meet our needs, the tendency is to withhold our love. This risks a cycle of punitive withholding between partners, which fosters an escalation of mutual dissatisfaction.

The partner is the special person we chose. In making that choice, was it our intention to love our partner in a part-time, intermittent fashion? To love the partner only when we feel that he or she deserves it instills a conditional nature to love which dries up stability and trust within the partnership.

7-28. Better Loving Through Chemistry

The couple reminisce about the moment their eyes first met. There was a spark. Upon learning that the attraction was mutual, both grew excited that they were part of a togetherness. One happily describes it as a "click" and the other, flush with warm remembrance, recalls feeling a strong chemistry between them. Their deep synchronicity felt magical. Thereafter, sex was frequent, passionate and fun; relating to each other was natural, easy and effortless.

The concept of chemistry, in love relationships, not science, is spoken of often when partners grieve the loss of relationship satisfaction. It is a special bond in which connection is deep and harmonious. When chemistry is present, relating is simple. It features as an important determining factor when choosing a partner. When chemistry is gone, however, partners are mystified as to why it is so difficult to recapture, when most lovers painfully long to feel it again.

Chemistry happens when our deeper part, our souls, are involved in loving. When both partners give this pure, nourishing love simultaneously, the magic of chemistry spontaneously erupts in a golden cloud that blissfully envelopes both partners. In this delicious state, partners are soul mates.

Despite the way the term is customarily used, the condition of being "soul mates" only has the potential to become a permanent condition. It is almost always a temporary state which, disappointingly, cannot be maintained. Each partner is a potential soul mate if deep simultaneous love is ceaselessly given. Wonderful chemistry is effortless in the beginning of a relationship, before the foibles of partner personalities exert their influence and bring the couple "back down to earth." Friendships are relationships with a lesser chemistry, which is easier to maintain because the emotional intimacy is shallower than in romantic relationships.

What makes it so hard to keep this chemistry alive in long-term relationships? When not living out of the deep soul, a partner's emotional wounds and limitations strongly and negatively grip behavior and experience. Old unresolved emotions interfere with freely giving or receiving love. Over time, hurt and disappointment cause toxic emotion to accumulate like snow in a blizzard. The vulnerability demanded by love causes most partners to synchronize in a dance of distancing and self-protection, instead of connection. A common pattern is for partners to swap blame for this disconnected condition, accelerating the journey away from deep connection.

A united chorus of disappointed partners complain about disconnection; "There just isn't any chemistry," they cry. The meaning of these words does not just speak of a temporary loss, but a belief that this is a permanent condition. In other words, the current partner is the wrong partner, and was a poor choice from the beginning.

Yes, when the chemistry is absent, a relationship is troubled, but just as chemistry was present and has gone, this disconnected state, too, is capable of being changed. Because of gravity, falling down is easier than climbing up. Similarly, it is easier to lose chemistry than it is to rebuild it. When gone, it feels, undoubtedly, like it can never be regained.

Yet chemistry is not some kind of magic that suddenly appears; it is deep within us all the time and can be revived, but to succeed, partners must dive deeply below the limitations of personality. The chemistry you crave is available the moment you and your partner use your strength and courage to mutually offer deep love.

7-29. A Thing Called Love

Beth admits calling her husband, Steve, a slew of demeaning and disrespectful names. In spite of her behavior, she says she loves him. Rick describes his latest passive-aggressive action: taking Lauren's car when she needed it. He refers to it as payback for Lauren divulging details of his sexual inadequacies to her best friend. Even though he sometimes hurts her, he says he loves her.

If Beth and Rick are serious about their feelings, then love is a very strange phenomenon indeed. Rather than strengthening and nourishing each other, these two behave more like two NFL football teams trying to pulverize each other at a Sunday afternoon football game. Their competitive, hurtful tendencies unfortunately characterize the mannerisms of many couples in love relationships. The divorce rate bears out the sad truth that people are not all that good at loving.

But what is it about love that is so hard? Love demands a multitude of strengths that most people do not possess, or have not yet developed. Many partners do not have the ability to control their angry impulses, and blindly and destructively hurling anger does little to warm the heart or encourage closeness. Love insists that partners and spouses learn not to hurt each other. Each can do a little good for their relationship until each learns to do little harm. This is the essential truth about love relationships, and is also their purpose. I see love relationships as a laboratory in which partners can learn to grow and love if they have sufficient will to do so, as the saying goes: "Change is constant, but growth is a choice."

Love requires that partners be willing to be open, so that a connection between them can be forged. This is the challenge of intimacy. It requires great strength to juggle the vulnerability of openness with the availability of closeness. To be seen clearly and closely by a partner, with all their flaws and weaknesses, is chilling to some and causes others to run away or to attack, pushing the lover away for safety. In doing so, insecure lovers prevent love from happening.

Many lovers confuse power and control with love. Too many couples remain locked in power struggles and control battles for years, mistakenly believing that their duel of domination is the connection of love. Forcing our partner to bend to fit our world does not encourage an open heart. Love is not about power. Love is simple; it is all that allows us to grow, to be stronger, to connect, and to merge.

> We must be less
> hurtful, but also
> be less easily hurt.

7-30. Loving Yourself

If you desire passion in your long-term love relationship, be aware that it all starts with yourself. The truth that we cannot fully love another if we don’t first love ourselves is often spoken, but not often described in detail. When it comes to intimacy, especially sexual intimacy, if we do not believe deep down that we are good and valuable then we will not be comfortable letting another person experience us deeply.

What does it mean to love yourself? How do you begin? Within our minds and thoughts, there exists an inner conversation that consist of two parts: one part speaks and the other part listens. It is the quality of the relationship between these two parts that determines our level of self-esteem. Each person is called an individual, meaning "not-dividable," but self-esteem points to inner divisions of “me” and “myself.”

The process of loving yourself results in these separate parts becoming more unified and integrated. Love melts away divisions and separateness. If your relationship with yourself is a positive one, you will possess good self-esteem or confidence, whereas in an inner conversation full of negativity, doubt, criticism, hurtfulness, and harsh language, your self-esteem level will be low. This also translates to a lack of love for oneself, which is the root cause of most relationship and sexual problems.

Improvement requires that positive and loving changes, also called growth, be made. If we alter our inner conversation so it possesses love and qualities such as kindness, patience, generosity, and encouragement, our inner relationship will be improved. If we change our choices so that our actions only express kindness and helpfulness and avoid hurtfulness, this too, will slowly improve the inner relationship. Our emotions are like a record of our history, but refusing to allow negative emotions to influence our choices will lead to improvement.

Poor self-regard may show up as a cycle of having a chronically harsh and disapproving inner attitude towards yourself, for example, inwardly berating yourself for mistakes. Being kinder and going easier on yourself is the fix for this problem. Others who go too easy on themselves by falling into a pattern of being lazy or irresponsible will instead benefit from the discipline of holding themselves more accountable. This wide range of response shows that creating positive self-esteem must be sensitive to balance; strong but not brutal and loving but not spoiling.

Feeling good about yourself contributes greatly to the development of effective self-regulation, an essential ingredient in personal success and loving. Coping successfully with intense emotion, by avoiding shutting down, and eschewing self-destructive and impulsive expression, will create the possibility of always putting yourself in a good position. Self-regulation becomes achievable when your internal relationship is self-compassionate, moderated by positive, supportive and accepting inner attitudes.

It is a universal truth that each one of us wants to be loved.

Being loved by another is only likely when we demand it first of ourselves. Only then we are we able to identify and choose another who is truly capable of loving. Other methods for increasing the love you have for yourself include: practicing assertiveness as a way of being true to yourself, avoiding hurting others, being strong and setting firm but balanced limits on your choices, learning from your mistakes and not repeating them, creating a satisfying and mess-free life, and making choices that cause you to grow. By loving yourself and living a good life, you have the greatest potential to be passionate and sexy from within.

Loving yourself doesn't mean liking everything about yourself. It is not about being perfect or flawless; it is about accepting yourself fully, human as you are. Love yourself by gradually cleaning the physical and emotional space you rent for a lifetime of all negativity, hate and darkness. Love, directed towards yourself, functions as the inner broom, mop and cleaning rag, making an inner space of peace, stillness, and love possible. You are the instrument through which you love. If you are not well tuned, the loving music you create will not be beautiful. Loving yourself is tuning the instrument so you may make life and relationships like a beautiful song.

7-31. Jealousy: Poisoned Love

Jealousy poisons many relationships while partners are searching for love's closeness. The jealous lover is gripped by chronic, irrational and unreasonable fears of future rejection and wounding. For the jealous lover there is never enough love from themselves or their partner; no control is enough to ensure safety from harm and insecurity. Even in the warm arms of love, the jealous lover can find no relief.

The source of jealousy is strongly related to its emotional cousins: fear, envy and insecurity. It develops out of feeling that one is inadequate: not powerful, beautiful or good enough. Jealous lovers, believing that they do not deserve love, fear certain rejection. Some come to be jealous through deprivation and others through injury, such as betrayal, in which trust has been damaged. Other lovers, who already have a propensity for fear, are malnourished in their relationship with a partner who loves poorly by offering insufficient affection, openness, or dependability, while the insecure are sure that past harm justifies the fear that they will be hurt again. In all cases, jealousy springs from the pain of unhealed past wounds that are repeatedly re-injured, provoking anger and acts of retribution. Regardless of its source, jealousy is a toxic emotion that defies easy solutions. Partners of a jealous mate grow quickly frustrated and react to their unreasonable demands in ways which may validate already intense insecurity. Trying to make an insecure partner feel loved rarely meets with success.

Jealous partners have difficulty trusting. Doubting their own worth and value, a jealous partner questions the sincerity of the others' love. When efforts to build trust are met with consistent suspicion and distrust, it is often, naturally, taken personally by the partner. The non-verbal accusations of untrustworthiness can seem incessant, and a partner who behaves deceptively, sometimes out of self-preservation, only solidifies and further validates the jealous partner's distorted emotional truth.

Distrust is like a deep well with slick, unscalable walls and a strong gravitational pull; any information offered is sucked into the well, trapped within, and provides no means of escape. Distrust spawns suspiciousness until any defensive explanation is viewed distrustfully by an insecure partner and is rendered suspect. Trustworthy partners find themselves defenseless against their jealous partner's irrational suspicion. Proving that the hurtful non-event a jealous parter imagines did not happen is an impossible task.

A suspicious mind functions like a detective. Questions are asked with obvious pre-formed doubt about any answer's truthfulness, so partners grow wary of, and seek to avoid, probing questions, knowing painfully well that they precede sessions of "20 questions." With the skill and tenacity of an interrogator, jealous partners will grill the other for information while accusing them, often without proof, of hurtful actions.

The fear and discomfort of jealousy are manifested by

repetitious worry-based thoughts that anticipate painful and catastrophic future events. These worries link in a cycle which builds momentum, forming itself into an obsession; a pattern of thought which the jealous individual feels powerless to slow or prevent. Fear has control of the jealous person, not the other way around.

In attempts to reduce fear and increase comfort, a jealous partner attempts to control his or her environment so as to decrease risk and increase safety from harm, this includes controlling the partner. If a couple is healing from infidelity or other harmful crisis, increasing control by an injured partner is appropriate to achieve healing and relationship stability. But if no recent betrayal has occurred, a jealousy-prone partner's chronic need to be in control, for safety and reassurance, incessantly violates the other's boundaries. Emotionally caging the partner is an attempt to prevent any risk of flight or attraction to another. Despite jealousy's attempt at control, the strategy backfires; the caged partner grows more distant and disconnected, less attracted, and wishes to flee confinement.

Jealousy and insecurity form a self-validating cycle; the greater the distrust, the more the distrustful partner will find justification for their suspicions. Insecurities defy easy change unless the root feeling of personal inadequacy is healed, which is a long-term task. Short of that, some behavioral efforts may soothe jealousy-based relationship problems. Rules similar to those that guide the introduction of evidence into a court of law are helpful to reduce the toxic power of suspicion. This is performed by the jealous partner using strength to reject suspicion if no solid, direct proof exists, and then by offering their partner the benefit of the doubt. Such discipline prevents the inflation of suspicion when it becomes married with imagination. Hearsay, or indirect communication from another, others' opinions, assumptions, and general interpretations must be rejected as unworthy evidence. By assuming a partner is innocent unless direct proof confirms his or her guilt, the build-up of poisonous contamination is prevented.

Additional practices may loosen jealousy's grip if sufficient emotional strength is used. A non-jealous partner can reduce the other's suspicion by practicing generous sharing of information and complete openness. Avoid violating a partner's privacy by snooping...evidence obtained this way injures and is tainted; it is sure to cause a nasty, difficult-to-resolve conflict. Use strength to resist the investigative obsessions of social media tracking and hunting. Asking for reassurance is more constructive than throwing hurtful accusations. Jealousy is poisonous. Love is not built from fear.

INFIDELITY

8-1. When Love is Given to Another

Affairs and cheating have eternally been a dark feature of the romantic landscape. In a perfect world, love would be shared consistently between faithful partners, but the world is not perfect. Casual talk of affairs neglects the extremes of soul-wrenching devastation felt by injured partners and the soul-uplifting bliss of new-found love felt by unfaithful partners. With the widespread relaxation of ethics and morals, affairs share a similar air of a romantic right-of-passage to the now-common divorce; both are indicative of insufficient partner strength to maintain a commitment.

After an affair has been revealed, an intense drama follows, which includes permanent, traumatic wounds to the injured partner and inward conflict including feelings of guilt, shame and loss in the unfaithful partner. Couples who are in the throes of the fallout will assign blame, renegotiate their relationship contract, and perhaps attempt to heal. They will endure storm after storm during the insecure journey of uncertainty. Healing and repair can be tortuously slow. Couples repeatedly face the possibility of dissolution during their crisis of truth. Whether the affair was purely emotional or became sexual, the pain of its wounding is just as sharp.

Many lovers warn the other early in the relationship that should the other cheat the relationship is finished; real-life circumstances cause a majority of injured partners to deviate by choosing the route of forgiveness instead. The quest to resurrect love amid the scars and wreckage is marked with predictable and painful milestones. Successful couples are rewarded with a healed relationship that may be stronger than before, with a renewed passion; an outcome that never justifies the infidelity.

The unfaithful partner has a responsibility to right the wrong, demonstrate sorrow, and pay the injured partner emotional compensation for the pain and injury caused. Sorrow must be expressed in a thousand ways and a thousand times, accomplished by simply loving sincerely once again. Reassuring the other that they are important through the practice of honesty, transparency, and care heals the partner and the relationship. The purer the love given by the unfaithful partner, the faster healing will occur. But rarely is the situation that simple. The burden is on the unfaithful partner to prove honesty and love so as to erase the strong negative message conveyed by the affair that the partner is neither loved nor good enough.

Affairs are typically experienced by unfaithful partners as intensely pleasurable and exciting. Affairs do not feel wrong; the heights of love feel like a birthright. A truth is that it is rarely wrong to love another, but simultaneously it is rarely right to hurt another. The unfaithful partner may be confused between contrary feelings. He or she may feel sorry and guilty for the deceit, but also experience grief at losing a passionate love, which was shared with the affair partner. Compassion and love for the injured partner conflict with anger and dissatisfaction from the unresolved relationship problems which pre-existed the affair. Having so much internal confusion, unfaithful partners may be hesitant to step up the loving and healing efforts, and their ongoing pain makes them impatient with slow progress of healing. Eager for release from probationary restrictions, they are tempted to express without compassion that the injured partner should "just get over it."

Wounded partners live with excruciating pain. The revelation of an affair rocks their world, putting into question all that was previously known and certain. They may suffer a profound and traumatic loss of self, in which rage, desperation and insanity may be mixed. Cycling through these moods can feel and seem crazy. Whether to fix the relationship or end it is a big question, as is whether or not the injured partner would be a fool to repair it. What felt like a secure floor has been pulled out from under them. Desperate to make sense of it and feel in control, an injured partner asks hundreds of detective-like questions to investigate the infidelity. Each question exposes the unfaithful partner to wave after wave of guilt and shame. Flare-ups of pain triggered by sometimes innocent situations can return the couple to ground zero.

An injured partner's anger is fully justified, but if it is chronically and repeatedly expressed in order to punish, the progress of healing will halt and may backslide. Couples who get out of the blame game and escape from the victim/criminal mentality possess a better chance of healing. The injured partner's difficult task is to allow the other to re-earn their trust and cooperate with the healing, a process that doesn't feel fair. Meanwhile, the unfaithful partner must unequivocally return to the loving track. As pain subsides, couples may begin to explore what went wrong that initially made the relationship vulnerable. Repairs are only achieved by loving in all its infinite varieties.

> Loving another is rarely wrong, but more importantly hurting another is rarely right.

8-2. Protecting the Faithfulness

Words are insufficient to express the enormous pain a partner feels when betrayed. Yet for an unfaithful partner or spouse, forming a new romantic connection is exciting, blissful and effortless. For a relationship attempting to heal from an infidelity crisis, it is anything but. Ask any lover who has been through it, and they will say that the best choice is to make the ongoing relationship or marriage strong and satisfying so an affair never happens.

Affair prevention is little different than effectively loving with all the fullness of the heart. A partner or spouse who is fully satisfied, whose heart is full of the love of the romantic partner is least likely to be interested in another. The need to have a loving connection is so powerful that even a highly moral person will violate his or her own values to fulfill their need for a loving connection. To protect an unfaithful connection, a cheating partner will act covertly and with unabashed deceit.

An affair is an emotional relationship, physical relationship, or behavior that violates the commitment to uphold mutual well-being and non-harm. The presence of harm to an injured partner is the factor that determines whether a behavior or connection to another is unfaithful, not whether it is sexual nor whether the connection was live or virtual. Most affairs are not planned, but occur when an opportunity arises for two people to be together and discover a mutual attraction and understanding, often an understanding that loneliness and relationship dissatisfaction are also mutual.

Is it any surprise that in a majority of relationships damaged by cheating, the love connection is dissatisfying for one or both of the partners? Love relationships by nature are intensely challenging. Great effort is necessary to solve problems that interfere with satisfaction. Unsolved problems, resentment and frustration accumulate to kill goodwill and the "loving feeling." Accumulated hurts and resentment render a romantic union vulnerable to the potential excitement that new love offers. In so many instances of betrayal, both partners are responsible for damaging the relationship and making it vulnerable, even if it is only the unfaithful partner is responsible for the choice to cheat. Partners who are most afraid of betrayal, either due to insecurity or past unfaithfulness, actually increase the risk of cheating when living out their fear by acting in controlling and distrusting ways.

Partner needs tend not to remain unmet for long, and a dissatisfied partner is one whose needs are not met. He or she will crave, even obsess, about obtaining a satisfying love connection, to the point where relationship tension will build and conflict may be provoked. Needs such as food, clothing and shelter, if missing, will result in death, whereas a partner need, if missing, will prevent a man or woman from being a good enough husband, wife, provider, nurturer or lover, and risk relationship death. In cheating, many partners experience the infidelity as a way of negotiating with the impossible, and even attempting to save the primary relationship. They fulfill unmet needs to maintain their relationship role, as immoral as that choice may seem. This is not dissimilar to the way a starving person justifies stealing food to survive. Put a person in a bind between needs and morals, and needs usually win.

The best solution is found through increasing partner strength...in growing, making changes and in loving. Strong partners express their needs while minimizing hurtfulness. Strong partners adjust quickly, are willing to grow, and are open to taking unmet needs seriously. Can the risk of infidelity be reduced to zero? Sadly the answer is no, but for romantic partners who are strong teammates, friends and lovers, the risk is very low. A heart that is not full will seek fullness. A heart that is full with the love of a devoted partner has little room for another.

8-3. Repairing Trust

Trust is an essential relationship ingredient, yet it is fragile; once damaged, trust neither heals quickly nor is easily repaired. The very task of repairing and restoring trust between romantic partners frustrates many who try. Re-earning and repairing trust can seem like an impossible obstacle course.

Whether trust is damaged by mistake, unfortunate coincidences or unrestrained impulses, the ability to repair it may very well determine a relationship's survival. The process of repairing trust must include growth. In addition to an apology, behavior change needs to be included for repair to be sincere and effective.

Distrust is similar to a pool of quicksand; once something enters the pool, such as information, a situation or a person, it is not likely to escape. Once within its grasp, everything gets darkly labeled as untrustworthy. Some partners have difficulty trusting, a condition which pre-existed their relationship, due to prior abuse, traumas, deceptions and betrayals. A trustworthy partner is quick to take lack of trust personally, but more common is a partner who made selfish mis-steps and wishes to escape the dungeon of damaged trust.

The process of re-earning trust varies depending upon the cause and severity of the damaged trust, from a minor failure of dependability or a small lie, all the way up to a large lie or an affair, covert chronic gambling or drug use. Each violation demands a proportionate response of compassion, apology, growing changes, openness, honesty and transparency. The discovery of covert behaviors may be traumatizing to an unsuspecting partner, while repair may seem daunting for a partner who has fallen too deep into a hole.

The impotency of words makes re-earning trust difficult. When within the shadow of distrust, words carry no value. Debating the details of past ethical violations is a harmful, ineffective use of words. Compassion for the pain caused is loving, and is the only kind of effort that really matters.

An untrusted partner will have to endure much discomfort to succeed at repairing trust. An angry, injured partner may express pain-filled accusatory words and be actively punitive, feeling that punishment is deserved, even though it interferes with healing; investigating obsessively and cross-examining the violator like a prosecutor are common. Distrust and fear produce a kind of blindness which can feel dangerously out of control. Without clear facts, the injured partner's pain combines with their suspicion and imagination into a toxic cocktail resulting in catastrophic speculations.

When trust is low, interactions may seem to feel more like the relationship between a probation officer and a probationer than between lovers. It is the burden of the untrusted partner to re-earn trust by humbly accepting restrictions and reduced freedom, if he or she wishes to succeed. Untrusted partners who succeed at making the issues "just go away" end up with a zombie relationship; they keep the relationship, but without the partner's heart. Openness, honesty and transparency generate good will and may be offered in many forms, including accepting cell-phone tracking, discontinuation of any text message and call log deleting, giving the injured partner advance notice of choices, associations and whereabouts. Video calls may be used to prove location. The generous sharing of information allows an untrusting partner to determine the consistency and congruency of the truth. For protection from specious accusations, untrusted partners may diligently maintain a daily journal, which can be helpful to resolve disputes about past events.

Time supports healing and is a friend to an untrusted partner, but only if no new hurtful incidents occur. Lost freedoms will gradually be restored if handled well. Importantly, openness, honesty and transparency will have to be continued as part of the healed relationship; it's what real friends do for each other.

COMMUNICATION

9-1. Do You Understand?

Couples who argue often are steeped in mutual misunderstanding. Partners who are emotionally disconnected don't truly hear each other, so it can feel impossible to get the most important person in your life to listen to you well. Getting better at listening, hearing, and understanding is vital to make relationships more satisfying, and partners who successfully maintain passion and closeness have a high degree of mutual understanding which creates a stronger connection.

After a verbal exchange, many partners assume an understanding has been created without testing if it is so. Later, upon learning that in fact a misunderstanding has occurred, the missed opportunities, failed encounters, unnecessary pain, and wasted time are common precipitants of anger and conflict. Repeated frequently over time, miscommunications accumulate, and the partners experience a widening disconnection and the feeling that they are not a good team.

There are numerous obstacles to understanding. Meanings are often made unclear and vague by poor or inexact choice of words, while a partner with a busy mind may be distracted by his or her own thoughts and may only partially receive the other's communication. During tense moments, such as during conflict, partners' attempts to listen or hear are complicated by the discomfort of anxiety, fear, and stress. Such emotions are stimuli which compete for the listeners' attention. In relationships where conflict is common, over time partners grow emotionally defensive and thus are only partially receptive, which is like trying to communicate through a brick wall. Quick-minded people tend to compose their responses before the other is finished speaking, as a result of which the speaker's final thoughts are never received, and some partners possess the poor habit of interrupting one another. Angry partners tend not to listen to the other as a way of passive-aggressively negating them. Understanding is simple to achieve, but simplicity is not always easy to achieve.

Being understood can make us feel like our partner "gets us;" we are part of a togetherness. Hearing and listening are vital skills in the quest to create understanding, but are not the only elements. In any communication, most of the intended meaning comes not from the words, but the attention-worthy emotion expressed in non-verbal ways. Attitude, tone, pace, intensity and volume of speech, and body movements all combine to add substantial meaning on top of the words expressed. These non-verbal elements may convey more meaning than the words themselves. Too often couples fail to create the proper conditions to maximize the potential for understanding. Poor word choice by the speaking partner is a limitation that excellent listening will not overcome. If words are hurtful, a partner is not likely to hear the message well, as they will focus their attention instead on defending him or herself. Communication, in general, is inexact at best, but if used skillfully, words may bridge partners' separateness. Words alone, however, will never allow us to fully share our direct experience. If expressed and received well, effective, rounded communication can allow two individuals to become one couple.

The "communication loop" utilized by police and the military maximizes the likelihood that understanding will be achieved, especially during "mission critical" events when coordinating in unison is vital and when misunderstanding can be fatal. At first seemingly clumsy and slow, the communication loop is quite efficient when compared to speedier communication which produces inefficient misunderstandings. In a communication loop, after the first partner speaks, the listening partner repeats back what was expressed. The speaker then confirms or corrects what was received. If he or she offers a correction, the listener repeats back the corrected version. Finally, the speaker verifies that the listener received the communication and the meaning properly. Only after the speaking partner's expression has been verified does the listening partner have a turn in the speaking partner role. The communication loop intentionally slows down the process of talking so that each step may happen carefully, deliberately, and successfully. Lazy communication frequently results in a misunderstanding when loops of speaking, listening and understanding are orphaned.

In addition to hearing and listening, receptivity and openness are also required for understanding. When we are open, awareness of ourselves is suspended; we become an open space in which our attention is fully focused upon receiving our partner's message. If we are attending to ourselves, we have failed to open a space and are preoccupied, hence a communication cannot be received and understanding will not occur. When we open ourselves to receive another's message, we are giving ourselves, our time and attention, as a loving gift to the other. Under-standing is joining to another, via a loving act of receiving. By receiving our partner, we offer the potential to build a bond and connection. The more understanding is achieved, the greater and deeper a bond between loving partners will be.

> We can often do more for others by trying to correct our own faults than by trying to correct theirs.
>
> *-François Fenelon*

9-2. Here Comes the Judge

Keeping a romantic bond close and positive is hard. With the rigors of daily stresses and partner differences, a satisfying connection gets tested constantly. How partners define a good-enough bond varies with each individual. While the human need to couple up is universal, nearly equal to it is the fear of getting too close. Opening up to another comes with risks that threaten individuality and personal adequacy. Pushing a partner away hurts those partners who prefer greater closeness, but fearful partners who are uncomfortable with too much closeness use many distancing techniques to ensure self-protection.

Judgement is one common method. It is an intellectually-based defensive strategy. Sometimes subtle, other times obvious, judgement often goes undetected as a hurtful distancing mechanism. Why does the use of judgement rarely get identified as a defensive tactic? Because once judgement is expressed, the recipient's intellectual faculties are engaged, effectively pulling his or her attention away from feelings. The partner is distracted when the pushing away occurs.

As an intellectual ability, judgement is very useful in the right situations, but it is destructive if misapplied or used in the wrong situations. When used within non-emotional, non-relationship settings such as problem-solving, judgement is essential and positive; it does no harm. But within love relationships, where maintaining a positive warm bond is characteristic of a couple's success, judgement severs the bond. Judgement is an evaluation regarding value, worthiness, or goodness. Yet from the perspective of love, our being can only be worthy. To be judged diminishes our worth. The list of intellectual gymnastic feats that make up judgement-based processes is lengthy, including a focus on accuracy, insistence on being reasonable, rationalization, deflection, criticism, comparing, and negating, to name a few. When utilized deftly, these practices take the focus of a connection away from the experiential and emotional.

When partner experience is shared and understood, the connection is strengthened, but the many forms of judgement challenge this personal experience and call into question its validity. Judgemental people frequently employ a "reasonable test" by which ideas, perspectives, and others are evaluated to determine if acceptance or rejection will be offered. Another form of judging is an insistence on accuracy instead of understanding. Judgement typically includes some form of negativity, yet no amount of negativity will produce a positive relationship. Judgement trumpets the intellect as a superior method and it rejects the value of the emotional process, but it is through the heart and emotions that couples build a bond and relate. Intellect does not love. By responding with judgement instead of compassionately receiving a partner's internal, emotional experience, an opportunity is missed to build connection. Judgement brings the head, but closes the heart.

Judgement, and intellectual exercises in general, temporarily provide self-protection from painful feelings. Placing our awareness in the head, the location of our thinking, allows us to flee from the physical location of our feelings, lower in the body; thus judging creates distance from the discomfort we feel when facing something that is unappealing, unattractive, threatening, or distasteful. But more than that, when judging others and their opinions and ideas, the "judge" always places him or herself in the higher, "safer" position, effectively lowering the other, so that a soothing fantasy of being elevated, of being higher or better than others is created. Two lovers can only connect when they live together on the same level.

Judgement reduces a person from a complete being to a quality or characteristic, evaluated and determined as worthy of acceptance or rejection. It hurts. On the surface, it appears to be intelligent, but dig a little deeper and its real motivation, an attempt to avoid closeness and discomfort, is uncovered. In the end, judgement is ineffective as a means to attain the goal of self-protection and avoidance of pain because it does not eliminate discomfort but only shifts its location into what becomes a disconnected, disappointing, and dissatisfying relationship. Judgement is closed, whereas love needs openness. Loving with the heart is effective, loving with the head just won't do.

> Criticism is to love
> what acid is to metal.

9-3. The Language of Empowerment

When stressed or frustrated, a feeling many of us experience daily, negativity easily develops. It may unintentionally creep into our talk. When in pain, most partners fall into negativity, yet expressing ourselves positively is far more beneficial. It is easier to listen to. It feels better. It is more effective when teaming up to get things done. And it is more constructive and offers a pathway to success. Most importantly, positive language supports and nourishes a loving connection.

The most commonly cited relationship problem is communication. When a loving connection has broken down, words often fail to aid in rebuilding the connection. When unresolved problems flare up again and again, the inability to repair them seems to be a breakdown in communication. The real culprit is underlying painful emotions, which most easily get expressed negatively. Positive language, however, has a unique quality of getting through pain-based obstacles so that meaningful and effective dialogue can happen, but romantic partners must use strength to employ it.

Negative expressions tend to push others away. As a self-protective mechanism, negativity builds isolation, which is useful if solitude is needed, but a poor choice for connection with an intimate partner. Whereas constructive problem-solving falls within the domain of positive communication, negativity expresses hurt, pain, and anger through criticism, blame and fault-finding, which all fall into the negative basket of expressions that cause hurt to others. Being around a chronically negative person is draining, so when couples fall into a rough patch, as discomfort and dissatisfaction grow, negativity grows as well. A vicious cycle forms where negativity follows hurt which leads to more negativity which causes more hurt. It is a signal that problems are accumulating instead of being solved. It is a sign that one or both partners are experiencing distress.

No amount of negativity will create a positive relationship. The language of empowerment is positive. Power is required to shift a romantic connection from troubled to healthy, from unhappy to satisfying. An empowered partner can express what he or she wants rather than what he or she doesn't want. When we focus on the negative, we create it. The most natural topic when venting frustration is what the other partner is doing wrong, an example of focusing on the problem instead of naming a solution. Negative expressions point out the breakdown, the failure, the error. Negativity focuses on a person's shortcomings. Thinking and speaking this way cultivates feelings of hopelessness and powerlessness, a pit into which couples and individuals can easily fall and get stuck. Negativity directs energy away from solutions in favor of dwelling on the problem.

Teamwork is an essential part of a successful love relationship. Partners working together for a common good energizes a bond through good communication, coordination, and synchronization. As a team, two partners work as one. Negativity erodes team-building while positive language directs teammates to collective success. For a relationship to be viable for the long-term, a couple must function as a good team for solving problems, a vital skill that is a weakness for many couples. Positive language, which is free of the words "no" and "not," is part of effective problem-solving and greatly reduces the possibility of hurt or conflict escalation. Staying positive is also accomplished by keeping the focus in the present and singularly upon the current issue. Everything can be expressed positively by simply saying what is desired and what the possibilities are, and suggesting a potential solution.

Positive language eases the path towards progress and success. It promotes a positive loving connection by resolving the problems that divide you.

> Nothing that you do matters...
> It only matters that you do it.
>
> — *Mahatma Gandhi*

9-4. Relationship Turn Signals

The way many people drive suggests that the use of turn signals is optional. Failing to use them is not only illegal, but is frustrating to other drivers, shows a lack of driving etiquette, and is also dangerous. A lack of communication from a leading vehicle that is planning to brake and turn risks harmful collisions. A similar pattern unfolds in love relationships when partners make unilateral decisions that affect the other without first consulting him or her. Feelings of being disregarded commonly result, while the act also robs an uninformed partner of choice.

Keeping the partner informed about upcoming choices is more than just polite; doing so demonstrates consideration and respect. Being informed of future experiences provides a sense of control over one's life direction, as well as security and emotional safety. Loving effectively includes taking care to protect a partner from being hurt, regardless of whether the hurt is major or minor.

The strength of a relationship bond, or "glue" between romantic partners, may be either weak or strong. Weak relationship bonds are often characteristic of a relationship in which hurtfulness is common. While failing to consult a partner tends to be on the less egregious end of the hurtfulness spectrum, and causes only annoyance and aggravation, a good and loving partner seeks to avoid and eliminate all negative impacts. While no one can be perfect at it, attempting to rid a relationship of disappointments and inconveniences is sure to build more relationship satisfaction, which is a good thing.

Where there is a constant repetition of insensitive unilateral choices, usually there is also a pattern of other kinds of hurtfulness. Each emotional injury does not exist in isolation, but joins with older residual hurts to generate an emotional "field" of pain. Each and every injury adds to the accumulation of emotional distrust, building an injured partner's truth that "I cannot trust you to protect me from feeling hurt." Failure to consult a partner about a matter by which he or she will be impacted behaviorally states, "You are unimportant." The pain is not softened just because its cause appears unintentional. An unfortunate relationship truth is that each hurt neutralizes at least a dozen loving gestures, so that a careless lover may effortlessly travel away from love in the injured partner's heart.

Many lovers avoid seeking input due to a concern that doing so will case them to give up control. "My wife is not my boss," or "I don't want him to run my life," are the worries raised by those who commit these lapses in care. How would this approach affect the New England Patriots if Tom Brady refused to tell his wide receiver which play will be run? The team would lose. Every couple is also a team that loses every time the partners are not on the same page of the playbook.

Greater communication will only become a relationship habit if the other partner avoids using instances of consultation as an opportunity to gain control. One who reacts to a request for input with criticism, or who hijacks the issue by telling the other what to do or how to do it, is sure to find that requests for input stop being made.

The suggested guideline is clear: if the partner will be affected by a choice, the safest, most loving practice is to seek consultation. Offering a chance for input is NOT asking permission, as in the way a child, who has little power, seeks permission from a parent. Seeking consultation is instead a considerate, loving effort to hopefully include the partner as an equal in decision-making. To say, "Honey, I am thinking of doing this; do you have a problem with it?" Or "What concerns do you have if I handle this situation this way?" Another option is: "I just want you to know that I am planning to...are you OK with it?" It is like using your turn signal on the road of your relationship.

9-5. Communication: More Than Just Talk

Time and again couples enter relationship therapy (marriage counseling to some) complaining of an inability to communicate. In most cases, both spouses have been English speakers all their lives. Spouses regularly demonstrate a fine grasp of language and communication skills, and indeed, many of those who cite communication problems are highly-educated professionals whose daily skilled use of language contributes to their successful careers. So what is really happening that means attempts at effective communication between intelligent people are rendered ineffective?

If love is to stay full and satisfying, maintaining a love relationship is the name of the game. The importance of maintenance is not unique to relationships; if a new car is not maintained it will soon run poorly and seem old. The trick to successful maintenance is identifying problems and fixing them while they are still small. Doing so is not easy. Partners must first identify a problem, talk about it, mutually agree that it is worthy of focus, and negotiate an agreeable solution. All those steps amount to a lot of communication.

Frequently, couples who list communication as their major problem are specifically pointing to an inability to negotiate and solve difficult, repetitive problems. When getting into a reoccurring issue that is not resolved, it appears that communication is the problem, whereas, in actuality, the poor manner in which each partner reacts to the other's pain and hurt feelings is what causes the issue to seem impossible. The intensity and pain of the moment make the challenge of problem-solving very difficult. Additionally, when emotional intensity is present, poor conditions for constructive dialogue, like fear and defensiveness, prevail. Consequently, openness is lacking, preventing communication from having any chance of solving the problem.

Love relationships and marriages are highly emotional entities. Through the trials of relating, emotions are provoked and over time these become a powerful, often negative, force of influence. When negative emotions prevail, normal communication is not likely to be effective. If couples routinely solve problems, less accumulated negative emotion is available to be ignited, like many dead branches on a dry forest floor; primed with plenty of fuel for a large fire.

Communication seeming ineffective in a given situation has little to do with the partners' communication skills, but instead is all about their emotion-based tendencies. For instance, the impulsive tendency to interrupt or talk over the other prevents good communication, but is not indicative of a lack of communication skills; it is more about a problem of impulsivity. The habit of being closed off to the partner by listening poorly is expressed by stonewalling, anger, and defensiveness, with a peppering of disrespect and contempt. Raised voices indicate mounting frustration, anger, and potentially rage. Words that attack a partner's character, or make threats, are more about an accumulation of anger, resentment, and an absence of impulse control, boundaries, and positive morals. This does not inherently represent a lack of communication skills.

That which is routinely labeled as a communication problem, at its foundation is about pain-based emotions and lack of discipline in following firm rules of non-hurtfulness, compassion and mutual respect. If partners would establish such rules and use all their available personal strength to stick with them...even when it gets tough, communication would likely be effective. Other vital rules that may support successful negotiation and conflict resolution include slowing down the process of speaking and listening and taking turns talking while concluding each partner's turn with confirmation that understanding has been achieved. The talking is just the surface, but the emotions underneath are what truly determine whether a couple seems to be able to communicate.

9-6. Offer Understanding Not Advice

There are many different ways to love. While all of them have value, each has a different purpose, like the tools in a toolbox, each tool has a unique use and may be the best choice in a specific situation. If a tool and a task are mismatched, failure and damage may result. Yet in love relationships partners commonly attempt to love by giving advice which, although well-intentioned, has unintended negative results. Providing advice tests the relationship bond by introducing a dynamic that strains the connection.

Giving advice at an inappropriate moment seems to be such a small error that it rarely gets corrected. The giver or the recipient may not be fully aware of the slight misalignment, but, as with so many other minor annoyances in love relationships, damage is not caused fully by any one instance, but instead by the frequency, repetition and accumulation of negative experiences. In response to poorly timed advice-giving, romantic partners grow slowly aware that the good feeling is draining away. A partner may have the increasing sense that the other just does not "get" him or her anymore. As time passes, a partner grows hesitant to share, not wanting to experience the awkwardness of another failed attempt to connect.

An intelligent partner may be motivated to display his or her intelligence by offering solutions. An eager partner may want to demonstrate helpfulness. Still another good-willed partner may wish to feel needed. Independent of the good intention, unsolicited advice violates a personal boundary and gives legitimate cause for building a wall of defensiveness. An often-repeated phrase, "The road to hell is paved with good intentions," points out that good intentions may not lead to good results. When loving another, positive results are all that really matter.

It is a general truth that unsolicited advice is received as an insult; the act of giving advice is often interpreted as a vote of no confidence, communicating, "I know better than you. I don't think you are capable of doing it for yourself. You are stupid." Just as damaging is the suggestion that the other could have made a better choice, a communication interpreted as saying that he or she is wrong and is not good enough. In the end, the giver of help or advice gets little or no appreciation for his or her intended, but misguided, generosity. When a partner is wanting to help, it may not be considered that each of us learns best from our own mistakes, an opportunity that is stolen when unwelcome assistance is given.

To illustrate the boundary violation, imagine if, late one night entering your kitchen from your bedroom, you found your neighbor, having entered your house uninvited, peering into your refrigerator. The neighbor announces authoritatively that you use the wrong kind of ketchup and that in the future you must use the ketchup that the neighbor prefers. Additionally the neighbor announces that you will be better off after switching to the new brand. How would you feel? More than likely: violated.

In our modern culture, a similar kind of disregard for boundaries is commonplace in social and marital conversation. Deep respect for personal boundaries is essential for positive relationships and the maintenance of emotional safety. Asking first if the recipient wishes to receive advice frees the exchange from the risk of negative outcome, so long as the recipient's answer is respected.

Understanding is a universal way to love. Rarely can it cause harm. Required qualities such as attention, listening, and acceptance, are all positive. When giving another our time by offering undivided attention, the recipient's importance as a human being is reinforced. A partner shares, not to be improved, but to be accepted and loved. Yet for those who are doers and fixers, understanding as a practice can seem weak. The truth is to the contrary; by being understanding, a powerful "doing" and the best kind of giving occurs, in which the bond of connection is strengthened.

> When arguing about
> who is right and who
> is wrong, the relationship
> *always* loses.

9-7. When it is Wrong to be Right

Is there a spouse or romantic partner who has not been told that he or she is wrong? For some bickering couples right/wrong arguments make up most of their communication. Any little slight is enough to kickstart a new round of bickering. "If you'd done it my way, you would have avoided that mistake!" Have your right/wrong debates produced good results? Probably not. When couples argue about who is right and who is wrong, the relationship loses every time.

When two people are first attracted to each other, and later learn that attraction is mutual, differences are good; they are the source of curiosity, interest and excitement. However, as relationships age past the thrilling honeymoon phase and into the routine of daily living, differences cause friction, annoyance and irritation. The fundamental truth of romantic partner differences energizes the negative dynamic of right/wrong conflicts.

The theory goes that if my partner does something or keeps doing something that annoys me, he or she is wrong. No one, in their own being, is actually wrong, yet defining the behavior as "wrong" countless times eventually solidifies into contempt. There is just as much responsibility to make ourselves less easily annoyed as there is for the other partner to alter his or her behavior. Each has a responsibility to avoid having a negative effect on the other and causing them harm, which we can never manage perfectly. Each also has the responsibility to make as many changes as their own personal strength allows in order to move towards a middle ground of good enough. In the cycle of discomfort between partners, expressions of contempt, a form of payback, form the interactions between them into an acutely destructive pattern. As a contemptuous quality creeps into even minor exchanges, partners make each other wrong with eye-rolling, criticism, dismissal, negation, invalidation, belittling, and pronouncements that the other is deficient and unreasonable.

The question each partner ought to ask is: "Does the way I act or react contribute to relationship distress or relationship success?" When a partner automatically acts however he or she wants, to pay the other back for some less-than-good-enough behavior, it just adds to the race towards the bottom of the relationship barrel. Real emotional strength is required to respond to problems in a noble, solution-creating way rather than compounding the problem by giving pain and conflict a longer life. Arguing about who is right and who is wrong locks the partners in a solutionless struggle that promotes bad feelings.

A variation on the right/wrong theme is the blame game. Assigning blame is an investigation into who is wrong. Even if the blame-worthy partner is identified, this results in at least one partner feeling bad. Blame always divides the couple, who are no further along the path to a solution than when they started. Blame is among the best ways to <u>not</u> solve a problem.

People cannot be wrong for how they feel. Yet when a partner feels emotions that lead to behavior that causes discomfort, the most common reaction is to state that he or she is wrong or deficient. Contempt finds a thousand ways to express “What is wrong with you?” Hence the effect of contempt is shaming, in which the value of the other’s very being is invalidated. A contemptuous partner adds to the relationship difficulties, instead of choosing a compassionate route to uphold the other's right to be him or herself. None of us is perfect, but a high level of contempt between partners correlates strongly with divorce and breakups.

It is better to seek progress in unity than victory in being right. The competition generated by right/wrong debates divides couples, whereas positive couples seek to unite. The method of shifting away from this destructive pattern includes refusing to be made wrong and refusing to make the other wrong. Every problem has a positive solution, which is arrived at by generating possibilities together, while using our strength to overcome challenges. By staying away from the zero-sum game of right and wrong, couples can feel much better while working as a team.

9-8. Assumed or True?

In Swiss cheese there are lots of holes, which are good and expected. But in an intimate relationship, holes in partner knowledge are damaging to a relationship. By "holes" I mean gaps in the knowledge partners have of each other. The fewer gaps, the better connection, intimacy and passion will be maintained. Poor relationships are riddled with such holes. Partners tend to fill these holes in their knowledge of their partner with assumed information. Most disconnected partners have a stronger relationship with their own assumptions than they do with their partners.

A husband, wanting to make his marriage satisfying again, was asked why his wife had been unhappy. He responded, "I guess it's because I haven't been very attentive for the past several years." The words "I guess" revealed the man's uncertainty about his knowledge of his wife. In fact, a large part of the reason why his marriage had been poor, and was getting poorer, was that he knew very little about his wife. His relationship contained large areas where he lacked information or was misinformed. Had he asked his wife directly about the cause of her unhappiness? No.

When making assumptions, the holes in partner knowledge are filled with unverified and often incorrect information. Forming inaccurate conclusions may give us a short-term illusion of comfort but are destructive in the long run. Yet some partners maintain a state of unknowing purposefully, out of fear and self-protection. The rationale is this: what my partner has not confirmed is probably about how I fail at being a good enough partner, and hearing about it will hurt, so it is better left unexpressed. Forming incorrect conclusions can be a convenient way to protect ourselves from what we acutely fear is a painful truth. In reality, assumptions serve only to allow our worst fears about ourselves to linger, rather than providing a path to freedom from them that more knowledge may provide. When making assumptions, we remain alone in a relationship with the worst of ourselves, and not with our partner.

It is important for couples to discuss their problems, but this causes potentially tense communication. Many partners avoid these discussions because having them is uncomfortable. Magical thinking, which can come to our rescue in stressful moments, attempts to convince us that if a problem is avoided, it might go away. Many partners feel ashamed as they assume that the problems are caused by their inherently flawed nature, which they feel powerless to change. Destructive assumptions block partners from developing greater intimacy and accepting each other's good and bad qualities by solving problems together.

Partners tend to fill in the knowledge gaps with their worst fears about themselves, and the unknown serves as fertilizer for these fears. Worrying that we are not good enough, leads us to assume that, if we don't know how our partner feels, then his or her malaise must have something to do with our own inadequacies. As a bad emotional habit, assuming keeps old wounds open and raw, while increasing the likelihood of a pattern of re-injury, so a negative emotional reality becomes the default plug-in for what we don't know. Like worry, in which only the most tragic outcome is feared, assumptions draw their information from an emotionally toxic pool. The darkness of the emotion inhabiting most assumptions is the active ingredient in their destructiveness. The rarer cousin, positive assumption, otherwise known as benefit of the doubt, is employed less frequently and can actually be beneficial.

Partners are rarely aware of the fact that they are making an assumption, but quickly trick themselves into certainty about what they believe. Within the consciousness, assumptions function so subtly as to make detection difficult, as difficult as identifying the negative self-beliefs which tend to keep us feeling bad about ourselves.

To combat the bad habit of assuming instead of knowing, try to notice the way you fill in missing information. Altering such a destructive a pattern is best accomplished by asking questions of yourself and your partner, such as: How do I know this information? Is this information one hundred percent true? Was it directly communicated and verified by my partner? All information, like evidence in a court of law, must be rigorously tested to determine veracity. A great situation in which to gain important but previously missing information is learning about the partner when he or she is upset or angry. The potential for a closer relationship will be the reward for developing the discipline of allowing yourself to not know something when you really don't know it. Let that hole remain empty, until you directly ask your partner for his or her verified truth. Know your partner better than you know your assumptions.

9-9. The Power of Mind Reading

A husband should tell his wife everything that he is sure she will find out, and before anyone else does. —Thomas Robert Dewar

Mind reading is a communication tool couples often unknowingly use in their day-to-day interactions. Even though in their personal beliefs they give no credence to any form of supernatural phenomena or ESP, they continue to base their actions upon what they believe they know that their partner feels or thinks, thus avoiding the need for any direct verbal exchanges. It is marvelous to be free of the miscommunication-prone spoken word, but only if this method is truly more effective. The sad truth is that most of us are not skilled enough at reading minds, and are more likely to do damage to our relationships.

When we read our partner's mind, by assuming we know what our partner thinks or feels, we run a great risk of getting it wrong. When we do get it wrong, and our choices are based upon what we mistakenly believe our partner wants, our partner increasingly feels misunderstood by us. Consequently, intimacy is eroded. Just as interest in a bank is compounded exponentially, so is the erosion of intimacy over time if real and accurate communication is not restored. Gradually this produces the condition in relationships where partners feel they do not know each other anymore.

Knowing your partner's thoughts and feelings is the basis for intimacy. Without an accurate understanding of your partner's inner experience, your relationship is destined to be distant rather than close, and conflict-filled instead of harmonious. So give up on assuming that you know anything about your partner without asking them. The only risk you take in doing so is that you might pester them too much, but they may be thrilled by your attention and excited that you are once again very eager to know more about them.

By assuming we know our partner's inner workings, we actually no longer know who they are. It is common in relationships that in each partner's mind the other is defined in some general way according to certain characteristics. After years of marriage to Julia, Steven (fictional characters) had drawn the conclusion that Julia was selfish. This did not mean he no longer loved her, but he accepted that this was one of Julia's limitations. During their interactions, because Steven had long been in the habit of assuming he knew the reasons for Julia's choices, he increasingly viewed her through his distorted filter of selfishness. Even during times when she displayed generosity, Steven could only interpret her actions as having a selfish motive. Julia withdrew from Steven, feeling that he no longer viewed her in a favorable light.

Dissolving the damage created by mind-reading is relatively simple: instead of assuming anything about your partner, ask them directly, and be honest and generous in sharing your own feelings and desires, so your partner will not have to guess or assume anything about you.

9-10. Conflict About How to End Conflict

Are we one human race or billions of separate individuals? Both are true, but the two states hint at our need to connect; to couple up, to form families, groups, neighborhoods, communities, associations, committees, etc. to challenge our singleness and to experience a greater wholeness. By our very nature, we tend to explore connection in varying degrees all the way up to complete oneness. Love relationships are a tiny but intense laboratory for connection. In love relationships, partners strive to form an optimal connection, so that each feels loved. Each partner, as unique as his or her fingerprint, has their own definition of what a good connection is. A struggle between partners about whose version of the connection is the goal, and how to reach it, is not unusual.

In addition to being a collection of billions of individuals, we are also divided into males and females. Each gender is distinct. The differences between sen and women are more than just physical; a deeper distinction is the opposite way men or women go about creating an emotional and sexual connection. Such opposing methods are most obvious when couples in long term relationships seek to repair a damaged connection.

Women build connections by opening up, by sharing emotions, by spending time with the other, and especially by engaging in conversation. Within a love relationship, women desire to have an emotional connection intact before engaging in sex. Men build connections by providing so as to fulfill a need. Within a love relationship, however, most men attempt to build an emotional connection by first engaging in sex. This basic difference in approach between men and women commonly places love partners in relational gridlock; the outcome of which is the destruction of the couple's sex life. This causes the predictable sexless relationship. Under these relationship circumstances, sex becomes the battleground upon which war is waged. The unfortunate partners are likely to be driven crazy by increasing frustration and decreasing satisfaction.

The very conflict is testimony to the dramatic differences

between men and women; a distinction so large that it almost prevents men and women from relating at all. If people were wheels, women would be wheels which rotate from right to left, and men from left to right. Each is the opposite of the other, but neither is better. The bind in which partners become trapped grows increasingly tense as each partner follows their natural tendencies. The woman attempts to increase communication, share her feelings, and invite her partner to spend more "quality" time together. The man attempts to initiate sex. The woman grows frustrated by her man's sexual attempts when she does not feel emotionally ready to be sexual. The man grows frustrated by talking about problems, especially those in which he feels criticized, without the sexual confirmation of his female partner's love.

The approach each gender takes to reestablish a healthy connection will seem to the other to be the opposite and incorrect remedy to what the ailing relationship most needs. Because of the great differences between men and women, each tends to view the other, and the other's methods, as simple, inadequate and childish. Yet both methods are adequate and valuable as a portion of the solution to restore a healthy relationship connection. The battle between partners is truly over whose method will be used first. Spending time together, opening emotionally through sharing, and engaging in conversation are as important as an active and passionate sex life. Neither method is poor; both are effective as a partial prescription. Once partners break through the gridlock to affirm the other's method of connection-building, reconstructing a deep and abiding relationship connection becomes easy. A renewed love connection will have some of the sweetness that excited partners about each other from the beginning.

RELATING

10-1. Pain Runs the Relationship

Romantic partners intend to love each other throughout the life of their relationship or marriage, an intention task that will only endure if their problems are regularly solved. But the problems that develop are always of the most persistent kind, because they arise from the partners' greatest weaknesses.

Problems also develop from pain. When a partner habitually avoids something due to discomfort, washing dishes for instance, the avoidance will anger and frustrate the other partner. With most couples, layer upon layer of unsolved problems accumulate, so that determining which action is triggering which problem becomes hard to figure out. When a problem remains unsolved, it causes pain. In such instances it is pain that runs the relationship.

Each couple wishes and intends that love run the relationship; when action after action expresses love, partners feel connected and nourished, and when it is like this, life is good and easy. Most couples are tricked by this illusion into believing that maintaining it will also be easy. However, when problems remain unresolved due to a combination of blindness, weakness, and holding onto resentment, the relationship and desired intimacy can feel impossibly complex.

Pain will always precede love, the way incompleteness always comes before completeness, and kindergarten will always come before high school. Each partner pulls or pushes for his or her needs to be met, but when those needs go unmet, pain results, and partners who are in pain do not open up to receive love until their needs are met. Fulfilling partner needs demonstrates that the other is important. Each problem pressures the couple for a solution, and will persist forever until it is solved, like a river that will continuously put pressure on a dam until it is overflowed. In this way, pain runs the relationship.

Imagine a tall stone wall made up of jagged boulders. Each

pain-generating unsolved problem is like a stone in the wall. A wall of problems gets built as unsolved problems accumulate. It separates the partners, just as a real wall would if partners were on opposite sides. When the wall is low, partner communication becomes strained. Over years as more unsolved problems make the wall taller, partners can no longer see "eye to eye." When the wall is high the household is inhabited by roommates, who may still function as a team, but are no longer emotionally connected as friends and lovers. The partners cannot reconnect so long as the wall separates them. In this way the pain runs the relationship.

After the problems have accumulated to become a very high wall, partners lose all hope. Problems coalesce so that no one problem is distinct, but instead they all seem collectively to be a large singular morass of pain. In this situation partners live in an environment where any move may spark an argument. Losing hope, partners question if they are right for each other by internally asking "Did I make the wrong choice in choosing this partner?" Arguments include threats to end the relationship. In this way pain is running the relationship.

It is not hopeless. Only someone from the outside is able to see each distinct problem, isolate it, and guide the partners in problem solving. Partner weakness prevents solutions. Even seemingly impossible problems have solutions, which may only be seen after a paradigm shift is forced by a crisis. Sometimes problems are not solved, but outgrown. Problem by problem, stone by stone, the wall of division may be dismantled. As problems diminish, pain is reduced. When the remaining pain is small, it is powerless to influence the couple. Only then can love alone run the relationship.

{ There is no love without pain. }

10-2. Teammates, Friends and Lovers

How good is a love relationship? A framework can be valuable in conceptualizing a relationship so that it can be more easily discussed, evaluated and even improved. Thinking of a relationship as made up of three distinct parts: a team, a friendship, and a love affair can reveal areas where positive change is needed.

To evaluate your love relationship ask yourselves, "How satisfied am I with how the two of us function as a team, as friends, and as lovers?" Each part must be strong and deeply satisfying for the relationship to be strong and satisfying as a whole. The way two partners function as a team is different from how they maintain a friendship. Most partners function best in one or two of these realms and are weaker in the others. Areas of weakness are opportunities for change and growth.

The parts of a love relationship can seem separate, but in reality they are not distinct from each other. Each "part" blends into the others and affects the others. For instance, if two partners do not function well as a team, the frustration of poor teamwork will harm their friendship. If partners are weakest in their sex life, a dissatisfied partner will eventually struggle to be a best friend. If the friendship is weak, many partners will not be as enthusiastic a lover, or try as hard as a teammate. Relationship parts are interdependent.

Functioning as teammates is the most thought-oriented and least emotional of the three parts. To be an effective team also requires the least emotional connection and closeness. In many poor and unhappy relationships, partners still function well as a team to parent the children, run a household and take care of daily needs. Being good friends requires more emotional sharing. A close friendship also requires more openness and a deeper bond, so partners who are less emotionally aware may be limited in offering good friendship, and angry and resentful partners cannot be part of a real friendship. Being great lovers demands the most closeness and openness. Intimacy is the most vulnerable of the three relationship elements and has the potential ability to heal early childhood issues by including partners' eroticism. Yet many couples maintain an active sex life without emotional connection. They participate in mechanical sharing; their bodies are involved but not their hearts. For most partners, this is a poor-quality love affair...a bit like a hot fudge sundae without the hot fudge.

Being friends is essential for the well-being of a romantic connection. The friendship is the core of a relationship. It functions as the hinge-pin between being teammates and being lovers. When the goodwill of friendship has evaporated due to a build-up of resentments or damaged trust, the relationship is at risk because the friendship core has been corrupted. A friend connection is fragile and easily frayed by the stresses and intensity of modern life. Partners who have lost their friendship no longer feel close, and experience emotional disconnection. Without the core, relationships are at heightened risk for infidelities, dissatisfaction, and dissolution.

By considering the status of these three components of teammates, friends and lovers, partners have a useful tool to use to better pinpoint relationship weaknesses. Each part offers a different way of loving. By being teammates, love may be offered in the form of support, thoughtfulness and making the other's day easier. In friendship, love may be offered through understanding, listening and compassion. As lovers, love is offered through deep openness, expressing passion, and sharing pleasure. So many ways exist to love. Your relationship or marriage will be most satisfying when love is expressed generously in all three ways.

> Most injuries are not caused by malice, but instead by ignorance.
>
> — *Anonymous*

10-3. Veterans of Domestic Wars (VDW)

When talking to a partner who has been in a twenty- or thirty-year relationship, the tale they tell often sounds more like a battle than a love story. The truth is that, while romantic relationships are intended to be about love, many end up being mostly about war. A widely experienced reality is that fighting is a normal part of a relationship. In many peaceful relationships, peace is only attained by holding inside feelings and words which may cause an argument; the relationship struggle is invisibly hidden within each partner. Love is the goal, but the journey is about fighting hate, making romantic partners veterans of domestic wars.

A paradoxical truth is that everything seems to turn to its opposite. Examples of this are teachers who value education spending time with the uneducated, police officers who enforce law and order spending most of their time with criminals, and doctors who promote health associating mostly with the sick. Similarly, lovers end up dealing with hate; hate for disliked aspects of themselves, hate for specific partner characteristics, hate for limitations which block infinite love, freedom, and satisfaction.

We would prefer our romantic relationships to be more like a beautiful dance than an ugly battle. Many couples don't find their way free of the relentless outward or inner struggles to make their relationship more loving. The ways a partner "drives us crazy" are evidence of the struggle. Partner differences commonly mark the flashpoint of combat. In a moment of opposition, when each partner feels right and is strong in their conviction, a control battle ensues, a competition in which a loving connection will certainly be broken. When partners compete for power, it is a war in which one partner may win, but the relationship *always* loses.

Craving to love and be loved is common and normal, but love possesses a dimension that is rarely acknowledged: Love also destroys. It is valued for its nourishing quality, but love forces change and transformation which destroys that which was before. It is like when hot water is poured on an ice cube. The hot water melts the cube's rigid form. The water that had been trapped in the ice becomes merged with the hot water. The melted ice water becomes fluid and flexible; in the process, the ice cube is destroyed. Love is like that, though it acts slowly with relentless patience. Ice cubes don't resist transformation the way people do. The resistance is part of the lover's war with hate. Love wishes to destroy us through transformation to make us soft, flexible, and pure in love. Because of this, love, at times, seems like an enemy.

Each one of us possesses a few natural qualities out of an almost infinite variety, but when the qualities we individually possess do not match what we prefer, or they interfere with living the kind of life we want to live; we develop hate for our own qualities; we hate ourselves. Any state other than love for ourselves will fuel a conflict within. Inner battles become outward battles with a romantic partner. To influence a partner, and deal with his or her resistance to change, sometimes a fight is required to impress upon the partner how important it is that they get beyond their limitations.

Outward acceptance and surrender to what life brings are part of the practice that leads to discontinuing a war-like stance. Inwardly diving deeper into your centermost place from where your love springs makes it possible to disengage. It is a life-long journey. Once peace in yourself has been attained, instead of war, love, peace, and harmony may rule your love relationship.

> Beware of making permanent choices when reacting to temporary emotions.
>
> — *Buddha*

10-4. The Quiet Man

Who is that quiet mystery man? He barely says a word. His icy silence offers few hints about what he thinks or feels. His wife complains about his lack of sharing. She feels lonely and disconnected. If only he would open up.

A chorus of wives and female partners complain that their men don't communicate. They keep everything inside. The female partners usually say, "When we first met, he talked a lot. What happened?!!!" Adding to their pain is the fact that women prefer building closeness and connection through verbal sharing; confirming the adage, "The way to a woman's heart is through her ears." So when a male partner falls quiet, the relationship bond weakens, especially for wives and girlfriends.

Generally, men and women talk for different reasons. Whenever generalizing about genders and relationships, a truth often applies but exceptions are common as well. Men tend to communicate for specific purposes, to get things done, whereas women talk more often to relate, or to gain or give support. Because of this, women use more words, while the male perspective on words is commonly, "the fewer the better." Adding to the confusion about male communication patterns, a quiet man at home may be talkative with non-intimate acquaintances and co-workers.

Differences in communication styles explain only part of the reason why male partners go quiet. Another complaint female partners voice is that, when their men do talk, they rarely share their feelings, the most valuable kind of sharing for developing closeness. Men and women differ in how they experience their emotions; unlike women who are readily aware of their feelings and whose emotions feature largely in how they identify themselves, men's emotions are buried below their moment-to-moment awareness. Louder in men's consciousness are their thoughts, opinions, and preferences. Generally, men are less "emotionally intelligent" than women.

Because love relationships are highly emotional entities by nature, less emotionally aware men gravitate towards relating through activity rather than through verbal sharing. Examples of this are men who make themselves valuable to their female partners by being a good financial provider, by being a helper, a fixer, an expert, or a guide rather than by being an emotionally expressive conversationalist. Given their inner make-up, it is far easier for many men to do than to feel. A man can fulfill his capacity within these "doing" roles, which are constructive, but his female partner will always wish for a more complete, balanced partner; one who can do these activities and can also talk, share, and express, since this is her preferred method to connect. Most male partners will never be like a woman's girlfriend, who naturally excels at free-flowing chat.

Men have just as many emotions as women, but are less aware of them. The volume of the feelings is quieter, which is part of the reason men do not prioritize their feelings as highly as women. Nonetheless, when men feel bad, their feelings also strongly impact them, but their strategies for coping with negative emotions differ from their female partners. Unlike women, who typically seek support by sharing with other women, men tend to isolate themselves while staying busy with non-emotional tasks, such as an active project or video game. Because women seek support in problems, a female partner may feel hurt and rejected when her male partner does not come to her for help with his troubles. Men are different than women in more than the obvious ways, yet many women expect and hope that men will respond the way women do.

When a relationship has become troubled, tension grows between partners. It is not unusual that female partners, conscious of discomfort, express what they feel and wish to verbally process problematic issues. Women are much more likely to react and express their emotional discomfort strongly. Male partners cope poorly with female partner expressions that are loud, sharp, disapproving, or accusatory. Men experience much discomfort at their female partner's unhappiness and the way it is expressed, but they possess no adequate response. Some men "shut down" in reaction, lacking the emotional confidence to mount a challenge or offer compassion.

Most men avoid expressing themselves to prevent unintentionally provoking conflict and the associated discomfort. When tension and emotionally intense discussions erupt, male partners do not experience a level playing field; most find that, when in conflict with their female partner, she repeatedly succeeds at "turning it around on them." Male partners are at a disadvantage because they are less emotionally aware in a highly emotional situation. Men prefer to use a rational strategy, so when a female partner expresses herself strongly, male partners often do not adapt well to an emotional, non-rational process. Feeling powerless and at a disadvantage, some men resort to the use of aggression and loud anger to level the playing field, a destructive and ultimately damaging method.

A male partner's reticence has many causes. Many men fear abrupt, negative anger, such as sharp reactions to momentary displeasure, which find them emotionally unprepared and confused. Men grow cautious and ill-at-ease when around female partners who have a history of sudden negative emotion; the same uneasiness that is at the root of many male sexual performance problems. These are the quiet men. They are wary of hurtful anger, negative or intense emotion, and cannot consistently predict when it may erupt or what may provoke it. To them, female unhappiness is frequently confusing and irrational. Men in this situation prefer the safety that is secured by remaining quiet.

Many men are not all that good at identifying their feelings in the first place, thus they are incapable of expressing what they feel when something is wrong. When asked by their female partners, their response of "nothing" may be true to their actual awareness. At other times, "nothing" is a deflection to avoid revealing an emotion that will make them feel vulnerable, an experience too close to weakness for most men's comfort. A man's silence may hide his inner pain and give outward justification to the common modus operandi, "If there's nothing good to say, say nothing at all."

Other men have given up on expressing their emotions after experiencing the prolonged feeling that their emotional needs are not listened to or responded to by their female partner. The male way of thinking and doing can appear odd and even wrong to women, but may be differently effective. After repeatedly finding that their voice has been disregarded, and their ideas, thoughts, and opinions dismissed, sharing feelings is a high hurdle over which many men do not want to jump. Opening up and sharing more may happen once a man is secure in the knowledge that if he does, he will be sincerely listened to and responded to.

"Just talk more" is not an effective prescription to increase male-partner communication and restore the way they spoke freely, months or years earlier, during courtship. To reduce tension and melt away the anger and other negative emotions that led to their female partner's sharp anger and harsh attitude, other channels of showing love must be utilized, because verbal sharing is not the only method of building a connection. Male partners are more comfortable with activity-based methods of showing love, even more so during times of relationship distress. Quiet men can benefit from the strengthening of their confidence and assertiveness. They ought to learn more about their emotions and practice putting words to them, while female partners should simultaneously attempt to soften the sharp edge when expressing displeasure. For the development of more sharing from male partners, couples being relaxed together with a lowered risk of conflict or negativity may get the job done over time. Even quiet men wish to share in order to be successful romantic partners. Doing so is important, because the way to a woman's heart is through her ears.

10-5. The Mirror Doesn't Lie

Every relationship has problems. Each partner views these problems and their causes differently. A majority of couples' problems are caused by both partners. However, it is a universal tendency for most partners to conclude that relationship problems are largely the other's fault. With a subjective perspective, each partner tends to minimize or even negate his or her contribution to problems, while magnifying the other partner's share of the blame. As time passes, the disagreement as to who caused the relationship's problems undermines the couple's connection.

The power of denial is absolute, a blindness in which a person doesn't know what he or she doesn't know. Partners are generally unaware of their own limitations when it comes to loving. Defensiveness, selfishness, avoidance, and insensitivity are some of the obstacles that make determining one's contribution to relationship problems nearly impossible.

Within love relationships, each partner functions as a mirror, albeit an imperfect one, reflecting back the other's qualities and ability to love, and the mirror always reflects some truth. Reflection occurs when a partner's actions are mostly a reaction to something the other person said or did, for example, a partner who gives back a loving gesture after receiving one, or another partner who acts hurtfully as payback for having been hurt previously. The cycle of action and reaction complicate the determination of who is the cause and who is the effect.

When problems develop within a relationship, partners often reject the feedback from the mirroring of the other person, and as problems increase in number and grow in significance, relationships take on a negative tenor. Consequently, the tendency to assign blame increasingly influences each partner's feelings and behavior. Now in a state of painful disconnection, each partner is rendered powerless in his or her inability to break through a wall made of painful unresolved problems; neither partner knows where to begin.

Only feeling his or her own pain, each partner is isolated like an island. Having far less knowledge of the other's pain, the view of the relationship and the partner grows distorted. Each partner is now looking through a filter of being the one who is wronged. When both partners feel wronged, little connection is likely. If partners choose a repairing conversation to rebuild their connection, just a minor assignment of blame, one that undoubtedly feels unfair, can derail the conversation. If one person's unhappiness is expressed in an extreme way that causes more hurt, the disagreement over who is the most at fault is further widened.

It is an obvious truth that relationship problems need to be resolved for a couple to improve their connection. Determining what each partner contributes to the problems is a necessary but complicated step in the journey to improvement. The painful emotions of both partners that play a large role in relating and in the rise of problems are not distinct like a physical object. Emotions are hard to quantify or define. Boundaries are defined "edges" where one partner begins and the other ends. Sorting out who is to blame can be as confusing as walking through a hall of mirrors in a carnival due to people's inherent inability to set boundaries. Without an objective third party, getting clear on one's contribution to problems can be futile. Hence, people in troubled relationships often seek a friend's or a therapist's input.

Each partner does possess some power to get clear about his or her role regarding relationship problems; a pathway that has been obscured by pain and anger. By self-correcting so that all behavior is consistently loving, and by using pure strength to prevent painful feelings from determining words and actions, a partner may remove himself or herself as a contributor to relationship problems. Partners who have been hurt rarely take this path, out of a sense of unfairness, but not doing so prolongs the suffering. Making positive changes in oneself is an effective way to softly influence the other partner and is also personally beneficial.

By being consistently loving, a partner becomes a mirror that reflects only positives. The other partner's negative contributions become exposed when he or she is the only cause. Problems are easier to solve when there is only one source. A relationship is refreshingly simple when each partner is clear and distinct, with well-defined boundaries. Loving is easy when both partners look in the mirror offered by the other and only love is reflected.

10-6. The Queen and the King

Upon checking into a five-star hotel, guests are quick to notice the royal treatment they receive. Attentive service that provides a high level of comfort makes us feel special and important. That is why it is expensive.

Similarly, we should treat our girlfriends and wives like queens. Maintaining the generous loving attention given to them during courtship shows a woman throughout the relationship that she is important. Simultaneously, husbands and boyfriends ought to be treated like kings.

When love relationships are successful, a key to that success is service. What we give, and the attitude with which we give it, either contributes to a loving environment between romantic partners or fails to do so. Yet each one of us, in part, believes that we deserve the best. Some call this entitlement, but it can also be called honoring the inner queen or king.

Giving your spouse the royal treatment is not spoiling him or her, as long as the giving is mutual. Service is about giving. The more attentive we are to our partner, the more we are likely to fully understand what will make our queen or king happy. Observing and studying our partner may help us better understand him or her.

Some confuse service with subservience — but being of service does not indicate higher or lower, better or worse. On the contrary, being of service elevates the one serving. Giving not only communicates that the other is important, it also expresses, "I am here to make your life better."

Treating your wife like a queen or your husband like a king embodies the values of honor, respect, reverence, loyalty, and adoration. At first glance, such treatment may appear to be too high a standard, but wouldn't you want to be treated this way? Living these values means that the best of us is given, which has the greatest potential to evoke the best in our partner and others in our lives. A couple's deepest potential is generated when both partners simultaneously respect, honor, and adore each other. The best in one lover triggers the best in the other; lifting the loving bond even higher. A kingdom of love and peace, a space of security and harmony is created in a frantic, sometimes unsafe world.

Most spouses and partners don't treat each other like kings or queens. The factor preventing us from building the harmonious and loving royal kingdom is that each one of us is unable to aim that high. Why? Because the reality in relationships is that the more intimately you know your partner, the more clearly you see his or her limitations and flaws. The longer you have been with your partner, the more you have been hurt or frustrated by his or her flaws. So as long as we base our loving efforts on the degree to which the partner "deserves" our love, a pattern is established in which partners are treated like paupers or prisoners instead of royalty.

In its purest form, love is unconditional. When conditions are placed on love, such as, "I will love you when you when I think you are good enough," the relationship will begin to devolve to a low state. Giving love at a high-level lifts both partners up so that behaving in a regal way becomes increasingly easier. Offering attention at a high level requires great effort, but it may take less effort and pain than living in a poor-quality relationship and trying to repair it after it has fallen apart.

Kings and queens do not just receive lavish attention. Mutual loving actions are one way to maintain the status of royalty, but behaving in a strong and responsible manner is another. Royalty must manage their sovereign domain well in order to succeed; history is full of the consequences of haughty or insensitive leadership. Scared people do not adore their king or queen. The ability to verbalize the need for change, to redirect resources to a place of insufficiency, and to act as a loving leader all support receiving the adoration due a king or queen.

Reciprocal and simultaneous royal treatment is the "secret" to a lasting, happy relationship. So go ahead, honor and revere your queen. Don't hesitate to respect and adore your king. Give each other the five-star service that lifts your love to the highest level.

10-7. Openness to Influence

Imagine if you need changes from your spouse or partner, such as spending more time together or eliminating an annoying habit. How wonderful would it be if you just asked your spouse and he or she replied, "Of course, if it would make you more comfortable," and followed up by making the changes quickly? What does it take to influence your partner? Powerful people are considered influential. The amount that a person may influence others is a measure of his or her power, but within a love relationship influence functions in reverse. A partner's willingness to be influenced without the use of power shows how important and loved the other is. Openness within a relationship is valuable as an expression of love, whereas power and force are harmful to love and connection.

Partners always seek to change the other; this is vastly different from the beginning of many relationships when partners experience each other as perfect. Over time, as a partner's limitations and flaws are revealed, the need for growth becomes apparent. Each of us has a varying appetite for growth, but none of us can avoid change, a sentiment that is well expressed by John C. Maxwell's quote, "Change is inevitable, growth is optional." With the passage of time, the cycling of the seasons and aging, partner needs vary. Due to partner differences, the need to negotiate for change is ever-present and requires constant adjusting and adapting. Whether partners may influence each other or not determines whether the constant and dynamic adjustments flow smoothly and easily or, instead, painfully with tension and friction.

To stay fresh and alive, a love relationship must adapt to new circumstances. Fluid and flexible adjustments are only possible when partners are open to each others' influence. Being flexible is a symptom of emotional health. Being open is a requirement of love. The tree that is flexible in high winds bends, the one that isn't breaks. Only when soft and pliable for each other do partners grow well together.

Some partners are "yes" people and others are "no" people. The "yes" people naturally react to a request for changes in a positive way. "No" people respond by opposing changes and negating possibilities. In terms of being open to the lover's influence, a "no" response abruptly silences the music and halts the dance of love, and a refusal to be influenced can be interpreted as a lack of love. Instead of "no," consider starting out by offering a "maybe." Choosing to think about a request or give a delayed response softens the exchange. Such a practice demonstrates greater openness to influence and the creation of new possibilities. A partner who always says "yes" may be seen as a push-over who is weak and without self-esteem. Agreements are cheap and dissatisfying if they are consistently achieved too easily. Balance is necessary. A well-negotiated change nourishes the growth of both partners.

How partners attempt to influence each other may determine whether openness is offered. If a desire for change is forced rather than requested, giving the other no choice, a reaction of resistance is likely. Force is the enemy of love and is best avoided; if a partner is flexible, force will never be necessary. In dealing with a chronically resistant, stubborn partner where attempts to influence have failed, the other is tempted to explore indirect ways to gain satisfaction. Pressure is necessary at times, and better than force to obtain agreement but should be used with care. Trickery, manipulation, and being covert and deceitful are tactics that may ultimately attain a goal, but pose a risk of hurt, damaged trust, and conflict. Being closed to influence will ultimately limit the relationship's potential.

Remaining open to a partner's influence is a non-verbal expression that the other is important. How do you influence your partner? Great openness communicates that the partner is so important that effort, accommodation and even discomfort is acceptable for the other's happiness and well-being. Relationships are about love; influence is the dance of love. When partners are open to the other's influence, the dance of love may be beautiful.

> MARRIAGE:
> Do it well and it is uplifting
> Do it poorly and it is bondage.

10-8. Why Do We Marry?

Why do we marry? It is a crazy thing to do. Talk to most married people and you will hear that the hardship is substantial. How many really happy married couples do you know? Beyond the happy faces couples put on when out in public, scratch the surface and you will learn of marital strife. All couples have their issues. Marriage has a bad reputation well expressed by the HL Mencken quip, "Marriage is a wonderful institution, but who would want to live in an institution?" Forty to fifty percent of marriages divorce well before realizing the ideal of "until death do us part." The average length of a marriage is about eight years.

What about the couples who remain married? The statistics don't suggest that they are happy; some stay together for the kids; some cannot afford to divorce; others don't wish to endure how it will look to others; still others value the package of house, savings and financial security over the uncertain future after a divorce. The relationships of unmarried couples, on average, end more quickly.

Sounds pretty bleak! And I am a proponent of marriage. It is almost as if we cannot help but couple-up; we are hard-wired to do so. Some couples serve as a sparkling example of wedded bliss, though they represent a minority. The delicious feeling we have when discovering that love and attraction are mutual always tricks us into forgetting the enormous work that follows in forming a bond of love; similar to how a beautiful store-front window pulls us into the store. Love truly is blind. We cannot help ourselves.

When we begin a new phase of life, celebrating it is common, for instance with the birth of a child, or when a student is accepted into college. An engagement is also on this list. A wedding ceremony is part a grand party honoring a newly bound couple. In each case the celebration heralds the beginning of a new kind of work. Work is hard. But unlike the obvious work of raising a child or studying for a degree, the work of marriage tends to be unacknowledged. When the work appears, in the form of marital difficulties, most couples are caught off guard. The denial disables couples from being prepared to cope elegantly with the sure-to-arrive rigor.

Hidden in plain sight is the reality that love relationships offer the possibility of tremendous growth. Some call it maturation, others call it being battle-tested. The growth arrives in the form of a deepened capacity to love. Patience, acceptance, unconditional love, putting desires in their proper place, and forgiveness are some of the loving ways developed when we practice love within a marriage. It is a universal but unrealistic hope that marriage will just feel good; that we may be "lucky in love" and experience no marital adversity. Because of the misconceptions of marriage when issues develop, which they almost certainly will, partners conclude that something is wrong with the marriage instead of realizing that a lesson in the normal process of growth is ready to be learned.

Marriages become deeply troubled and stuck when problems are avoided and growth is resisted. However, extreme solutions must be considered in response to extreme situations, such as when a partner is violent, abusive, self-destructive, and resists all attempts to outgrow dysfunctional patterns. In such an instance, growth for the healthier partner may come in the form of loving oneself through self-protective measures.

The strong boundaries of a committed relationship provide a self-imposed containment which ultimately forces partners to face painful personal limitations and weaknesses. The loose structure of non-committed relationships allows partners to easily avoid uncomfortable tests of character rather than face them. Having no choice but to find a solution creates a dire situation that promotes a potential paradigm shift of exponential growth. Once teamwork, friendship, and intimacy are established within a marriage, the work of marriage is to maintain them.

Compared to the fantasy of marriage, the real experience stacks up rather poorly. When the glories of growth are considered, marriage becomes an important part of a life worth living. The inability to adjust, adapt and change constrains a relationship to live within dissatisfying limits. We all must change, and this is called growth, which, in its essence, means progress and improvement. When growth ceases within a couple, the spark of love dies. Until we as a society sing the praises of marriage for its true deeper purpose of growth, marriage will remain vulnerable to the unrealistic expectations that doom it to high levels of divorce.

10-9. Driving Each Other Crazy

Many couples bicker and fight about driving. It is high on the list of argument-causing activities, above loading the dishwasher, folding the towels or properly making the bed. But neither folding towels nor loading the dishwasher carries the risk of injury like driving. Driving is complex and partners may experience and evaluate good driving in very different ways. The issue is further complicated by how divergent a driver's and a passenger's experiences may be.

Some drivers are cautious while others are aggressive. One will take greater risks, while others may be timid or generous to other drivers to a fault. A partner may look upon the other's driving not as a matter of style, but rather of more or less skill; and judgement and criticism can hurt. Differences in driving can become the source of a power struggle over whose influence determines how driving happens. An anxious, uncomfortable partner, when feeling threatened by a roadway situation, is likely to sound off in sudden, accusatory and critical ways. Tensions are heightened when in a moving vehicle.

While driving, vision, emotion, sense of speed and distance vary widely. We each literally "see" distance differently. The comfortable stopping distance for one may feel completely unsafe to another. While driving on a crowded highway, a safe enough distance from the car in front is highly subjective, but the experience seems much less safe to a passenger who has no control. Partners who have been in car accidents, have trauma in the past, or who live with problematic anxiety find driving situations particularly unnerving. In the passenger's position discomfort is magnified.

A medley of driving-related issues, many about distracted driving, spark conflict and tension. More now than ever, differing levels of comfort with driver cell-phone use is a contested point. Eating and drinking, or fiddling with the radio, may also cause trouble. Reacting with road rage to inconsiderate drivers who fail to use a turn signal, or following being cut-off, is sure to become a relationship problem. Repeatedly taking eyes off the road, or sudden braking, accelerating, and cornering will all draw passenger complaints.

When lost or in an unfamiliar area, guessing the right highway exit is a moment primed for extreme tension. The way in which a partner's anxiety is expressed may make the difference between a calm adjustment, an ugly argument or a deadly accident. Accusations, attacks or abrupt criticisms such as, "You're driving too fast!" or "You drive like a maniac!" may not only create a high risk of an argument, but also interfere with safe driving. We will never know how many accidents have been caused by driving-related arguments between partners.

The politics, or division of power, is clear between a driver and a passenger. The driver who has control of the vehicle also has the power of life or death. Much like the captain of a ship, the driver is fully in charge, but in moments when the first mate attempts to usurp power by telling the driver how to drive, also referred to as "back seat driving," tension and conflict are likely. Does the power distribution when driving accurately reflect who is most in control in your relationship?

The degree to which the driver changes their driving technique for the passenger's comfort can make all the difference between a tense or relaxed ride. Doing so is a loving effort. Resentful partners take pleasure in the roadway torture of a troublesome passenger, but an uncomfortable passenger can show love by practicing restraint when it comes to negative or critical commentary.

The ultimate judge of driving skill is not a partner's opinion, but the driver's driving record. If a driver has very few or no speeding tickets, moving violations or accidents, then this driver is a safe one, whether or not his or her driving style meets with the other's comfort and approval. Nevertheless, a multitude of factors make driving a hot-button issue for relationship conflict.

10-10. Pain in the Relationship

Even this past hour may have been marred by worry, the discomfort of stress, the throb of a headache, or a bumped elbow. Pain and suffering are part of our daily life experiences. We can't escape pain, though sometimes we may avoid or delay it. We live with and around it. For some, such as those with chronic physical pain caused by disease or injury, pain is far more acute. For others, emotional suffering from mental illness or unhealed trauma makes each day seem interminable. Less frequently acknowledged is the chronic emotional pain established in our lives' first days, born out of insensitive, unstable or insufficient loving. It is pain so pervasive that, like white noise which fades into the background, it is long forgotten in its ever-presence. It has grown to be part of what is normal, and is therefore cast into the unconscious. Pain runs our relationships.

Pain is, in many cases, an initial cause for a relationship's formation. Out of the pain of loneliness or lack of fulfillment, many a partner was sought and accepted. Incompleteness seeks completeness. The quest to love for many is launched as an attempt to soothe a form of emotional pain, the aching emptiness of inadequacy in which a lover validates worthiness. Relating offers the possibility of having togetherness in the pain; understanding opens the possibility to further vanquish suffering's aloneness. The exceptions are those inevitable moments when it is the partner who hurts us, amplified when we judge ourselves as not deserving of love.

Our success in loving another is determined strongly by how well we manage our pain. In the process, we run headlong into a paradox: loving requires openness, yet to endure our personal suffering the pull is strong to become closed off in self-protection. The wounded animal hides securely in a hidden place to lick its wounds. As much as togetherness seems to soothe, it coincidentally aggravates pain by hooking onto the remnants of very old early-life injuries sustained before our memory was formed.

In reaction to our relationships, old pain, but not always its associated memories, rises into awareness. Ghosts from our beginning days are set free into our current consciousness. Most lovers shadow-box with these ghosts while firmly believing it is their partner doing the misdeeds. Innumerable partners are punished due to the others' pain. It is almost automatic, when in pain, to make the other wrong, expressing, often non-verbally, "If I am hurting, it must be your fault!" Patience is barely a hair's thickness while suffering; it is easily snapped by even a well-intentioned partner.

Shame-based pain is toyed with when teasing and taunting. Competitive bickering can be exciting, but underneath it forces fearful partners to hide their authenticity like buried treasure. The relationship's loving potential goes down along with it. Partners urgently seek relief from shame in activities that are temporarily soothing, but which quickly become extreme in obsession, while injuring the other along the way. Anger and subsequent hurtfulness are provoked by sharpness, while frustration voices a low-grade form of the same thing. Countless lovers keep their best selves out of view due to the painful fear of rejection. The myriad paper-cut-like hurts from insensitivity are uncountable.

The environment in which love thrives is contaminated by

the effects of pain. Negativity blocks out the sun of love. Being made to feel wrong by accusations forces us into defensiveness, a seemingly impenetrable wall in the path to connection. Belittling a partner passes on the pain from past disrespect. Irrational, futile hopes of improvement and repair energize partner battles. Couples in pain turn away from each other to feel relief in the short run, as distance gives the illusion of freedom from tasting the other's pain. But the can of pain is only kicked down the road upon which they soon will travel, to be tripped over again later on.

My pain is no less valid than yours. In a couple, all pain is OUR pain. We live in this suffering together. It is hard to remain open while resisting the urge to push away or run away from the important other. Listen to what is underneath many of your loved one's expressions and observe his or her suffering. It deserves a compassionate response, offering togetherness in what otherwise can be very lonely pain.

10-11. Just Not Feeling It

When loving another, emotions play a large and vital role in how relationships develop and function. In some cases, emotions are used like antennae, as a vital way to gather information for making choices. Emotions are referred to in order to gauge a relationship's success. However, at other times, for the relationship to function at its best and be most satisfying, emotions must be controlled, limited, and even rejected as an influence.

An example of where emotions play an important role is when it comes to feeling loved. If a partner does not feel loved, the amount the other actually loves him or her makes little difference to relationship satisfaction or stability; how we feel forms our reality. Love may be abundantly present, but if it is expressed in the wrong way, it will not be effective. Each one of us is unique, as is our way to be satisfyingly loved. To be effective, love must be delivered in the right form, in line with the beloved's preferred way. For instance, if a partner feels most loved by hearing the words "I love you," but the other shows love by being dependable and reliable without verbally expressing love, the first partner will not feel loved.

Many actions are loving, but not all are appropriate for a specific person or situation. Knowing one is loved is vastly different to feeling it, which is far superior for relationship satisfaction. If affectionate touch is the action through which a partner feels love, buying him or her nice gifts is not bad, but it is not the proper action to cause the other to feel loved. Let's hypothesize that you have two pets, a dog and a fish. In caring for them while wishing for each to be healthy and well-fed you give the fish dog food and the dog fish food. Each will quickly grow sick, because both are getting the wrong kind of nourishment; love is a form of nourishment. Only the right way of giving, well suited for your unique partner, will result in the all-important feeling of being loved. The right efforts need not be a mystery, just ask and your partner will tell you which actions feel most loving. Loving in the right way is most effective if hurtfulness has been eliminated.

Being of service is a central practice in many spiritual traditions. By loving our partner the way he or she wishes to be loved is an example of service. For the best results service must be given in the right spirit, which includes letting go of personal preferences and expectations of return. Performed well, giving service fosters growth and honors love's essence, while simultaneously satisfying the partner.

As much as feelings are an integral part of relating, they can also prevent relating. Negative and toxic emotion, usually from unhealed past hurts, causes partners to avoid closeness and seek self-protection. Negative emotions, a natural by-product of long-term relating, if not resisted, are just as likely to cause partners to want to end the relationship as positive emotions are to encourage getting closer. Long-term partners, if they haven't done growth work, are likely to not feel good, not just within relationships but generally in life.

Making the effort, even when you don’t feel like it, is part of successful relating. The effort known as "fake it until you make it" is increasingly seen as a pejorative term, having developed a meaning of being insincere and selling out one's true feelings. On the rise is a belief that making efforts that defy one's emotional state is synthetic, non-organic and unnatural. Such an attitude devalues the importance of making the right efforts. Emotions are not the sole element in determining what is best. Among the hardest parts, not only of being in a romantic partnership, but also of being an adult, is that we cannot do whatever we want, whenever we want; on the contrary, we often must do what we do not feel like doing. Individual strengths must be manifested at times with adherence to integrity, morality, ethics, and responsibility; all of which take effort and oppose emotional consideration.

When a relationship has fallen into a rough patch, feelings cannot be trusted to guide partners to improve their togetherness. Painful emotions typically call for self-protection and defensiveness, actions which will not rebuild a damaged connection, but instead encourage further deterioration of the loving bond. Difficulties generate negative emotions, which feel bad and which, if acted upon, can easily lead to the end of relationships or marriages. Instead, if we are committed to our partner and value all that we have invested in the relationship, we do what does not feel good...we fix the relationship and work to improve it. Such efforts may be contrary to our feelings, but satisfy our deeper values, a case where the emotions are not valuable in guiding our efforts, but instead are opposed to such efforts. Emotions interfere with success at making positive change, growth, and learning; the bad feelings must be fought by choosing to do the right thing even when we are just not feeling it.

> The present moment is where life actually happens. Stay in the present to fully live it.

10-12. No Time Like the Present

The past is riddled with hurtful events, and the pain from any event has only fully passed when it is emotionally complete. But for many of us, past events remain incomplete and the pain from unresolved events lingers, contaminating our present. For many couples, their history of unresolved hurts is a lengthy narrative holding them back from enjoying the fullness of love, a condition that thrives in the freedom of an uncontaminated present.

Daily, we weave together an awareness of past, present and future. But of these three, the present is magic in a way the other two are not. Our "now" is the place where we really live. It holds the key to our well-being and balance. When having fun, all self-consciousness is gone and living completely in the present reigns. The present holds the key to happiness, and love relationship satisfaction. The past and future are danger zones; the past is a place for regret and unresolved hurts; the future is unknown and therefore is the cause for fear and worry. Thousands of years ago, the Taoist wise man Lao Tzu, wrote, "If you are depressed, you are living in the past. If you are anxious, you are living in the future. If you are at peace, you are living in the present." Our now is an emotionally safe place where we have the power to make a positive difference in our lives, the power to solve problems. Love lives in the present, a place of simplicity and peace. Couples who fully attend to their experiences of the present are better able to relate deeply and safely. In the present, we are most in control.

Resolving problems, healing hurts and repairing damage is optimally done quickly, thereby minimizing the risk of collateral damage. For many couples, the pain from past hurts has accumulated to become an easily ignited reservoir of explosive emotion. Old, unfinished hurts trigger conflict, where partners are strongly prompted to express old anger once that monster has been awakened. If addressed in the present, an issue may more easily be resolved non-hurtfully, without latent toxic emotions spoiling another day.

Negativity is a signal that a painful past is polluting the present. In the now, life is ever evolving and becoming as developing events happen. Expressing negativity, in addition to being unattractive, is toxic and brings forth old pain. Negativity forms a defensive wall of protection against fully experiencing life in the present. For many, the present moment is lived only a little bit. Living only in the present is a very difficult, but worthwhile, skill to master.

Forgiveness and acceptance function in the present, they are gifts to ourselves that melt lingering pain. They are practices of letting go. Forgiveness is often confused with "letting someone off the hook." Seeking retribution, revenge, or wanting payback signal holding onto the past; being stuck in pain and anger from the past is the result. Forgiveness and acceptance do not include forgetting, they are about allowing love to trump pain by not allowing it to pull us into the past.

Couples can escape the harmful habit of allowing their painful past to steal the joy of the present by practicing a variety of useful efforts. Holding onto anger and withholding emotion are negative habits that keep a painful past alive. Better to speak up the moment a problem arises. By using language of the present, the current moment is accentuated. While difficult to do, because our culture celebrates the past and future as much as the present, turning up the volume of the present is a worthy effort. Past events may be the source of unresolved pain, but the pain itself and its associated emotions are lived in the present. If, in discussion with the partner, the emotions that are presently experienced are shared without introducing the originating past events, the injury at hand is much more likely to be attended to and resolved in the present without defensiveness or conflict.

Few places in our lives require more forgiveness than our love relationships, where hurts, hopefully unintentional, occur regularly. The closer we are to another, the greater chance we will be hurt by them. Resolution of these hurts must happen in the present. When hurt, the more quickly repair is accomplished, the less chance that an unresolved hurt will fuel additional problems. Partners do this by speaking up soon after a hurt has been felt with a request for an action to complete the repair. Wants and needs exist in the present. "I want an apology; I require to be understood." What can be done to solve this now? The plan of action, in word and deed may resolve an injury.

Partners too easily follow the path of redressing past wrongs by repetitively listing all their old injuries. In doing so, the accumulated painful emotion is pulled with force from the past. An accused partner, facing an onslaught of recriminations, will usually grow defensive, hurt, and angry. While arguing about the past, and often debating about whose version of the past is more accurate, partners escalate their tensions while adding another negative chapter to their dissatisfying relationship history. Far more productive, albeit less dramatic, is to request an appropriate current remedy. The present is where positive change and growth bloom. Love happens in the present.

> Hold onto the past
> and your NOW
> will be contaminated
> by it.

10-13. Strong and Loving

It takes two strong partners to make one strong love relationship. Of the two essential ingredients in a relationship, love and strength, love is the most valued, while strength is the most often overlooked. In a successful relationship, the strength of partners is one of the less romantic qualities, but without it, a couple is not likely to maintain a successful relationship.

Without strength, a person has difficulty loving another well, no matter how loving she or he is. Love only lasts when hurtfulness is minimized, and weak partners often unintentionally cause harm. Strength is required for a partner to achieve balance, and hurts occur when a partner strays too far into an extreme, away from that balance. Examples are numerous; a partner who devotes too much time to work and not enough to the partner, a partner who fails to control spending, one who habitually speaks before thinking, a partner who expresses sudden explosive anger, or the partner who doesn't control a drinking habit. It is far easier, in the short run, to avoid a tough issue than to use strength to make a positive change. However, in the long run, being weak has a high price. Of the two, strength and weakness, strength is more rare. Strong partners take responsibility both for their actions and for producing results, whereas weak partners avoid or deflect responsibility.

Loving another is difficult; it always tests lovers in their weakest places. During moments of adversity, painful emotion is provoked. A strong partner is able to tolerate discomfort while maintaining the integrity of values. Loving another includes accepting differences between partners. Living with differences causes tension and friction and may also activate old, painful wounds. Without strength, a partner may avoid the risk of a conflict, a necessary evil to resolve differences.

Two elements within a relationship, unless balanced, cause opposition. Each partner is simultaneously an individual and a part of a united couple. Balancing these two is a juggling act that cannot succeed without strength. Each of us is born separately, so both individuality and connected togetherness must be honored. At times, being strong means setting limits and boundaries so that individuality can thrive, yet, at the same time, partners are part of one couple. Relationships demand openness in which individuality is temporarily surrendered.

A strong partner is able to tolerate the risks and discomfort that openness and vulnerability require, whereas a weaker partner avoids them by emotionally shutting down. Loving another constantly demands using strength to manage discomfort. Examples are: using strength to assert and vocalize needs, expressing anger without hurting the other, tolerating the risk and vulnerability when requesting greater sharing, openness and connection, and risking conflict by raising an unpopular but important issue.

Love alone, without strength, is not useful or effective. Children who are generously loved, but without strong consequences for misbehavior, become spoiled. Paint alone will not beautify anything unless it is applied to a surface. Light when traveling through space is invisible; it only shows up when reflecting off an object. Love is similar. Without strength, love will not produce wonderful results; combined with strength, this is possible. Strength is a turn-on. Without strength, the respect and attraction between partners may quickly fade away.

Most partners dream of everlasting love. Each relationship is a hope for a lifelong union. Committed partners verbally declare their intentions by stating, "Till death do us part." Long-term relationships are marathons, not sprints; without the strength of endurance, partners simply will not have what it takes to make a relationship happily last. Being strong means loving even when angry; facing fear when it rises up and remaining open even when hurt. The journey of an everlasting, ever-loving relationship will be long if both partners possess strength in addition to love.

10-14. Gridlock: It's Knot Love

Romantic couples have a bad habit of getting tied up in knots. Each partner influences the other with the intention of giving love or being loved in a satisfying way. Partner differences, which early in the relationship are a source of attraction, if unresolved, can years later become the energizing force in the ever-tightening knot of gridlock. Every partner wants to be loved, and typically feels loved in the beginning. So within a relationship, if this feeling of love fades, which it normally does, a partner attempts to solve this problem in his or her natural way, a way that they believe will maximize the possibility of success. Yet partners consistently fail to consider that the other partner functions differently and therefore must be influenced in a way that feels loving to the other partner, otherwise the effort will fail to produce the desired result. A successful solution always requires love.

Gridlock is an ever-tightening relationship knot that grows more and more uncomfortable. Tension builds, misunderstandings increase, conflicts become more frequent, disconnection becomes normal. Some couples stay in this miserable stand-off for decades while pretending to the outside world that all is fine. During moments of elevated hope, partners push and pull at each other, intending to loosen the knot of gridlock, but men and women build connections in opposite ways, a difference that often contributes to the formation of relationship gridlock. Opposing strategies result in a kind of tug-of-war, with each attempting to effect positive change using a method that is ultimately dissatisfying to the other. As each pulls, the knot grows tighter.

Imagine you are wearing laced shoes, and at the end of a long day, you are eager to get your shoes off. So you pull at the double-knotted lace hoping it will unravel easily giving immediate relief to your hot and tired feet, a high-risk maneuver. Instead, the knot refuses. With frustration, you pull again with more force, and again the knot does not give. If you then do what romantic partners do, with mounting frustration you pull again and again with even more strength, the knot clenches even more tightly. Pulling the lace was the wrong effort, and repeating the same action with more force only made it worse. Only a change of strategy, a rethinking of the problem, will solve the puzzle. Trying a new strategy, that is focused and careful instead of forceful, is like patiently finding the part of lace that will start the loosening process, it will cause the knot to unravel and lead to success.

Romantic partners in gridlocked relationships tend to repeat the same efforts, like pulling at the shoelace again and again. It is the wrong kind of effort to begin with, but each time more force is used with anger or resentment, and it continually fails. When the results are disappointing, partners distance themselves and withdraw their love.

Unilateral efforts are less likely to be part of a successful solution, and tend to increase frustration, because satisfying relationships are made from both partners loving simultaneously. One partner's effort to loosen the knot may succeed if it is guided by the understanding that you can only change yourself and not your partner. A second vital strategy is based on the truth that every effort, in order to be successful, must feel loving to the other, otherwise it will be rejected. An old knot will not immediately respond to new loving efforts. Before the knot of gridlock begins to loosen, patience and the passage of time are required while the right loving efforts are repeated at the right intensity. Only after the right kinds of love are flowing simultaneously in both directions between partners will the gridlock be gone, replaced by the positive feeling of togetherness.

10-15. Honey and Money

Money joins sex and parenting in the top three most common issues about which couples argue. Money, the lifeblood of our capitalist culture, has a substantial influence on individual partners and couples. How we use money expresses our fundamental values and emotional truths, and also reveals partner differences. Used well, money can fund our hopes and dreams, but more fundamentally, it also procures security and status. Loaded with importance and meaning, money complicates our love relationships.

Money contributes in a significant way to self-determination and self-expression. Autonomy and self-esteem play important roles in all life choices, and our most deeply held values show up in our spending habits. Money, therefore, reflects differences in partner values. If one partner cherishes security, while the other craves asset growth, the differing tolerance of risk will show up in money-related conflicts. The priority of planning for the future versus spending money to enjoy today is a common generator of partner tension.

Money is an energy storage container. The energy and intelligence devoted to work are stored in saved dollars, and may be released later when those dollars are spent. The link between money and power is absolute; with more money comes more influence, choice, and freedom. When partners are not aligned, money accentuates partner differences the way MSG enhances food flavor. Within couples, the distribution of power is commonly unequal, and when one partner unilaterally manages the money the resulting power imbalance can undermine goodwill between partners.

Couples who communicate and coordinate well about money benefit from a brighter future in terms of reaching goals and realizing dreams. Successful money management requires discipline and self-control, both practices that build strength of character. Unchecked, money-related problems will infect other relationship areas, harming a loving connection for example. Regular gentle, positive, and honest conversations about the state of the finances may help to protect a relationship from a power imbalance.

In general, people invest much time, energy and money into soothing activities. When partners are anxious, stressed, or depressed, seeking ways to feel better is a universal pursuit. Products, events and activities which provide pleasure are susceptible to becoming out-of-balance compulsions and addictions, and financial dangers. Alcohol, drugs, and gambling are the obvious culprits, but other "guilty pleasures" such as shopping, collecting, food, video games, online sexual activities, sports betting, and fantasy leagues can easily become habitual and expensive. Impulse-spending is also a financially dangerous behavior pattern. Enjoying pleasure in itself may not be harmful, but these activities, which are often used to make the partner feel better, offer no long-lasting solution to emotionally-based difficulties. When a partner spends money to soothe emotional discomfort, the chances of financial problems occurring are high.

When money is scarce, all money-related differences between partners are magnified, as is the potential for money-related conflict. Consequently, it is easy to assume that people who have money in abundance have no problems, but with wealth come unique struggles. Those who have limited access to money commonly wish for wealth as a solution to their woes, yet many who suddenly receive wealth through a lottery or inheritance find the windfall to be disruptive and destructive. It is hard to live a dream, but harder to live without one; wealth brings a heavy burden and may rob an unprepared beneficiary of motivation and life purpose.

Wealth does not eliminate difficulties or emotional pain, in actuality, it replaces common money struggles with other worries; guilt, fear, and distrust. A wealthy person developing new relationships may worry about whether a new friend likes them or their money more. In couples where one partner has a financial abundance and the other has little money, issues can be divisive.

Money, integrated tightly into our everyday lives, has a strong influence on our individual health and love relationships. It is among the most common sources of conflict between partners because money's use reflects our values, strengths, weaknesses, and emotional discomforts, but also magnifies partner differences. Money itself will not solve emotional problems, even though life is easier with it than without. And, of course, money will never buy love.

10-16. Powerful Understanding

What does it mean to be really understood? People and partners often say they understand, but saying so neither confirms nor proves that they do. The power of full understanding is great, such as the satisfaction and excitement we feel when someone really "gets us." Many crave to be fully understood; being misunderstood is painful. When two people form a deep connection, they share a world view in which understanding feels complete and a deeper life purpose is validated. Without understanding, relationships deteriorate.

Understanding literally means "standing under", as in “supporting”, the way a foundation holds up a house, keeping it upright and stable. When great compassion is offered in conjunction with understanding, agreement is not necessary; we can acknowledge another's pain or joy without agreeing with them. Offering understanding is a form of loving in which listening is the active loving ingredient. Attentive listening occurs when the listener hears not only the speaker's words, but also the experience expressed underneath them. In complete understanding, our pains and passions are completely received by another.

Much of the pain of life comes from the separateness of individuality, a painful condition that is lessened by enjoying others' company and by coupling with another in love. Romantic togetherness typically soothes the separateness for a number of years before differences overshadow similarities. The opportunity of understanding, if rigorously practiced, builds bridges between separate worlds. The connection offered by deep understanding, even without agreement, creates a shared experience. Being understood chases the clouds of aloneness away. When two people are in complete understanding, it is as if they are of one mind.

The personal worlds of romantic partners diverge when a relationship is troubled with problems. Understanding is among the right tools to repair the rift, but to do so, skilled listening, free of defensiveness, must be offered. Certainly, it is a huge challenge for partners where both are in pain. Understanding begins with the openness necessary to learn about the other's experience. When defensiveness is present, the reception of sharing, from which understanding is built, is blocked. Judgement is a form of defensiveness that is one of the many obstacles to understanding. Eliminating defensiveness is key to problem-solving and connection building.

Problems, of which misunderstanding is a common one, generate anger. When we are misunderstood, it is a painful rejection or abandonment. And the opposite is true as well, understanding reduces anger the way water puts out fire. Understanding comforts anger and pain by non-verbally saying, "Let me join you in your pain; we will bear it together." Where there is deep understanding, there is little anger, because there will be few injuries.

More than being simply a way to resolve difficulties, understanding is one of the materials from which a loving bond is built, the stuff of relationship hopes and dreams. Being close, having a sense of connection, and being part of togetherness all require understanding. Words give hope that being warmly connected to another is possible, while a subsequent action proves whether that hope was well deserved. Behavior that is consistent with a verbal understanding shows that this understanding is complete. After all, action has the potential to show that the phrase "I understand" is more than just two words. In action, an understanding partner demonstrates "I get you."

When the connection between two people has deteriorated, deliberate problem-solving discussions may rejuvenate closeness. Positive, solution-oriented language with respect for the other's perspective creates an environment in which understanding can grow. Great care practiced by both partners protects the potential for getting close again because, just as the winds of hurt can easily blow out the flame of love, careless hurtful words chase all possibility of understanding away.

10-17. Valentine's Day Duty

Dozens of red hearts adorn walls in kids' classrooms; the pharmacies are filled with Valentine's cards and candies; Valentine's Day requires action. On the day, most people will express their holiday-imposed love for their lovers and important others who fill their lives. In unison, many will do their best to avoid the hurt and relationship complications that forgetting to do their Valentine's Day duty could cause. Even when the romantic connection has been polluted with resentment, anger, and disappointment, expressing love is still necessary.

When it comes from the deepest place within our hearts, love can never be insincere, but on the surface, inauthentic love acts as a non-nutritious placeholder for the real thing. How many partners long for a sense of real closeness and intimacy when in their daily life they are enduring a cool stand-off? Valentine's Day can be a painful reminder of what is missing. It captures dissatisfied partners in a bind; either be inauthentic and make gestures of love to keep the peace, or do nothing and make the loudest silent statement that their feeling for the partner isn't what it should be, while also risking hurt and conflict. How many Valentine's Days have been damaged by the failure to adequately live up to the expectations?

Love relationships are difficult, especially lengthy marriages in which the marathon of decades severely tests warmth and passion. The awkward discomfort is raised into awareness on Valentine's Day, when the expected love expressions must coincide with the resentment, disappointment and anger which block access to real love felt deeper in the heart. The longer two people have been in a relationship, the more time has elapsed for irritating behaviors, habits, and personality differences to accumulate into large amounts of resentment and bitterness.

Most couples possess a handful of intractable difficulties that could be accurately called perpetual problems. Through the decades, perpetual problems defy every attempt at a solution, usually because their source is deeply formed personality characteristics. Relationship connections are tested regularly by the frustration that perpetual problems create. Loving connections between partners devolve to the point where they are just unromantic roommates, as passionate feelings are doused with the poison of bitterness. Hopelessness swells as the saying, "Can't teach an old dog new tricks," paints a bleak picture of future unhappiness; not the situation in which a Valentine can be shared authentically.

Change happens every day, even dramatic change. Unfortunately, such a change usually develops in sudden response to an emergency by which normal routine and security are deeply threatened. Amazing results become possible when a person dives deep into his or her being and when what is most important is risked. It is said that a problem cannot be solved on the same level on which it was first created; instead, a jump occurs onto a new and higher level, and this is known as a paradigm shift. From the perspective of personality and love, a paradigm shift represents an expansion of personality and the expansion of the capacity to love. Each one of us is capable of spontaneously creating such a shift if the quality of our life, relationship, and love are important enough.

Each one of us may avoid the need for abrupt and catastrophic change if we use our strength to make many small incremental adjustments. If partners practice a willingness to make minor changes, by adjusting to love a little bit each day, large painful changes are unnecessary. Practicing giving love regularly allows each Valentine's Day to be an opportunity to express love that is genuine and feels good.

10-18. Honesty Between Us

"Honesty is the best policy," is a phrase which has been repeated for generations. Yet in our love relationships, most partners are not very honest, and indeed, within a relationship, honesty may not even be the best policy. An episode of a television show comes to mind in which the two main characters, a man and woman who were intimate at times, were suddenly graced with the ability to read each other's minds. Beyond being comical and entertaining, the newfound honesty caused visible hurt, as each character became aware of the way the other viewed and judged them.

Dishonesty has several tiers of severity, from kind to cruel. Have you ever told your male partner how good he was at something, even when you were not so impressed by his accomplishment? Have you ever told your female partner how beautiful her new hairstyle was, when in reality the style was not immediately to your liking? Have you ever reassured your partner how deep your love is, when at the moment you are just not feeling it? Many dishonesties are offered with the intention of being kind, offering reassurance and keeping the relationship harmonious.

Withholding feelings is a different kind of dishonesty to the direct telling of lies, but builds inauthenticity into the relationship partner. Other untruths are fear-based, they are about self-protection, about discomfort with self-revelation, or the wish to avoid conflict, since many partners will go to great lengths to avoid conflict. Other untruths are more insidious and selfish, they are about hiding something that will hurt the other partner and could rob them of choice or self-esteem, like the hiding of drug use, an illicit affair, the unilateral discontinuation of birth control pills, or gambling with joint money.

Those things that we call "honesty" are really unflattering thoughts, feelings, and opinions that, if expressed, would likely cause hurt. Painful, uncomfortable and awkward issues fill this category. Our partner never has to fear being told about his or her virtues and strengths, but when talking honestly about a problem or problematic partner trait, appreciation is unlikely. Typical reactions include defensiveness, emotional shutting-down, argumentative denial, or even counterattack. Other partners build strong defenses to ensure that certain kinds of honest sharing never occur. There are myriad defensive methods partners use to put up large emotional stop-signs, signaling that the other's honesty is unwelcome. Many partners silently dance around each other's vulnerabilities by choosing against honest sharing. Negative responses cause an honesty-seeking partner to wisely remain quiet.

Relationships where honest sharing occurs only within the intensity of a heated argument are not uncommon. In this instance, honesty is used as a weapon, its sharp edge employed to intentionally wound. In these relationships, honesty is strongly associated with pain. How good is honesty when you are bludgeoned by it? When combined with the poor impulse control of an excitable partner, honesty creates an emotionally unsafe relationship environment. Partners fear sharing their real selves due to the concern that what is shared will be used as a weapon against them at a later time.

In theory, honesty is great. If romantic partners are completely open, the relationship has greater potential to be very loving, deep and real. A gentle but honest conversation may be cleansing to a relationship, clearing the accumulation of years of emotional discord in just a few minutes. Honesty can be powerful. But in the politics of intimate relationships, openness is often feared and avoided, due to the risk of vulnerability. Unless partners possess great sensitivity to each others' safety and well-being, such vulnerability puts partners at risk of being harmed, controlled, and abused.

How much of our real, honest feelings and perceptions may be withheld before we become inauthentic? Too many partners hide their real selves within their relationship. Avoiding conflict by regularly choosing safety over authenticity results in the loss of self-respect and a passionate connection. Deep loving includes never putting the other in the position of having to make that self-deprecating choice. The possibility of relationship dissatisfaction and an accumulation of resentment increases dramatically when honest sharing is emotionally unsafe. Partners who cannot be true to their individual uniqueness are powerless to love themselves or to create a loving, alive and vital relationship.

Love relationships are a machine for growth, and honest sharing may be regarded as the teeth on the gears of that machine. Romantic partners first need to be secure in love and acceptance, before they can look past the harshness of honesty and see its usefulness. Each incident of honesty is a request for change which simultaneously sends the message that in some way the partner is not good enough. A relationship's growth potential is damned when honest sharing is rejected, which it will be if it is too painful.

Striving to have high levels of honesty in a love relationship requires that honest sharing be consistently greeted with patience, positivity, and good impulse control. If it is not, honesty will feel too unsafe. When structured with disciplined diplomacy, honesty allows the sharing of deep, important feelings that forges a special intimacy, but a lot of strength is required. How much honesty can your relationship bear?

At its root, honesty is about being real; allowing the authentic you to be shared and to be loved. However, honest sharing will be disregarded and rendered ineffective if it is delivered hurtfully. The care and compassion of practicing to avoid causing harm is of a higher order than honesty, which is not always the best policy. Sharing honestly in small doses, while also practicing care and kindness may allow for authenticity. It is important that your truth is shared, but more important is that it is shared lovingly.

> You do not have the power to change your partner, but you do have the power to change yourself.

10-19. Marriage: To Stay or To Go

In disappointment and hopelessness, an unhappy spouse considers divorce for months or years before finally deciding to end the marriage. The process of decision-making is uncomfortable, as the spouse suffers vacillation and dissatisfaction. Being miserable within a marriage can cause one to feel crazy, since within the debate to stay or to go, a spouse must weigh opposing issues of great intensity. Many an unhappy marital partner is paralyzed by the enormity of the choice, which can devastate the spouse, children, family, community, and the quality of life thereafter. Tremendous inner conflict may also play into decision-making paralysis, as deeply held core values are in conflict with shallower, but nonetheless influential, emotional dissatisfaction. There is no simple, easy answer. The core values support staying together for a lifetime and honoring that commitment, yet the prospect of a lifetime of dissatisfaction is hard to bear. It is difficult to argue against divorce in a marriage in which violence, infidelities and addictions have killed all hopes of love; remaining married amounts to living in a house even after it has burned down. But even in unions which are not unhappy to such an extreme, the dilemma of staying or going is made unresolvable by spouses who fail to enact the growth and change necessary to provide relief or repair.

Broader society, too, is in conflict about the merits and morality of divorce. Promises and commitments receive lip service from good people, but integrity and honor are routinely and publicly abandoned by corporations, politicians and others seeking competitive advantage. Contrary to the spiritual ideals referred to in most marriage vows, it is not all that long ago that divorce was shameful and stigmatizing. An internet search of divorce statistics reveals that since the 1860's, when divorce was rare, there has been an almost continuous increase in divorce rates, so that now divorce ends about 50% of marriages. Divorce, now viewed as awkwardly normal, is so common that an adult is just as likely to have experienced divorce as not.

Due to the way our society has changed, divorce seems almost like a normal developmental transition that most adults routinely go through at common points of age and relationship stage. If not for the damage to the kids, (children of divorced parents are less likely to have life-long marriages), we might look at the prevalence of divorce as suggesting that society is progressing towards a more fluid and flexible attitude regarding love and relationships. The idea that marriage could be a time-limited contract in which both partners agree to re-evaluate and re-up at predetermined intervals seems to fit with how marriage is actually being lived. Yet couples who have children tend to stay in their marriages longer than childless ones. It takes a child eighteen to twenty years to mature sufficiently for successful independence, yet the average length of a marriage which ends in divorce is approximately seven years. Such divorces interrupt parenting before the job is finished and provide society with damaged future generations. We may be witnessing a cycle that is accelerating.

We are challenged to journey away from the reality that divorce is a failure. It is painful. It is destructive. There are wounds and losses. It is the breaking of a sacred commitment. Divorce is a triumph of ego over the spirit. Marriage vows, traditional or not, use language and concepts that are spiritual; referring to the eternal in "the rest of our days," and being unconditional in loving; promises of absolutes such as being by each other's side through good times and bad. Marriage vows point to the promises of human growth and the potential of pure love. Most couples, in the honeymoon phase of their union, experience in the bliss of new love the eternal and the perfect; they want more of this. The spouses who opt for divorce have concluded that this promise of complete love has no chance of fulfillment. Many a spouse has contributed to the hopelessness by failing to love deeply enough.

The commitment to strive for this potential and stand for each other's well-being (to honor and cherish) is the catalyst that forms a secure and stable environment well-suited for raising healthy children and transforming incomplete love. The huge increase in the frequency of divorce suggests that many perceive the commitment in marriage as optional, depending upon whether or not happiness is maintained. This appears to be an unreasonable expectation due to the hard work required to maintain a marriage. Millions of spouses experience the promise of transformation as empty and unattainable; unhappiness, partner failings, and poor quality of love prove that the early promise of complete love is unlikely.

The culture in which we live has gotten better at encouraging the flourishing of our desires, while also convincing us that the satisfaction of our desires is life's purpose. Buying into this message, unhappy spouses feel increasingly justified to pursue happiness by divorcing rather than doing the challenging marital work which requires holding tight to deep core values. Indeed, ancient spiritual traditions suggest that the transformation we crave, the one referred to in our marriage vows, is accomplished by rigorously holding tight to core values.

Divorce does not deliver the sought-after happiness, though it may provide short-lived relief. Statistics support this by showing that second and third marriages fall into divorce at a higher rate than first ones, also implying that divorce does not teach ex-spouses to love any better. Simultaneously, those same statistics do not suggest that spouses who stay married are any happier, so could happiness, fleeting by nature, be a misplaced goal?

Regarding the question to stay or to go, there is neither a right nor wrong answer. It is a certainty that a spouse caught between these options will suffer. It is a choice. Leaving an unhappy marriage and being true to oneself may bring short-term relief from emotional distress. Staying, and using strength and grit to remain in line with eternal values, part of the journey of the soul, is hard. Both choices will ultimately provide the necessary life lessons. There are no shortcuts to growth. Both roads will have potholes and steep grades, but also beautiful vistas.

10-20. That's Close Enough

There is an assumption made by most who wish to establish a romantic partnership that the union will lead to a satisfyingly close connection. Closeness is not deeply considered because it is seen as automatic; love relationship partners are naturally close. If asked about his or her ideal relationship, most if not all partners would indicate that "real close" is preferred, as in, "We're real close, we share everything." Unlike our fantasies, which are cleaned of real-life complications and irritations, achieving real romantic closeness is not so simple, and is sometimes impossible. In theory, “very close” sounds good; in reality, the preferred amount of closeness by partners varies along a broad spectrum from continuous constant togetherness, to barely communicating or being in the same place at the same time. Within many couples is a battle over closeness.

During the honeymoon phase of a relationship, idyllic closeness is easily achieved. Neither a partner's true capacity for nor comfort with closeness is demonstrated during this "trial" phase of loving; it is instead revealed much later, roughly one to three years after the relationship has been fully established. Closeness is not always a good thing, for example, avoiding closeness with a hurtful partner, due to a justified need for self-protection, is wise. Also, as relationships age, closeness is commonly reduced by partner distancing, a patterned reaction to unresolved issues, accumulation of anger, bitterness, and resentments as well as the normal maturing of individuality.

Not all partners value equally the different actions and efforts that build closeness, and which are considered normal parts of a love relationship. Affectionate touch is universally cited as important for health and relationship satisfaction, but some partners are uncomfortable with it. Cuddling and snuggling are craved by many, but those residing at the lower end of the closeness spectrum find that these forms of togetherness trigger a claustrophobic reaction. For as many partners who love kissing, there are many others who would rather avoid it. Closeness may also be generated by sharing thoughts, feelings, experiences, ideas, etc., but a great many people prefer to keep much of this hidden inside, a habit that accentuates individuality over togetherness. With the passage of time, partner differences regarding a preferred level of closeness often spread to polar extremes.

Unresolved differences with closeness cause a build-up in tension between partners, an issue which might appropriately be titled, "The battle over the relationship thermostat." How "warm" should a relationship be? A close relationship is regarded as a warm one, whereas a less close union is considered cool, or even cold. In couples where partners prefer a different relationship temperature, each partner advocates for his or her preferred level, much in the same way that one partner who prefers the house warmer might turn the thermostat up, while the other secretly turns it down. In a cycle where the thermostat is repeatedly turned up and down, tension and frustration build, just when warm and cold air meet in the weather outside, storms may result.

How much closeness is ideal? The best answer should include a delicate balancing act, where individuality is eclipsed by closeness as little as possible, but individuality does not prevent closeness. Partner satisfaction is maximized while each partner is challenged to grow. The paradox is that two strong partners, who can each assert themselves, but who are also secure enough to surrender to the relationship union, may develop the greatest closeness. Partners who do not possess individual strength and confidence tend to have trouble building and maintaining positive and stable closeness.

The individual characteristics which inhibit healthy and balanced closeness are varied. Partners who crave intense, extreme closeness tend to be troubled with insecurity and crave love to obtain validation of their own worthiness. For some partners like this, no amount of closeness is enough. To those suffering fear and anxiety, great closeness with a partner feels soothing and comforting. Any extreme need from one partner will provoke an opposing and balancing response from the other.

At the other end of the spectrum there are those who react in the opposite way to inner self-doubt, by avoiding closeness and promoting separateness. Such partners flee opportunities to connect by sharing little and choosing activities which take time and energy away from the togetherness, sometimes to the point where no real relating remains. Staying away from closeness reduces the risk of emotionally "losing oneself" in the relationship, or of really being known.

No good comes without a cost. The cost of closeness is vulnerability. Connecting with another and sharing ourselves cannot happen without opening the door to let the other in. The risk and subsequent fear of vulnerability, and how partners try to keep it at low levels, often rules relationships. Among those who desperately avoid vulnerability are partners who have previously been hurt or traumatized. Partners attempt indirect efforts to keep risks of closeness low, including bickering, criticism, negativity, avoidance of risk, and sabotaging behaviors such as lying, cheating and making unilateral choices that may directly or indirectly keep closeness and its associated vulnerability at bay.

Each one of us is born separate, yet simultaneously we are part of a single unified humanity. The challenge to surrender our individuality in favor of a union is a universal struggle, whether it be on a grand scale of merging in spirit, or the smaller scale of a human union of love. The emotionally strong partner can tolerate the vulnerability of love and closeness; it takes two strong partners to make closeness satisfying.

10-21. Growing Together

Growth is a part of the natural order. Each tree grows for years to reach its full height. Rivers flow relentlessly to their final rest in the sea. Love relationships form nature's preferred way to encourage our growth. When two people, in their attraction and chemistry for each other, join their lives in love they participate, consciously or not, in the natural process of growth.

Conventional wisdom says do not try to change your partner, but this goes against the natural order. Every partner in every relationship, functioning as nature's agent, urges, even insists at times, that his or her loved one grow beyond their limitations and imperfect love. Each lover wants the other to grow towards completeness, to fulfill the dream of a complete partner who is strong and whose love is deep and transformative.

Our intense thirst for growth and completion is almost equally balanced by our fear of, and resistance to, that very same progress. Within love relationships, there are challenges, and each individual lover is tested. The relationship and love raise issues ripe for positive change, but wherever love exists it creates an arena for growth. Nevertheless, loving another is extremely difficult; causing the weakest places in partners to be exposed. Relationships are full of problems, although they are often hidden from public view; these problems are evidence that growth is needed. The problems are the growth lessons.

Most partners, acting as comes naturally, will pressure, nag, coerce, bribe, beg, and even force the other to overcome their limitations. On the surface, the purpose of a wish for change is to alleviate individual frustration and pain, but on a grander scale, it functions as a push for growth as a part of natural progress. Romantic partners in a couple simultaneously request growth in each other, offering mutual reflections of imperfections by targeting areas where love is incomplete. A byproduct of the work of growth is the negative reputation earned by relationships and marriage.

When a partner's influence is ignored, or rebuffed with a refusal to grow, the long-term harm to the relationship is considerable. When a river is dammed, water builds up under stress until an alternative way forward is patiently found, and any obstacle will eventually be worn away, even if it takes a million years; think of the Colorado River and the Grand Canyon that it formed. Partners are not so patient. Love will not be denied its growth, even if the relationship fails as a result. In reaction to resisting growth, tension builds between partners. The openness that is so necessary for love to flow begins to close up, anger or resentment accumulates, conflicts erupt, and pain and contempt pollute the connection. Growth is a necessity within a loving union. There are certain kinds of fish that cannot breathe and will die if not moving forward; relationships are like that. If they are not growing, relationships stagnate, and the spirit of love dies. An exception is a codependent relationship where partners mutually support each other's avoidance of growth; an intentional eddy that temporarily escapes the river's flow towards completion in the sea.

Change is constant, but growth is a choice. Each one of us will change, like it or not; for instance, we all age effortlessly. A superior alternative to change is growth, when we deliberately respond to a challenge by opening and expanding instead of shrinking from an issue. Growth always leads to opening, not just to a partner, but to deeper parts of the self, love and life. The many difficulties that confront a couple represent opportunities for each partner and the couple to grow. A love relationship is like a growth machine; it constantly presents each lover with evidence of personal obstacles, so the opportunities to grow are repeatedly faced.

For all its benefits, growth is not easy. Just as when ice melts into water the ice must lose itself, as we grow we become different, and who we were is lost. To grow means first looking at ourselves without blinders, and acknowledging that we could be better, more complete. When unresolved injuries block the way of growth, sometimes healing must take place. Courage and effort must be mobilized to advance towards improvement.

The most common reason that partners oppose growth is a wish to avoid fear, discomfort, and pain. The strategies used to prevent growth are many, including avoidance, defensiveness, irresponsibility, blame, and denial. Every method of hiding from growth only delays the inevitable. Just as a serious weightlifter will increase the weight on the barbell to the point where it is almost too heavy to lift, our love will challenge us up to the point of our tolerance.

Growing requires that we leave our comfort zone by accepting discomfort. When growth is chosen, pain is also chosen, but to refuse growth is painful too. Exercising regularly, keeping to a diet, succeeding in business, maintaining sobriety, getting that college degree, eliminating a bad habit, improving one's attitude, and loving in the right way are all hard. To do so, however, increases our capacity to love ourselves, others and life, which will not end life's suffering, but will facilitate the development of pride, self-satisfaction and a positive love relationship along the way.

Built into a love relationship is the expectation of growth. Your partner is your personal growth agent, who hopefully delivers the growth lessons in a loving way. The ecstatic connection most couples enjoyed early in their union may be recaptured as a reward for growing. Cooperating with nature's design for our growth allows love to flow.

10-22. Too Stressed Out

Couples who seek to improve their relationship consistently underestimate the negative influence of stress on their togetherness. Just as when we breathe, we rarely think about air, the impact of stress tends to be minimized by many. Yet modern culture, the environment in which couples function, is fast-paced, rushed, always-on with never enough time. Stress is produced in abundance by the countless demands placed upon us. Families, and the couples who head them, are unprotected from being overwhelmed; unhealthy levels of stress magnify problems and make resolving them more difficult, and when the burden is too heavy, balance is impossible to achieve. The prevailing stressful environment is hostile to healthy intimate relationships.

When water is stirred in a barrel, once the paddle is removed the water continues to spin. Our emotions are like that; once stressful events cease, our emotions don't calm immediately; many partners do not have sufficient time to calm down before the next set of unsettling demands arrive. As a result, many people seemingly lose the capacity to relax, and chronic anxiety and agitation result. With ceaseless demands, romantic partners have less than enough time together to maintain their intimate bond, and when partners do find time to be together, each remains stressed, anxious and exhausted; not the centered qualities necessary to enjoy a strong and passionate connection.

Our modern technologies, such as cell phones, offer the convenience of anywhere, anytime communication, but also mean that we can be reached almost anywhere at any time; they interrupt undisturbed down-time. Choosing to be available is a thing of the past; the modern twist is choosing to be unavailable. In other words, by default the assumption is for constant availability, and we are under exhausting pressure to be "always on."

A good friendship is hopefully at the core of an intimate relationship. It is nourished by having enough together-time, while sharing enjoyable, relaxing interests and challenges. When stress and demands are too high, relaxing and enjoyable activities are commonly deemed inessential and are allowed to fall away. Under such circumstances, core friendships grow malnourished and die. When demands are unreasonably high standard values of integrity, commitment, and dependability break down, but for trust to remain a solid relationship cornerstone, these vital values must be maintained.

Under the burden of great stress, partner differences are magnified and grow intractable. Personalities distort and tend towards the extreme; partners fall back on simplistic, often infantile ways of coping; these undermine mutual respect. The challenge of loving, already very difficult, becomes nearly impossible when stress is too high. Stressed partners are defensive. To survive the continuous onslaught of insensitive and unfriendly demands, defenses are raised for self-protection. Chronically raised defenses, employed to keep out the worst effects of stressors, are not selective; they also keep out partners. Stress is draining. Partners look to each other for much needed emotional nourishment, but a drained partner has little left to give. When both partners feel this way, friendship and connections fail.

If left unchecked, chronic stress produces physical health problems such as heart disease and a weakened immune system, increasing our susceptibility to disease and illness. Emotionally, too much stress increases our vulnerability to anxiety disorders and depression. Exhaustion mimics the symptoms of depression, and sleep problems are common among those harmed by our hectic lifestyle. An ability to be emotionally available is essential to be a good partner, a quality that unhealthy and unbalanced conditions impair. Furthermore, stress erodes one's capacity for patience; irritability, negativity, and a quickness to anger result.

Protecting ourselves from the harmful effects of chronic high levels of stress is essential to keeping a relationship satisfying and long-lasting. When it comes to the quality of life, less can be more. By living simply, we grasp the opportunity to live more freely with a lower stress level. Couples make many good choices in pursuit of fulfilling dreams, but good and bad choices equally invite unhealthy levels of stress. Getting another pet, buying a vacation home, joining another club, or allowing a child to play multiple sports are seemingly good choices, but may add enough stress to tip the scale from manageable to unhealthy, especially if stress is already high. Collecting possessions is easy, but few consider the cost that responsibility and ownership add in terms of expense and stress. When facing choices, consider the long-term effect on your economy of stress. By keeping the quality of your life and relationship as the highest priority, instead of money or time, you may be protected from the trap that has fatally ensnared many failed couples.

Stress is a problem of contemporary life that no single person will solve, but the following efforts provide some protection from its corrosive effects; regular exercise creates a protective layer of resiliency, meditation nourishes increased compassion, self-compassion, and overall well-being; good nutrition increases vitality; getting enough good quality sleep is protective, but is the first to disappear when stress gets too high. Maintaining a positive attitude combined with positive thoughts will help. Select life options that maximize the number of future choices, because stress that is chosen is healthier than stress that was imposed upon us. Lastly, when together with your partner, make specific periods of cell-phone-free time to give each other undivided attention.

10-23. Stop the Hurt

Some efforts build a loving connection, while others destroy it. For a couple seeking to improve their relationship, ridding their togetherness of harmful actions is the quickest route towards improvement. Negative actions destroy a relationship far more quickly than positive ones improve it, a simple but seemingly unfair reality. The negatives rule the quality of your relationship.

Each negative or hurtful action neutralizes many loving efforts. A general guideline is that one hurtful action eliminates twenty loving ones; a minor incident provoking disappointment or annoyance may only negate five positives, whereas a betrayal may destroy the accumulated benefit of hundreds or even thousands. If the hurtful act is a repetition of one about which complaints have already been lodged, the number of destroyed loving actions increases.

To earn trust, the deep trust that safely encourages a partner to be him or herself and completely open and vulnerable, takes years to accomplish. Actions that negatively impact the partner degrade emotional trust gradually, or prevent it from being earned in the first place. A large hurt may wipe away the trust that took years to build. Emotional trust is a fragile bridge that is easily damaged or destroyed.

The nature of this seemingly unbalanced economy traps many partners. A partner who loves a lot may grow frustrated that his or her loving efforts do not accumulate and manifest in relationship improvement, a possible reason for this is the continual repetition of minor but hurtful behaviors. In the economy of love, he or she may still be running at an emotional deficit if minor hurts chronically occur. Due to the disproportionately large negative impact of "minor" hurts, frequent loving efforts count for little, which may seem unfair. A frustrated partner may come to believe that the other is unreasonable and impossible to please.

In the world beyond relationships, a similar dynamic exists in which negative events are more impactful than positive ones. Examples abound and highlight the same interrelationship. Falling down a mountain is fast, but climbing back up happens slowly, one small step at a time. Negative events are far more likely than positive ones to make the news. In school, a high grade point average is lowered more by an "F" than it is raised by any "A." If your employer arbitrarily chooses to not pay you for a week's work, the negative hit to your trust in the employer will be very high, but each week you get paid only increases your trust marginally. Not getting paid for a week of work will probably motivate you to begin a job search immediately, whereas each week of pay is not incentive enough raise your diligence to win the employee of the year award.

Hurtful actions between partners automatically trigger defensive reactions, signaling that emotional walls are being built. People choose to avoid others who cause them pain or discomfort, but if the hurtful person happens to be the intimate partner, a difficult person to avoid, emotional barriers are the protection of choice to minimize the negative impact. The defenses provide safety, but simultaneously prevent connection. Long-term relationships where hurtfulness has not been eliminated are more characterized by distance than closeness due to the partners' need for emotional protection.

Some of the sources of hurt are subtle while many are obvious. Because long-term relationships are more like marathons than sprints, minor but chronic hurts have a large cumulative negative effect. A dripping faucet, if not repaired, may cause large-scale destruction over the years, even though no single drip is large. Unresolved differences cause chronic tension; criticism erodes goodwill; negativity tires the partner; unrelenting resistance to a partner's influence creates romantic disconnection; weakness sponsors contempt.

Much more benefit is achieved by making efforts to reduce or eliminate negative impacts or hurts within your relationship. Bailing a leaking boat may lead to exhaustion if water flows in steadily, but if the leak is patched, bailing becomes more effective. Commonly, romantic partners direct their energy towards increasing loving efforts. This choice is not bad, but if negative interactions continue, any accrued benefit will quickly neutralize the possibility of real improvement.

When attempting to improve your relationship, your energy is best spent working to eliminate the negatives and hurts first. Identifying the source of hurts in a relationship is easy, but discussing them constructively is not. Anger, intensity, and blame can quickly derail positive efforts, so using great care is essential. To this end, let each partner take alternating turns to receive complete attention regarding the fulfillment of his or her needs. Partners will benefit most if the desired changes are shared, instead of each criticizing the other. Listening well while only offering positive changes will lead toward success.

> Choose to be angry
> or choose to fix the problem.
> You cannot do both.

10-24. Fair Fighting Makes Togetherness Safe

If it weren't for marriage, men and women would fight with total strangers.
—Anonymous

A relationship without conflicts is unusual and may even be unhealthy. While conflict is uncomfortable, it is also normal. It signifies that each partner in the relationship is strong enough to assert his or her own will. Of course, this is all a matter of degree. There are various patterns of relating in which conflict is avoided or reduced, but often at a high emotional cost; where one partner gives up on equally sharing control or power in order to keep the peace.

Each couple have their own unique way of beginning and engaging in a conflict. The amount of resentment built up and their personal individual histories determine the "temperature" of that personal connection. There are couples that are "hot" and only need a small spark to detonate an explosive confrontation, while other couples seem only to smoke and smolder without ever entering a real argument. Conflict generates anger; anger does not need to be hurtful.

The challenge is to have a conflict where the opposing positions are clearly stated; a resolution is reached with some degree of compromise, and no permanent damage is done to either person or the union between them. Each healthy conflict is like a single word in an ongoing negotiation between partners, ever rearranging their togetherness as they change and hopefully mature. So controlled conflicts should not be avoided; they propel couples forward in growth, provided the conflicts are safely resolved.

The following 11 rules, if followed, help to keep arguments constructive, safe and under control:

1. No name calling, threatening remarks, or violence are allowed.
2. No put-downs or personal attacks are allowed.

3. No threats of ending the relationship are allowed.
4. Take turns. Listen attentively, without interruption when the other is talking.
5. Try to enter into conflict when the problem is still new and small.
6. Stay focused only on the issue that caused the conflict.
7. Stay in the present without bringing up past events. One issue at a time.
8. Stick to positive, constructive language that expresses what is wanted or needed.
9. State what you want to be different.
10. Develop a plan of action.
11. Create a standing agreement that if things get too hot, you two will separate for a predetermined length of time. This should be no longer than an hour. Return precisely at that time, ready to discuss the issue more calmly.

Enter conflicts boldly. To become skilled at fair fighting takes practice.

10-25. Let the Games Begin: The Games of Courtship

At the beginning of a new romantic connection, the negotiation between potential partners can feel an awful lot like playing mind games. What is actually happening is that negotiations are underway as to how the relationship should proceed. Each person is also being careful to present as positive an image of themselves as they can, in order to increase their power of choice while decreasing their chance of rejection. This negotiation is about topics like power and control, who accepts what responsibility, and what understandings will be in place for behavioral expectations in the future.

This is the development of the "invisible unspoken contract." Be aware that your choices and behaviors at this early point in the relationship determine how it will go later on, should it last. So if the interactions are not to your liking, or if this other person does or says things which make you uncomfortable, this is the easiest and most effective time to speak up in terms of making changes.

Early on, after meeting someone to whom you are attracted, it is wise to keep in mind various important considerations:

1. Be aware of any old relationship patterns or patterns in your choice of previous partners. Also note any patterns within those relationships. Be mindful that the one to whom you are now attracted will also be part of this pattern. Try to determine what problems occurred in past relationships, and how you may have contributed to their formation.

2. Deliberately slow the relationship's development. The faster your relationship is going, the less control you have. Imagine yourselves in a car, speeding down the highway at eighty miles per hour. The view along the side of the road is a rushing blur, so if there is a beautiful flower on the side of the road, you will not notice it, let alone appreciate its beauty. Now imagine yourselves walking along the road. It is unlikely that you would not notice the flower. It is much easier to stop and appreciate its beauty when you are going slowly.

There is no need to rush; you have the rest of your life to get to know this person and determine if he or she is the right one for you. The beginning of a love relationship is among the sweetest times of your life; savor it slowly, the way you would delicious food. If you take it fast and allow sex to begin quickly, this sweetness will be over too quickly. Taking it slow will give the relationship the best chance of being healthy. Going slow helps you to notice and address problematic situations early in their growth, when they are still small and more responsive to change.

3. Keeping the relationship's development slow prevents your destructive unconscious patterns from asserting themselves. If they do, the old negative patterns that contributed to the

problems in your past relationships are more likely to be repeated once again. These are the choices that either cause you to behave in destructive ways, or cause you to accept destructive behaviors in your partner. Take it slow! Make your actions and choice conscious, not unconscious!

4. Determine your potential partner's intentions. Ask lots of questions. Consider this metaphor: You are traveling to a distant location. You go to the train station to catch a train to take you to where you want to go. You quickly board the nearest train. The train is about to roll. Then you realize that you are uncertain if the train is going to your desired destination. Isn't it best to determine if it is the right train as soon as possible, so you will have the opportunity to get on the right train? When a new person is invited into your life, make sure the new person wants what you want. This way you will avoid becoming attached, only to break-up later because the two of you want a different kind of relationship.

5. Look for "red flags." While getting to know a new person, it is wise to keep yourself alert. Pay attention to all your senses, your thoughts and feelings. Do not let this other person talk you out of your feelings; value them as you would a message from your wisest advisor. Your feelings are your antennae in a love relationship. If you have feelings of discomfort or disrespect, if things don't add up to you, or if something confuses you, trust these feelings! These are warning signs that all may not be right with this person. Proceed with caution. Be on the lookout for red flags: characteristics, situations, and occurrences that do not fit with your values, which reveal character flaws or weaknesses in your potential partner. After weeks or months, if there are no "red flags," or very few, but only minor ones, then you are probably safe.

It is wise to be cautious if this new person has financial troubles. If they ask you for money, let this be a strong warning to eliminate this person as a potential partner. A good partner is one who can be strong, self-sufficient, and responsible. If this person seems to be in a financially bad position and does not ask for money, do not lend them any. To do so is to encourage a dependency, which would prevent them from learning a lesson, and would put destructive pressure on the relationship. If you have grown to value this person and they do have financial problems, let them know that this is a problem, as soon as you are aware of it, and suggest ways they may learn to fix them.

If he or she is not receptive to your observation, or does not take action, you may consider moving on to find someone who is strong enough to be in control of their finances and their life. Finances are one of the issues about which couples argue the most, but lack of integrity is also a major red flag. A good partner's words and actions must match. If a person makes a promise, they must keep it, unless there are reasonable extenuating circumstances. If these kinds of extenuating circumstances seem to occur frequently, then this is a red flag that hidden problems exist, and you should probably stay away. You must practice integrity as well. Lack of honesty and lack of respect for you and others are major red flags.

6. Again, ask lots of questions. If your potential partner does not want to give you answers to your questions, their silence should be a red flag of caution. What is this person looking for in a relationship? What needs do you want to be met in a relationship? Are you ultimately looking for someone to share a committed marriage with you, or are you seeking something more casual? It is of utmost importance that you ask this person about their intentions early on.

Ask about the person's past. Learn about their past relationships and struggles. How did they solve problems in the past? A good problem-solver will be a good "teammate" for you. What kind of people does this potential partner choose as friends? Do these people share your values? How open is this person to seeking outside help should a difficult problem develop? If the two of you do create a long-term relationship, how willing is he or she to fix a problem, no matter what it takes? How do they treat friends and family members? How do they handle money? Is this person willing to be influenced by you and your needs? If not, this is a red flag. Questions, questions, questions!

They do not need to be answered all at once, but these answers are vital to your safety and to your success at choosing a good partner. The process is challenging, but no more challenging than being in a bad or dangerous relationship! Consider the kind of life this person leads. If they have many problems, be aware that by joining your life with theirs, their problems become yours.

7. Arrange it so that the first times spent together are safe and highly informative. Your first few dates are probably best spent in public settings until you have determined that the candidate is trustworthy and safe. For men, realize that female partners may be fearful of spending time with you in unfamiliar or isolated settings. Act in ways that make it easier for her to feel safe and to say yes to your invitation.

Talking is nice, but words deceive more than actions can; you will learn more about this person through their behavior than their words. In a getting-to-know-you situation, each person is on their best behavior, which limits your ability to get to know their true self. Choose an activity that allows you to learn as much as possible about the way a person carries him or herself. People are more likely to relax in situations where they are able to focus on a shared activity, rather than a more direct face-to-face situation. Some good choices are physically active and challenging pastimes such as bowling, tennis, miniature golf, going for walks in a pleasant public place, eating messy foods, and challenging activities.

Activities that are new to the candidate allow you to see this person when they feel awkward or frustrated. While it may be slightly uncomfortable for that person, it allows you to see how they behave when they are not at their best, a predicament in which they will often find themselves if your relationship should last a long time. This kind of togetherness can also provide ample opportunity for laughter and fun, as opposed to an interview-style restaurant dinner. If a person refuses to enter a new kind of situation, consider why; if they cannot handle their anxiety, how will this person be able to handle the anxiety provoked by deep intimacy, an essential for a good relationship.

8. Delay sex as long as you can; this helps to rule out potential mates whose main interest in you is motivated solely by gaining sexual gratification. You should not be having sex with a new person with whom you are still uncomfortable talking about sex, asking about their sexual history, and asking if they have a sexually transmitted disease. If you would be uncomfortable sharing your sexual history with this person then you probably do not know them well enough. Remember, the two of you can talk about sex without being sexual. Doing so can add deliciously to the exciting build-up of sexual anticipation. Sex can be talked about as a way of determining if this new person may be sexually compatible and share similar sexual values.

While single, and while exploring the possibility of a relationship, masturbation can be not only a pleasurable relief from the build-up of sexual tension, but it can also be valuable practice to get to know your own sexual response more fully. This will better enable you to teach your future partner how to please you. During your single days, try to learn to be the best lover you can, for when that time arrives. If you are a woman, you might practice Kegel exercises so as to improve your sexual responsiveness. If you are a man, you might practice developing strong ejaculatory control.

If sex occurs too early, the relationship will speed up dramatically in its emotional intensity, reducing your ability to choose what happens. Once sex has been experienced, your emotions will become more fully involved, causing you to be much less rational, and therefore less able to be aware of all that is happening. Old unconscious patterns assert themselves more strongly after sex has become part of a relationship. If your partner wishes to be sexual and you are not ready, this person will demonstrate the depth of his or her of love for you by waiting. If all seems right between you and this special person, let the sexual tension between the two of you build until it is driving both of you crazy. Let it build to fever pitch.

Undoubtedly, once the relationship is much older, you will

look back and view this sweet, early time as all too brief. There are many exciting ways to show you care, without including your genitals. If this person is truly great, and the two of you make a good match, there will be plenty of opportunities for great sex in the future!

Good luck with loving yourselves, loving life, and being loved by others!

10-26. Touched by a Partner

We would have died if not touched routinely after our birth. Being touched is equally important to the well-being of our adult love relationships. Lovingly applied, physical contact literally nourishes us and helps to keep us emotionally and physically healthy. Each loving touch is a small but essential building block, all of which accumulate to become trusting connections. Touch is the medium through which love may be delivered, but it also has the capacity to communicate a wide range of feelings.

The full spectrum of touch expresses the whole range of emotions from cold to hot. Examples of emotionally cold touch are violent strikes intended to cause pain, touch used as a method of delivering punishment and discipline, the utilitarian touch required to provide rudimentary care, and the civil touch of a business-like handshake. The withholding of touch also sends a message. Meanwhile, a friendly hug, a pat on the back, and a warm, accepting stroke reside at the warmer end of the touch spectrum. Distinctions may be made between different kinds of love-based touch, such as affectionate touch, loving touch, sensual touch, and sexual touch. The loving kinds of touch, if applied appropriately, may facilitate healing.

Each time you touch your partner, or are touched by your partner, something is communicated. Words are the language of the mind; touch is the language of the body and emotions. Each touch bypasses the mind and directly influences our emotions. It communicates feelings. What are the messages you communicate to your partner through touch? Each kind of touch has its appropriate time and place. For instance, if a sensual touch is given when a friendly touch is best, a negative reaction will result.

Touch is a language all its own. Not only does the kind of touch express a sentiment, but the frequency of touches does as well. We each need a certain amount of physical contact; an amount which is unique to us and which will either nourish or deprive the partner and relationship of love and a strong connection. Each touch between lovers is like a single note in a song, where the pressure, length, and speed of the touch create the pitch and tone. With too few touches, the song becomes simple and boring, but when touch is frequent and varied, the song may be beautiful. How often and in what way do you touch your partner?

Lovemaking is a nonverbal conversation. Varying and generous touching in a sexual encounter determines the quality of the soothing, pleasure, arousal, and excitement. Here too, the various touches are like the notes which determine the nature of a song; romantic, deeply intimate, or passionate. Each key must be touched correctly on a piano to produce the sounds of music, just like your fingers on your lover.

Many partners are not generous enough in giving loving kinds of touch, yet it costs the giver nothing. Some partners make the mistake of giving the wrong kind of touch at the wrong time, for example, many male partners are guilty of giving sexual touch when their female partners are in need of loving or affectionate touches. A sexual touch may communicate sexual desire, but is best given when a sexual opportunity is truly available. Female partners generally offer too little affectionate touch to their male partners, especially in moments when an appreciation for kindness is warranted. Your generous, loving touch is a way of building a stronger, more positive bond with those you love.

10-27. Saddled by Expectations

We come with a whole lot of baggage to our love

relationships. One of the bags is filled with unrealistic expectations about love and what a satisfying love relationship is. People cling to the fantasy that in a good relationship, partners simply and easily enjoy one another in continuous pleasure and bliss. Exceptions may exist, but for the most part the reality differs greatly; troubles are normal, just as storms are a normal part of the weather. In our fantasy relationships we escape the rigors and challenging reality which, to many, represent disappointment. It is troubling that this fantasy has replaced the harsher reality in most people's minds. A healthier approach would be for new partners to understand and accept that when a new relationship develops, a "hard work" phase is soon to arrive. Be ready to work hard on yourselves and your relationship. Every living being must work to maintain its life. The cost of love is pain, and relationships are not immune from this truth.

Our love relationships eventually push partners to their emotional limits, forcing each to grow or face the prospect of a breakup. Most often, if a relationship is easy and harmonious all the time, then partners are not living fully by pushing themselves. Couples who never argue may be couples who avoid conflict, a habit that exacts a high price later on. We sell ourselves out by choosing to not assert our needs. Mounting unresolved problems that are not allowed to be expressed in tension or conflict form a pattern of kicking the can down the road. Eventually, the bill comes due.

The work required by love is slow and often painful, not the stuff we dream about. Love demands that we push beyond our personal limitations. Two main tasks divide peoples' lives, careers and relationships, and both are necessary to create a complete life. Our jobs mostly utilize the strong intellect of the head, while our love relationships require more from the emotions of our hearts.

There is no expression similar to "lucky in love" for the realm of careers. Few people expect to have an effortless job that pays them well. When one starts a career after job training, it is expected that the job will include hard work. It would be unreasonable for an employee to say, "I can't believe it. My employer expects me to work hard."

But this is just what happens in the sphere of relationships. Despite ten thousand years of human society and billions of relationships, many people do not expect a love relationship to be hard work. Yet it is hard work; emotional hard work, and this is perfectly normal. It is unlikely that people who do not want to grow, or who are emotionally lazy, will contribute to a good relationship, just as people who don't want to exercise will not maintain a healthy body. When a relationship has troubles, an expected and normal occurrence, it is a sign that love is demanding growth, attention and effort.

Unlike the career track, no formal training exists for love relationships and marriages. The work that must be done is work of emotional strength, maturity, and living by love-based values. Most get into a love relationship completely unprepared, and with unrealistic expectations. Without any previous training, save that of one's family, many of which are dysfunctional, a relationship then becomes the arena in which this training takes place, and it is hard. It is like on-the-job training. Once the hard work of this training begins, many partners believe something is wrong because the real experience does not match their unrealistic, Hollywood-fueled expectations.

Long-term love relationships take daily hard work. This is normal. But the fantasy is that being "lucky in love" is possible, meaning that we have escaped the hard work. Because the "private face" of couples is reserved for behind closed doors and the "public face" is the one without problems, the universal belief has developed that a problem-free relationship is normal. Notwithstanding, some people do win the lottery and escape the hard work of earning money. But it is the exception, not the rule. Many of those people's lives are ruined by their windfall. Many end their relationships because the reality does not match their expectations. Others end their relationships because their partners are not ready to do the real work required by love.

Consider the differences in attitudes towards these two aspects of people's lives...in one they expect work and in the other, the sphere of the relationship, they do not. Yet life is a struggle, and our relationships are a subset of life and not immune to its rigors. It is unrealistic to expect that a relationship will be more perfect than the two imperfect human partners who constitute it.

{ Avoid avoidance. }

10-28. Build-up of Toxicity in Relationships

To keep relationships alive and healthy (and satisfying), special work and attention are required. This work is mostly emotional in nature. Without the right kinds of efforts, the very conditions that made the relationship feel "right" in the beginning are transformed from seeds of love to seeds of destruction. The partner who was found to be amazingly beautiful is later the cause of strong feelings of jealousy, because that beauty also attracts others. The partner with the gentle and sensitive nature becomes a source of frustration, because gentleness now appears as weakness rather than strength. The partner whose humor was so attractive seems pathetic, because their humor is transformed into a constant reminder that their pain is no longer well-hidden.

> "Keep thy eyes wide open before marriage, and half shut afterwards."
> —Benjamin Franklin

In these scenarios, the partners have not changed, but the qualities they possess now are viewed as part of the totality of their imperfect personality, rather than as a singular characteristic. As we come to know our partner more intimately, we also grow increasingly aware of their flawed humanness. This inevitable process in the early years of most relationships gives credence to the saying, "familiarity breeds contempt." Early on, just knowing our partner existed gave us hope that our own imperfections and discomforts could be healed. The disillusionment caused by the discovery that our partner is incapable of this healing seemed to transform them into a burden, and our relationship into a kind of worldly prison.

> "Take it from me, marriage isn't a word; it's a sentence."
> — King Vidor

Without the right kinds of work to counteract this degenerative process, partners tend to distance themselves into protective, emotionally separate camps. Each one wisely avoids further hurts, sensitive to the reality that the relationship will not provide the unconditional love that seemed within their grasp in the beginning. The remaining relationship does not contain the intimacy or love that each partner seeks. It becomes stagnant. The interactions between partners become a defensively defined dance with rigid and unchanging patterns.

> "For two people in a marriage to live together day after day is unquestionably the one miracle the Vatican has overlooked."
> —Bill Cosby

When this pattern stays in place over a long period of time, real communication no longer occurs. Each partner is increasingly viewed by the other through distorted, prejudicial filters. An example would be a person who does not feel loved in their relationship, and who has noticed that this feeling is especially acute when their partner does something for themselves. They would be likely to define their partner as selfish. Over time, this becomes solidified, since every action by that partner is thereafter perceived as some form of selfishness. Steps are taken to defend against the hurt caused by this selfishness, and communication then ceases to be effective because it is being attempted between people who have become inaccurate shadows of the people they used to love. Meanwhile, the hurt grows and mounts in both hearts.

Busy, stressful lives provide an added poison. Stress itself can be dangerous to our health when we feel we cannot control it. It is equally dangerous to our relationships. If our relationship is troubled, when there is increased stress, the frustration of any already-corrosive problem is magnified.

As time passes, and real communication does not occur, the partners lose awareness of each other. It is common that in place of communication, assumptions are made of the others' needs, desires and intentions. Even genuine attempts to please each other often fail miserably. The partners don't know each other anymore, they know only their preconceptions of each other. They know that their partner is someone who doesn't understand them, is someone who doesn't take the time to love them, is someone who makes them feel bad, and is someone who repeatedly hurts them by their seeming insensitivities.

Resentment builds. As time passes, the resentment grows more and more poisonous and bitter. It is not uncommon to meet couples who have been together for twenty years or more and are bitter towards each other and life itself.

"Edith, stifle yourself."
—Archie Bunker

That is all the bad news. While it is common that this pattern plays out through the years, it is not inevitable. Some partners possess a resiliency that defeats their relationship's erosion. Partners who communicate well are much more likely to avoid the build-up of resentment. People who are not afraid to voice their disappointments have a better chance. To be aware of one's feelings and to share them in a kind manner will go far to prevent distance from destroying the closeness.

Many partners did not have happy parental marriages to learn from, thus many relationships do not innately possess the qualities necessary for survival. Partners need resources on which to draw to learn how to maintain their connection with their partner. Oil changes and other routine maintenance need to be done to maintain the usefulness of a car; and routine physical exams, proper diet, and exercise are important to maintain a person's health. It is likewise vital that, for the longevity and health of a relationship, deliberate work is done to maintain it. It is necessary to meet with a psychotherapist and establish a relationship with them before there are real problems, as a way of preventing problems from becoming unworkable. It is certainly possible to heal long-standing problems, but it is a wiser course to prevent problems before they begin. Other steps which help are:

1. Establishing guidelines for emotional safety.
2. Establishing rules for safe conflicts.
3. Making regular time and effort to openly communicate feelings.
4. Making the commitment and expending the effort to maintain the relationship by making stress-free time together a priority.
5. Finding a couples' psychotherapist to meet with regularly.
6. Using the psychotherapist more frequently when seemingly unresolvable problems are causing tension.

10-29. Re-igniting the Flames of Passion

When a couple nervously walks into my office for the first time, the chances are high that they will describe how the passion has disappeared from what used to be an intense, hot love affair, characterized by frequent episodes of wild sex. Disappointment and desperation color their faces as each partner shares his or her theory as to why. The partners may even tell about their many attempts to resurrect the heat between them, by taking a vacation to Aruba without the kids, following the latest Cosmo advice, or buying frilly intimates at Victoria's Secret. Yet here they are, frustrated and tense in the marriage counselor's office. The attempts to recapture the romance either produced only momentary sparks or failed completely.

As the dreaded "last hope" marriage counselor, among the most pleasant of my tasks is to assure the couple that there is hope. Little did the partners know, when they floated into their romantic relationship on clouds of dreams and hope, that they were flirting with one of the most challenging exercises a human being can undertake: love. We are duped into believing, during the first few "golden months" that the love and excitement will last forever. Like a dream which is outside of ordinary daily life, when we are in love, we believe it will last forever. Like the moth attracted to the flame during a warm summer evening, when drawing near, it experiences not just the brilliance of light, but also the destructive burning of the flame. So it is with love.

It is human nature to be drawn into a love relationship, but life's plan is to demand that our growth is the burning price for companionship. Love demands that we extend beyond our limitations, otherwise the flames of passion dwindle. We grow when we strengthen our ability to handle the discomfort produced by letting go of ourselves, a necessary effort when seeking to make another feel valuable and loved. If we cooperate with life's process by doing the work insisted upon by our relationship, we will grow. In the process of being with our partner, if we are adept at balancing being true to ourselves and letting ourselves go to love our partner in genuine sincerity, our passion will not die. If we sell ourselves out, our passion will fade.

There is no shortcut. Sexy lingerie is not a substitute for lovers learning to be true to themselves. No amount of flowers will replace the passion-nourishing efforts of making the other feel deeply loved.

10-30. Making Love Throughout the Day

In our quest to create the kind of love that is deep and

soul-satisfying to us, it is common knowledge that sex is important, but sexual activities only account for a tiny percentage of our waking time. However, the remaining hours are not wasted, but time well spent in improving the quality of our lovemaking. Be aware that much of the potential satisfaction that can be experienced in those precious bedroom moments are but the mountain peak that must be supported by the middle of the mountain.

This mountain middle is formed of the essential, but often mundane, communications and interactions that occur during our daytime rush, while getting business done. In the way we go about our myriad tasks, there exist potentially hundreds of tiny opportunities to show our partner our love. Ask a lover what makes him or her feel loved, and it is likely you will hear, not about grand arrangements that include a limousine or dozens of long-stemmed roses, but instead about thoughtful gestures that signify "You are important to me." It is the brief kitchen shoulder-rub when reaching for the bowl; taking her car on an errand and filling her gas tank; thanking him for completing a task that had long fallen into the taken-for-granted category. These gestures fuel the fire and maintain, while also strengthening, an emotional connection.

When sex becomes routine, the misguided knee-jerk reaction is to search for a new sexual technique to spice things up. While doing so may heat things up for a few moments, once lovemaking is done, the temperature cools just as quickly. The way to get the "most bang for your buck" (no pun intended) is to make real the truism that lovemaking is best when the emotional connection is deepest; essentially the difference between having sex and making love. A deep connection frees the passion. Let your love be expressed frequently in many tiny efforts throughout the day. This is a different, and equally important way to make love that resonates deeply in the heart and echoes loudly, under the sheets.

10-31. Vive la Différence

Men and women are different in obvious ways; emotionally, intellectually, socially, and spiritually. Men and women are also different in less obvious ways; ways that are much more difficult to quantify. In love relationships, these differences are the sources of great fascination, eroticism, joy, and pleasure, and also of conflict and misery. There is no place where the differences are more noticeable than during a sexual encounter. One of the biggest problems is that the differences between men and women often produce such friction and acrimony that neither partner ends up feeling like having a sexual encounter.

There are many couples out there that don't have sex. Such couples fall into all categories: older, more mature adults who have decades of bitterness under their belts, middle-aged empty-nesters, and the stressed couples who are raising children. More surprising is that this problem also infects even the young couples, the newlyweds, and couples who are just engaged. Ask many newlywed couples about their honeymoons and, if they are honest, you will hear about many honeymoons in which the "do not disturb" sign was not used even once. The differences among us, if negotiated well, result in our growth, strength, and well-being, but if coped with poorly, create tension, conflict and anger. The challenge of differences is so difficult, that it tends to be only a minority of couples that negotiate it well.

Nature has played a trick on us. Among the differences between the genders, most women need to feel emotionally connected, loved, and valued before they're likely to express themselves sexually, but most men wish to form a deep connection through sexual activity, in order to feel loved and valued. It is not surprising that these differences are in opposition, and without goodwill, partners are unlikely to resolve this difference and the living room couch is likely to be frequently used.

The solution is in the building of goodwill. Love, the

commitment to the other's well-being, growth, and nourishment, is to be offered with sincerity, and must be given without the expectation of return; otherwise it loses its magic. Sex without love, while it can still feel good, is a bit like tinny music which has no powerful bass. So long as partners give freely and demonstrate a commitment to the other's well-being, the gridlock caused by nature's trick will be melted away.

10-32. Kids Are Bad for Marriage

There. It's out of the bag. Now I am an easy target to be attacked and accused of being a lunatic. Why would I make such an unforgivable statement? Because it's true!

Marriages change once the children are born; often for the worse. Please do not think that I am an opponent of children. I am not. Children are vital for the future of our species. Couples desire to have children and are usually wise to do so. We love our children. But let us not deceive ourselves. Children are bad for our love relationships.

Consider what children need in order to thrive: a great deal of our time, attention, energy, and financial resources. Now consider what we devoted to our partner before we had children: time, attention, energy, and money; the same resources! Good parents fulfill the needs of their children first. Nourishing the love relationship between partners usually falls off the bottom of the priority list and becomes a victim of other, overwhelming demands.

And what about sex? What often was a robust, passionate and lusty sex life gets designated only the little bit of energy that remains after an exhausting day, if anything at all. As children grow, the privacy required for a good sex life disappears. Mothers of small children commonly have little desire for sex, and most mothers who have been nurturing children all day long have little interest in nurturing their partner sexually. Mothers gain more pleasure from having alone time than having sexual time.

Does this picture sound bleak? It isn't. The truth about raising children while simultaneously trying to have a great and passionate love relationship is that it is difficult, but not impossible. However, those factors that are necessary to nourish your love for each other are slightly counterintuitive. Your relationship must rotate into the number-one-priority position at least once each week for two or three hours, with just the two of you. Sex must not be allowed to fall away, even if it is less desired. More than ever, couples with children are best to emphasize respect, etiquette and generous communication.

Give your kids the most valuable gift you can: a good marriage.

10-33. The Invisible Unspoken Contract

My Rules

If you want to marry me, here's what you'll have to do:
You must learn how to make a perfect chicken-dumpling stew.
And you must sew my holey socks,
And soothe my troubled mind,
And develop the knack for scratching my back,
And keep my shoes spotlessly shined.
And while I rest you must rake up the leaves,
And when it is hailing and snowing
You must shovel the walk...and be still when I talk,
And—hey—where are you going?

—Shel Silverstein, "Where the Sidewalk Ends"

Shortly after two people first meet, find that they share a mutual attraction, and seek to know each other more deeply, a process of negotiation begins. Partners start to establish ground rules for a potential future relationship. Partners also launch a process of determining if the fit between them is right and if each can, or is willing to, fulfill the other's conscious and unconscious needs. Unconscious is a fancy word for mental activities that we are not aware of. During the early phase of a new relationship, as much unconscious as conscious work is being performed.

As new partners get to know each other, an invisible unspoken contract is created. The words invisible and unspoken give a hint that it is primarily created by the unconscious minds of the new relationship partners. It details an agreement between partners about the expectations for each partner's behaviors, attitudes, reactions, hopes, and dreams in the context of the relationship.

Simply stated, the invisible unspoken contract details that "When I do this, you do that." It also defines or fails to define limits. A partner who does not assert himself or herself when the other behaves in a hurtful or inconsiderate manner is solidifying a clause in the contract which states that such behavior is acceptable. A partner who requires great closeness and does not let this need be known early on, tacitly agrees to a more distant relationship than they would prefer.

The time to craft the contract wisely is in the early days of the relationship, when it is fluid and flexible. As time passes the contract is solidified; with each passing week, the contract will be more difficult to change as partners come to accept what is in it. Every aspect of the relationship is detailed in its invisible wording: communication, secrets, expectations, attitudes, values, role assignments, distribution of power and labor, gender-based values, the future dreams of children, of sex, of money, of work, of living arrangements, and more.

The strength and maturity of each partner determine how well the contract is negotiated, and thus how long it may serve the relationship well. A partner with little assertiveness is less likely to set limits and insist that the contract includes certain provisions. An assertive partner will express early in the contract's formation what he or she will or will not accept, hence a behavior or situation will be included or excluded from the contract.

The contract is neither permanent nor unchangeable. However, when it has stood for years, more strength will be required to propose a change, and repeated efforts may be needed when facing partner resistance. Over time, the inevitable changes of growth, aging, and family development mean that the contract will undergo many small alterations. But during times of large change, such as a crisis, a job change, a house move, or sending grown children into the world, the contract faces great pressure.

Some kinds of growth and change may force the contract to be questioned. If one of the partners gets additional education, a new job or career, develops a new interest, or adopts a new group of friends, this may require that the contract be overhauled. Mid-life crises and large developmental shifts may be similarly influential. If important features of the contract are challenged, a partner may invalidate it entirely, thus placing the relationship in jeopardy. Partners are tested by new developments; their strength and love will be put on the line each time the contract is renegotiated or renewed. The stronger and more loving a partner, the greater ability he or she will possess to create a satisfying contract that will stand the test of change and time.

10-34. Sooner, Rather Than Later

> "Married men live longer than single men, but married men are a lot more willing to die."
>
> —Johnny Carson

> "The trouble with some women is they get all excited over nothing and then they marry him."
>
> —Cher

Monica and Will (fictional names) showed up on time for their first marriage counseling appointment. After initially seeming nervous, they visibly relaxed as they began telling the story of how their marriage had deteriorated to the point where they were willing to take the desperate step of calling a marriage counselor. Their story revealed that they'd been unhappy with each other for the past eight years of their twenty-two year marriage.

After only a couple of months in counseling, the tension between the two had greatly dissipated, they communicated more freely, and each was feeling loved by the other. They both admitted that the quality of their relationship probably would not have grown so bad had they sought help years earlier. Most couples do not enter marriage counseling until the possibility of divorce is looming on the horizon.

If you are married or in a long-term relationship, you will probably need the help of a relationship therapist sooner or later. Please let it be sooner. It is unlikely that you'll go through years in a relationship without difficult times. The odds of fixing a relationship where the problems have snowballed for years or longer are poor. There is deep sadness when two people who still love each other despite the years' accumulation of resentment, anger, and disappointment, have no hope left for satisfaction in their relationship. Save yourselves regret, heartache, and grief. Addressing your relationship's problems while they remain small will allow you to enjoy years of togetherness rather than emotional torture made up of misunderstandings, rejection, and anger.

Very few people are capable of loving unconditionally. Thus, human relationships are rarely forged without emotional strings attached to the love. Add to this the fact that our attraction for our mate is generated by the flaws we experienced in our relationships with those who originally taught us about love; our parents. These relationship truths suggest that our primary relationship will test us emotionally where we are weakest, bringing out our worst. Marriage and commitment both have bad reputations for this reason.

Avoid martyrdom and living a life of quiet desperation. If things are bad between you and your partner, without outside help, they will probably only get worse. If you have cancer and ignore it, will get better on its own? For the sake of the quality of your life, and the happiness of those you love most, get help sooner!

10-35. Emotional Safety

> "Marriage is a wonderful institution. But who would want to live in an institution?"
> —H.L. Mencken

It is easy to make jokes about marriage, but the pain of a troubled union is hard to get past. Consider the following scenario: you've been married for years. You are painfully aware of your spouse's habits, which have repeatedly reminded you of how he or she does not understand you, is insensitive to your needs, and is unaware of the pain you continually experience.

At some point you were brave enough to speak up about how you felt. You took a risk and finally shared your honest feelings. To your surprise and satisfaction your partner actually made changes, which felt good and empowering. Then you watched as your spouse's old habits slowly returned, and with them, your feelings of dissatisfaction. Your hopelessness sank to a deeper, darker level than it had been before. How could your spouse possibly love you if he or she behaved in this way? Could you ever trust them again? Could real closeness ever be possible again? In reaction to your disappointment, you pulled away emotionally. Damage had been done to your marriage.

The relationship described above has become emotionally unsafe. Instead of being a place of security and support, it has become a place of pain. It does not contain any overt forms of abuse; the difficulties described are caused by interactions more subtle than abuse, but they are just as damaging. In this example, the connection between spouses had been eroded over time by poor communication, laziness, neglect, selfishness, and insensitivity.

Emotional safety is a vital element found in healthy relationships. It is defined as a condition where each partner can express him or herself genuinely, without fear of invalidation, criticism, ridicule, disrespect, rejection, or abandonment. Put more simply, and in positive terms, a relationship is emotionally safe when each partner feels affirmed by the other. This means being valued, listened to, and supported.

Answering yes to any of the following questions suggests that you experience your relationship as emotionally unsafe to some degree: Does your spouse often disappoint you or hurt your feelings? Are you frequently angry with him or her? Do you avoid sharing your honest feelings with your spouse to avoid a conflict? Do you make lists of your spouse's disagreeable actions so you can prove his or her wrongdoings at a later date? Do you tell a friend about your relationship troubles or your spouse's shortcomings rather than voice your concerns directly to him or her?

A relationship is an emotionally safe place when each partner can trust the other to provide the care and support required for personal growth. To repair a relationship that has grown emotionally unsafe, both partners need to be committed to making positive changes. Including a third person in the process of repairing a relationship is invaluable. The longer a relationship has remained emotionally unsafe, the more difficult it will be to repair.

> Loving with sensitivity dictates that if a choice or action will impact the partner, he or she must be consulted.

10-36. Conflict Need Not Damage Love

The wife's face twisted in pain. Not knowing the situation,

one would think a knife had been thrust into her back. But no. Her husband had just sworn at her in a demeaning, disrespectful way; his typical reaction to a moment of disagreement. She would admit that she is equally as skilled at verbally assaulting her husband. This is the way of things for many couples; spontaneous conflict shatters a tense harmony.

Conflict is a normal part of every love relationship. Relationships are the arena for growth and change, and conflict is its engine. However, not all conflict is the same. Some conflicts are productive in creating positive change, while others are not. When the same issue repeatedly generates conflict without resolution, it is a sure sign that an important issue is being addressed in a non-productive manner. For couples who are proud of their lack of conflict; not so fast! Harmony may not be a reliable indicator of relationship health. Difficulties in these relationships may go unexpressed. Some constructive conflict helps to foster passion.

Being attracted to and choosing a partner occurs with an underlying need to solve certain emotionally based challenges, which were cemented in our personalities during our early formative years. Loving another, especially after making vows of commitment, activates these usually unconscious challenges, providing both partners with great opportunity for growth, but also for hard-to-resolve conflict.

The growth-benefits of conflict are lost once it is expressed in a hurtful or emotionally unsafe manner. Hurtfulness injects tension into the partnership, in which wounds and resentment may pollute the togetherness by casting a long shadow of emotional distrust.

An agreement between partners to institute rules of conflict not only helps partners to vocalize their grievances safely, but also aids them in developing healthy impulse control. Making these rules when partners are at peace provides the best chance of success. Safe conflict is a necessary precondition for achieving constructive resolutions. In their frustration, many couples deteriorate into destructive rather than effective conflict.

Some useful rules that help conflicting partners from "hitting below the belt" are an agreement to avoid profanity, to avoid frightening physical gestures, to exclude threats about breaking up, to avoid shouting, to speak about what is desired or needed, to stick with the issue that started the current conflict and to exclude attacks on the partner's character.

Intense anger may vent tension, but it does not contribute to problem-solving, instead it prevents the conflict from being resolved. An agreement that each partner can stop the discussion if anger escalates out of control is a valuable safety valve, as long as the partner calling the time out promises to re-initiate the discussion after a short, specified duration. Installing these agreements helps partners develop impulse control while also making conflict safe.

If what you want is a close and passionate love relationship, then protecting it from the potential destructive force of conflict is necessary. Ultimately, conflict is more about negotiating, listening and understanding than hurting. Intimacy and passion are fragile qualities that cannot bear the hurtfulness that conflict can generate. Make love not war; by fighting fairly, couples can make conflict more about loving than warring.

> The aim of an argument
> or discussion should
> not be victory but progress.
>
> *- Joseph Joubert*

PERSONALITY AND EMOTIONS

11-1. Selfish versus Self-Full

Many people are generous. Overwhelmingly, generosity is good. However, sometimes people give to avoid being seen as selfish, which has become a high-level sin. If a person is perceived as selfish, he or she is viewed as a bad person. Deeply rooted in our culture's religious foundation is the concept of selflessness, in which others' needs are prioritized and one's own needs are overlooked. "It is better to give than to receive," according to the old saying, but both giving and receiving have their proper place and time.

Yet giving and generosity can be out of balance. The value of it may become distorted. Certainly, in practice, giving and generosity can be kind in the right situation, but our culture has mistakenly installed a selflessness-based practice, despite most people still having a sense of self. Selflessness is a high spiritual state in which the ego has been transcended and little sense of self remains, such is the case with those who are regarded as saints. Ego-based actions derive motivation from a different source, a need to prove self-worth. To avoid being viewed as selfish, many give and give. Secondary motivations for generosity are to be liked by others, to overcome feelings of guilt and self-doubt, and to be viewed by others as good.

Many people, in an effort to cope with guilt and shame, act like giving machines. Their chronic generosity places others' needs and happiness ahead of their own, a pattern based in self-deprecation. These are good people. We all know somebody whose efforts appear superhuman. Outwardly they seem saintly, but inwardly, on a deep level, they feel ashamed; they doubt their own worthiness. No amount of giving and generosity will solve the problem of self-hate. But emotionally, such a person is convinced that if a little giving will not make themselves feel better, more giving is sure to do the trick.

A lot of moms are like this. They give and give to the point of exhaustion. Sadly, many fathers collude with the mom's journey to exhaustion because of their own emotional limitations and outdated gender roles. They avoid full responsibility and allow the mom to do too much and become an exhausted solo super-giver.

Chronic giving results in becoming drained and exhausted. It is unsustainable. Having demonstrated goodness, givers often hope for validation from others, but when it is not forthcoming, resentment builds; "I did all this, and no one even acknowledged it." Or if the giver is in a situation of need and giving is not reciprocated, he or she is hurt and feels slighted, suggesting that the giving has not been altruistic, but instead was motivated by the ulterior motive of bolstering the ego. The giver eventually becomes a burden to partners, loved ones and family due to an accumulation of resentment and exhaustion. Being resentful and negative interferes with loving; it is not the spirit of true selfless giving. Chronic giving is like living in a decrepit shack while helping the neighbor build a mansion.

Giving is good, but giving for the right reasons is better. It produces good results without generating the side effect of additional future problems. Each one of us has a self. Our first responsibility is to take care of our own needs, support our own well-being and improve our small space in this world by filling it with love. Self-care and self-compassion are part of a practice that might be called self-fullness as opposed to selfishness. If energy is left over after one's needs and one's family's needs are fulfilled, then the remainder may be distributed to others. If everyone took good care of themselves, far fewer people would be poor and needy.

11-2. Emotional Hibernation

Some partners suffer unfulfilling relationships in silent desperation. How likely is it that a partner will speak up about the causes of dissatisfaction? Many barely say a word or speak only indirectly by hinting at how they feel. Togetherness functions as a trial, testing whether vulnerability is safe. Subtle remarks indirectly request understanding and a compassionate response; if neither is offered, the pain of disappointment is sharp. In a relationship without dynamic change, painful emotions hibernate. Partners in pain wait for a sign that they are valued. Painful feelings remain in hibernation, waiting for the cold winter of insensitivity to pass and the warm spring of love to arrive.

Hibernation becomes a habit within a relationship where partners react to one another insensitively, harshly or with inaction. It takes just a few instances of receiving unloving responses to pain for a partner to choose to limit their sharing. Vulnerable feelings are stored safely within, where little risk exists of triggering an unfulfilling response. Yet the dissatisfied partner longs for a caring ear that will hear the depths of their pain and lovingly act to alleviate it. Feelings of loneliness, being unimportant, being hurt in any capacity, needing more attention or affection, and craving to be understood all are examples of pain-based unmet needs that often hibernate.

Look upon any strained or unhappy relationship and you will see an emotionally unsafe connection encouraging many hibernating feelings. Many partners are unaware of why the connection between them has grown toxic, because the degree of sensitivity required to maintain an open and safe relationship is far higher than many partners realize. They are not bad people; they are just oblivious to of the impact of their words and actions. They are unaware that how they respond or fail to respond can result in mild, subtle, and sometimes substantial hurt. An inconsiderate response to vulnerable sharing encourages an open heart to close down and choose silence. When emotional hibernation is actively engaged, it is part of a relationship system in which partners are partially or fully closed. An essential aspect of love is openness. Many of us grew up in family environments where love was incomplete, and this has resulted in love being defined by a lower standard.

The exchanges that lead to emotional hibernation are none other than normal everyday communications, but qualitatively they sever closeness and often signal partner unimportance. Defensiveness makes the issue about oneself instead of the other, and puts up an emotional barrier. Being defensive also chooses distance instead of the closeness of compassion for the partner's pain or need. Judgement and criticism diminish a partner's value. Failure to listen and intellectually process the partner's meaning is a repetitive pattern that non-verbally demonstrates the other's unimportance. Sudden and high-intensity reactions leave partners cautious. Counterattack and blame produce an atmosphere in which opening up becomes too risky. When previously shared needs, feelings and experiences are later used as a weapon to gain an advantage, it strongly encourages emotional hibernation for safety and security. Within relationships where large arguments erupt, many feelings and needs are withheld to simply reduce the chance of conflict.

As children, many of us were scolded to be quiet, a pattern that is easily replicated in our love relationships when the possibility of being threatened, dismissed or invalidated is high. The painful feelings that hibernate are stored seeds of essential solutions, having great potential for partner growth and a deeper relationship. When it is unsafe to share, opportunity after opportunity for relationship repair and improvement are painfully missed. As more time passes without problems being addressed, relationship crises such as separation, infidelity, and divorce draw ever nearer.

11-3. Never Quite the Same Again

In a split second, an unexpected event triggers a cascade of terrible feelings, transforming a loving person into someone darker, afraid, angry, and out of control. A sight, a sound, or a few insensitively chosen words may unleash the inner terror; the eruption of painful feelings from remnants of unresolved trauma long past. Too many have been hurt, and the aftereffects of violence and terrorizing threat may linger for a lifetime.

What is trauma and why do its effects linger so long?

Trauma results from life-altering experiences in which one loses control and at the same time anticipates or sustains painful harm. Soldiers live through it in war. Car drivers experience it in a major accident. Victims survive it in horrible moments of violence. This is the stuff of nightmares, beyond the sufferers' ability to cope. During a traumatic experience, extraordinary psychological measures are taken to endure; measures which forgo future well-being in exchange for current survival. Not all violent, terrifying or injury-causing life experiences result in what is known as PTSD (Post-Traumatic Stress Disorder), a bundle of painful fear-based symptoms that linger long after the traumatic event has passed. What causes PTSD in one person may not in another.

To escape the intense fear and pain during a traumatic event, a survivor psychologically retreats inwardly, splitting off from his or her body to create safety. But this extraordinary measure has an extraordinarily high cost; the psyche and the body remain split apart long after. Thereafter, the body is the custodian of the horrible memories and is perceived as toxic to the psyche. Rejoining the two is a difficult healing process for most, and seemingly near impossible for some. The name PTSD suggests that this emotional condition is a disorder, whereas in fact the condition is a normal response to an abnormal experience.

Rough estimates indicate that one in three women and one in four men experience abuse-related trauma, many of these people were harmed as children. To cope with enormous pain, some trauma survivors repress painful memories, burying the painful, and often shameful, traumatic memories in their subconscious so that they will not be experienced during daily life. The traumatic event just seems to be gone. Common symptoms of PTSD may include anxiety, panic episodes, nightmares, chronically heightened vigilance, sudden intense and disturbing memories, episodes of rage, obsessive and compulsive thoughts and behaviors, being startled easily, avoidance of situations similar to the one in which the trauma occurred, and distancing from vulnerable closeness.

Relationships that include a traumatized person suffer from trauma as well. The emotional openness needed for a strong love relationship can be fear-provoking for someone who has experienced deep hurt. In addition, the self-blame and shame felt by most PTSD sufferers, and their attraction to risky behaviors, complicate romantic connections. Certain situations normal to a loving partnership can trigger strong emotional reactions such as panic, flashback memories, or avoidance. It is not unusual for traumatized individuals to be unclear as to the cause of their strong emotional reactions. The link between confusing behaviors and attitudes and old trauma is not obvious. In some instances, previously repressed memories of old trauma will abruptly surface into a partner's consciousness, like a bubble rising from the deep, and this can thoroughly transform their personality, turning them into someone troubled and significantly different.

The intensity common to love relationships can also traumatize a partner or re-awaken old trauma. Large conflicts and those that escalate to violence may be traumatic. Partners with traumatic sexual abuse histories may dissociate in intimate moments, a way of mentally "going away" to avoid the discomfort associated with the past. Threats of abandonment, insensitive dominance, aggression, cheating, and breakup may all traumatize a partner, negatively impacting a relationship for years.

Regular talk therapy alone is usually not effective at healing deep injury. If it includes a re-living of the traumatic event it may actually re-traumatize the sufferer. For a treatment method to be effective, it must delve deeper than the conscious mind and into the more primitive body-consciousness, where traumatic emotions are stored. Healing is possible, however it is not easy. Offering a trauma sufferer patience and compassion is always a loving practice while individuals and couples travel the journey towards healing.

11-4. Becoming More Conscious

We can be a mystery to ourselves. When trying to figure out why we behave the way we do, it's not uncommon to say, "I don't know." This acknowledgment is the admission that we only have limited control of our own lives. Making choices consciously and deliberately is most effective, yet unconscious factors strongly influence many of our important choices and behavior patterns. In the journey towards becoming more conscious, learning about the unconscious is a great way to start.

The word "unconscious" can seem mysterious and formidable. The opposite of the conscious, the unconscious simply refers to those parts of us about which we are unaware. Unconscious factors would not be a big deal if we did not have a habit of burying hard-to-endure pain from difficult experiences in our unconscious. Positive, good experiences are not stored (or repressed), because we have no difficulty coping with, feeling and expressing emotions that feel good.

The unconscious becomes the emotional garbage can of rejected life experiences. When a situation or feeling of shame is too difficult or painful, we automatically repress it in order to distance and protect ourselves from the pain. If only the pain would stay nicely in its place. Instead, the unexpressed painful emotion continually seeks expression by fighting our intention to keep it below our awareness. When unconscious pain does eventually find its way to the light of conscious awareness, it influences our feelings, attitudes and behaviors. Overwhelmingly negative, most unconscious impressions wreak havoc on choices and relationships. When your intention deviates from your results and forms a negative pattern, you can confidently bet that unconscious forces are responsible.

Unconscious factors seeking resolution influence to whom we are attracted and who we choose as a partner. As relationships age, the deepening of love activates old, unresolved unconscious patterns, changing partners' personalities, sometimes dramatically, from what they were like early in the relationship, before these patterns awakened. The changes are typically negative. Unconscious emotions often result in repeating parental habits and attitudes, despite an intent to avoid doing so. A partner who grew up in an unaffectionate family may demonstrate much affection before old patterns are awakened, then become cold, distant, and avoidant afterwards. Abused as a child, a partner may start to be aggressive as the relationship deepens. When asked why they are behaving this way, the partner is sure to say, "I don't know." The cause is unconscious.

Within the unconscious mind are remnants of unfinished business; emotional injuries that have not yet been healed. Some typical examples of how unconscious dynamics are expressed are a fear of abandonment, powerlessness, conflict avoidance, laziness, aggression, patterns of disrespect, dependency, self-neglect, criticism, inability to trust, and inability to tolerate vulnerability. Powerlessness, and variations of it, are the most common theme, formed during childhood when life was without power.

Of greatest concern are those unconscious forces that are expressed in self-destructive ways. A large amount of buried pain may result in self-hate, causing partners to make choices that are not only not in their best interest, but are actively self-sabotaging and relationship sabotaging. A partner who is about to arrive at an achievement such as a college degree or promotion may abandon success by choosing irrational and misdirected options that destroy the opportunity. Partners who have successfully formed a romantic bond with a positive, loving and devoted partner, can push the other away or risk the relationship with carelessly concealed infidelities. A sabotaging individual, when asked why they behave in this self-destructive way will say, "I don't know." When we look back and label our choices as "stupid," unconscious emotions are at work.

Eliminating negative unconscious patterns is not easy. Sigmund Freud, the father of modern-day psychology, summed up the process as simply making the unconscious conscious. Psychotherapy is an emotional version of looking in the mirror to see your appearance. Therapy allows a person to metaphorically see their unconscious make up, with some ability to alter it. The more deeply buried the unconscious impressions, the harder they are to change or resolve, but sharing deeply held feelings and beliefs in a non-judgmental environment can help heal some unconscious forces. By becoming more conscious you have greater power to live and love the way you intend.

11-5. Nice and Strong

Often-used sayings become often-used because they contain a seed of truth. The saying "Nice guys finish last" suggests that nice guys are losers, at first glance it seems to be a criticism of nice-ness. Upon deeper inspection, it is really highlighting that nice guys are also usually weak guys. Within life and love relationships, weakness is a large problem. There is nothing inherently wrong with being nice, so long as when strength is required it can be applied successfully and appropriately. For men the issue of strength and weakness has an added vital dimension of being the primary attribute in the masculine identity.

It takes two strong partners to make one strong love relationship, and multiple areas of partner weakness make a relationship vulnerable to mounting problems. Weaknesses are the pattern of avoiding, or failing to bring sufficient action to a situation where action is necessary for effective completion. Weaknesses cause conflict and pain between partners by producing chronic failures. Men must possess strengths to be seen as a “man" or they risk losing self-esteem and the respect of others. One aspect of strength is the capacity to face adversity without surrendering intention, values, and morals.

Strength, as the core value of the masculine ideal, is contrasted with beauty and desirability, the core values of the feminine ideal. When lacking in strength, whether determined by self-regard or by others, the basic value and worthiness of a man is diminished. All people, male and female, need strengths, but demonstrating and acting from strength proves a man's masculinity and "manliness."

The core values of strength and beauty operate as a pair of dynamic polarizing qualities. Much like the positive and negative poles of a magnet, when similar they repel and when different they intensely attract. Men who possess many strengths such as intelligence, perseverance, sincerity, humor, and loyalty are seen as having a strong character and thus are viewed as attractive. Muscular strength and the physical appearance of power is strength in its most obvious form, but even more vital is the strength of assertiveness, the ability to express oneself without the need to control or dominate. Real strength is confident, not boastful. If a male partner demonstrates sufficient strengths, his female romantic partner will experience him as attractive. Strengths are a turn-on.

In its many forms, strength shows up as a solidness of being that confidently declares determination and self-authority. It may be demonstrated by moving directly towards goals. Weakness is characterized by avoidance, hesitation, failing to show up, and insufficiency. Niceness seems good, and at times can be positive, but it lacks the determination, perseverance, and mental toughness that uphold masculinity.

To be strong, a man must possess many specific spheres of competency. If significant weaknesses live among his strengths, his masculine value and attractiveness will be diluted and possibly destroyed. Some weaknesses function as a fatal flaw, the way a weakness in the middle of a steel beam makes the whole beam useless. Strength is needed inwardly, to control impulses and cope with painful emotion, as well as outwardly in the form of assertiveness, self-advocacy and perseverance. Strength is cultivated by facing and challenging fear, one tiny bit at a time.

Being nice, while pleasant, not only shows a desire to please others, but is also a practice of placing one's own feelings and needs at a consistently low priority. If this is an inflexible pattern in which strength and assertiveness cannot be expressed, then growth, maturity and the development of a stronger sense of self are needed. Strength is not mean, though at times using it may feel so; it is not aggressive, though it can have that incorrect reputation. Niceness at times can be good, but it does not contain the drive and determination to consistently get the job done, which ultimately demonstrates effectiveness and earns the attraction of romantic partners. Because of this, nice guys, without strength, finish last.

11-6. At Work and At Home

Partners, especially those in struggling relationships, use other relationships as a basis for comparison to gauge their relational abilities. In doing so, they hope to find the source of their troubles, and ultimately some solutions, by looking in an "emotional mirror" to determine the degree of their contribution. Talking to friends to get an objective perspective is one way, but doing so often garners opinions, or supportive but one-dimensioned and unhelpful agreement. Partners are strongly tempted to point to their successes in other kinds of relationships, such as friendships and work-related connections, to deflect responsibility for troubles in their primary intimate relationship. Such evidence is used to support the assumption that the other partner must be at fault.

Many a partner will point to their success in friendships in this way; "My friends all think I'm a good person, why don't you?" Using friendships is not a helpful strategy to gain a clear reflection of one's emotional self. It is like using a distorted carnival mirror when attempting to get an accurate sense of the shape of one's body. It will not be helpful because it is misleading. Friendships do not contain the intense need to merge, or the deep level of intimacy, even though very good friendships do share a high degree of openness. As a result, having the ability to develop and maintain friendships is not an indicator of one's strengths as a romantic partner.

But even more than friendships, workplace competency is the most often cited evidence that a partner does not contribute to relationship problems. "If I thrive in my work, have positive relationships with my coworkers, demonstrate strengths and abilities, then that proves that my relationship dysfunctions must be due to my partner, not me." This fallacy highlights a great difference in how individuals function in vastly different ways in the two primary spheres of our lives, at work and at home. The degree to which a person can excel at one but struggle within the other can be startling. The most frequent pattern is for an individual to excel at work, but stumble within a love relationship. How many extremely successful people have had multiple marriages?

Within our human make-up, two processes contribute to our functioning: the intellectual and the emotional. Often unequal in strength, the two capacities do not always work together, like a team with a strong offense but weak defense. Because the strengths and tasks required by most jobs are intellectually based, emotional limitations may not interfere with workplace success, but will definitely interfere at home with relationship success. Jobs require much intellectual horsepower, usually honed through rigorous, lengthy training and years of education, whereas relationships function in an emotional sphere without any formal training. Prior love relationships, failures, and family relationships during the early developmental years serve as the informal training ground for romantic partners.

In the world of work, employees function within a role that is clearly defined by a job description specifying particular duties and responsibilities. Workplace positions are designed for efficiency and success, to increase the possibility of profit for the employer. The boundaries of job duties, such as where the duties of one employee end and those of another begin is also, typically, clear. The longer an individual holds a job, the more he or she becomes an expert within the position and may enjoy a high degree of control. After performing a job for a long time, and repeating responsibilities numerous times, expertise comprised of familiarity, comfort, control, and competence is the natural outcome.

In contrast, the dynamics of love relationships are characterized by the sharing of emotion and risking openness. By its very nature, intimacy is the open sharing of partner feelings on a deep level, as an expression of a partner's sense of self. Spontaneous but safe emotional expression builds a love connection. Relating is not structured by any external agency, though it is bounded by moral obligations that dictate we should avoid causing harm, instead, role boundaries are negotiated between partners based upon what is comfortable or uncomfortable. Partner success is determined by the strength of what has been named "emotional intelligence," the awareness of feelings, the ability to express them well and employ them effectively amid the intensity and vulnerability of love relationships.

Our love relationships are undefined, but are spontaneously created moment-to-moment as partners react to and reflect emotions. Unlike a job, where an employee may develop mastery, partners in love relationships often experience less control with the deepening of intimacy and the simultaneous reactivation of old wounds which cause discomfort and out-of-control feelings. The challenges of long-term relationships tend to bring out the partners' worst. The well-known saying "familiarity breeds contempt" accurately sums up the dynamics, because the closer partners grow, the more visible partner flaws become. Sudden romances reflect only surface qualities, while long-term relationships show the true challenges. Success in a love relationship, as defined by the partners, may be about closeness, happiness and harmony, but life seems to define a relationship's success by partner growth in the capacity to love. In real life terms this means the most intense unresolved issues will be activated, and this produces discomfort.

There is no relationship that is similar to a love relationship. As a result, within no other kind of relationship will we receive a mirror reflection that informs us accurately about how we function within our intimate relationship. Our partner knows us best, even if our troubled relationship may not seem intimate or satisfying. By consistently treating your partner in loving ways, the reflection you get back will grow more and more favorable.

> If you allow fear to control you, you will never have a good life.

11-7. Bringing Fight to Fear

Fear is a potent adversary. The fear that we will be harmed is common. Fear does not play nicely; it does not easily go away when the risk of harm goes away. In our high-stress culture, fear-based emotion has become a way of life. Many people who are raised in anxious families are developmentally trained to be afraid. The fear-based emotions of worry and anxiety are as common as dollars and cents. When saddled with fear, romantic partners are emotionally disabled from loving well.

Contrary to popular opinion, fear, not hate, is the opposite of love. Within a love relationship, fear has the same effect on love as water has on flames. When one partner within a couple is chronically anxious, imbalances form that have negative long-term effects on the quality and longevity of the relationship. A partner who chronically worries, or is prone to panic, tries to feel better and gain security by controlling the other partner and violating his or her boundaries of autonomy. Other partners react to fear by distancing themselves in a dance of avoidance to reduce discomfort.

Fear is a future-oriented emotion that takes advantage of the unknown future to predict and assume hardship, tragedy and catastrophe. The roots of this pattern are usually in past experiences of loss, disappointment and trauma. Those who live in fear imagine a bad life before they have a chance to live it. Repetitive thoughts of a scary outcome inflate the intensity of fear. Often criticized as irrational, fear seems particularly inexplicable to those not feeling it, yet when gripped by terror, fear is completely real to the one experiencing it.

Fear-based emotions show up in many forms and with a wide range of intensity, severity, and degree of debilitation. A characteristic of the fearful person is a loss of control. Fear appears like a separate outside force; unchallenged, it takes more and more control of the emotional experience. To the worrier, worry does not seem like a choice. A traumatized person, who obsesses over repetitive thoughts, feels a loss of control over this cyclic mental pattern. The victim of panic attacks lives in terror, not knowing when the next episode will suddenly occur.

Other fear-based disorders include: Generalized Anxiety Disorder, a chronic state of fear that is not a response to any specific incident; Panic Disorder, episodes of intense debilitating fear which may arrive unexpectedly and are often confused with a heart attack; and Post-traumatic Stress Disorder, or PTSD, the aftereffect of extreme and harmful events suffered in the past beyond an individual's control. Jealousy and relationship insecurity can be associated with an unresolved past loss and are expressed as chronic fear of abandonment; and phobias are intense fear with a specific focus, such as heights, bridges, or spiders, which provoke terror and emotional paralysis.

The more that fear and its illusions of harm are indulged, the larger it grows, like putting fertilizer on weeds. Anxiety about flying in an airplane may progress to panic if the fear is fueled, and ultimately develops into a phobia if the fear is indulged by consistently avoiding that which is feared. Worry is the least productive kind of thought, offering no benefit while enticing the worrier with a short-lived illusion of control. It advances the cause of fear.

Franklin Roosevelt said there is nothing to fear but fear itself, a deeply true statement. Fear is an insidious emotion that encourages predictions of pain, loss, and catastrophe, which increase the likelihood of a negative future. When we challenge fear by facing it head-on and say no to it by fighting it one worry at a time, one fear-influenced choice at a time, we can do anything, despite our fear. Our love relationships cannot reach the heights of love and connection when darkened by patterns of worry and insecurity. Take back control from fear, confront it, and vanquish it by bringing your fight to fear.

11-8. Letting Go of Anger

Daily life events commonly cause anger, but love relationships are like anger-generating machines. Daily interactions are bound to produce wide-ranging anger-based feelings. The repetitive nature of partner interactions is the greatest challenge. Anger-provoking exchanges don't just happen, they keep happening. The ability to let go of anger is so important for well-being and relationship longevity. Anger signals that a problem needs fixing, but it is optimal to let go of it after upsetting events have stopped. Once a problem is effectively addressed, continued anger serves no purpose.

When angry expressions are larger than the size of the initial cause, this shows that anger is still just below the surface. Letting go is simple in concept. The majority of efforts require doing, letting go is not a "doing," but is a "releasing." Letting go is doing less. It is similar to relaxing or falling asleep, when less is more. For those who have habitually held on to anger, such as those who grew up in families where internalizing anger was part of the family culture, attempts at letting it go may initially seem baffling. Without an obvious action or doing, letting go leaves those unpracticed at the art feeling like it is an impossible task.

We are healthiest and happiest when living in the present, a state in which we are fully engrossed in what is happening now, and are not self-centered. When the present gets contaminated by old angry feelings, life doesn't feel good. When holding onto anger, past problems and emotional injuries remain unnecessarily active. Even though an upsetting moment is in the past, internalized anger prevents the anger-provoking incident from full resolution. By holding onto angry negativity from the past, we guarantee the creation of a negative future. Holding onto anger is like stockpiling explosives in your house; the more you store the less room you have to move around and the greater the risk of a destructive explosion.

Holding onto anger is a self-protective choice. It forms an emotionally closed state in which the ability to connect with others is reduced. Internalized anger builds isolation, depression, anxiety, and negativity; a poor environment in which to maintain a satisfying relationship. Anger attempts to stop hurtful actions from happening; it is a limiter. If they are angry all the time, a person is closed and unable to enjoy love, which requires openness. By holding onto anger, an angry person does him or herself a great disservice.

Anger is a powerful and necessary emotion, but in order to be an effective tool, it must be used in the right situation. If you need a screwdriver for a job but have a hammer instead, it cannot do the job, it is useless. To get better at letting go of anger, start with becoming conscious of when angry feelings arise, how long anger is felt after an upsetting incident has passed, and how it is buried within. It is best that anger is let go within minutes of being triggered. Learning to effectively address problems as they show up prevents old anger from lingering and new anger piling on top. The practices of acceptance and forgiveness facilitate the transition away from habitually internalizing anger. Acceptance allows the present moment to be what it is. Forgiveness is a gift to yourself of letting go of old anger while also letting go of the past.

11-9. The Cage That Loves Us

In some way, each one of us is caged. Living with limits is a normal part of the human experience. Equally, part of our life is to chafe against the limits, to push against them and strive for greater freedom. The cages in which we live are bounded by bars composed of the parts of us that are closed, negative and unloving. We are the very material that jails us. We push against the bars, hoping to get through them and escape from confinement. We hate the bars that keep us limited and stop us from getting what we want, yet the more we oppose our limits, the harder and closer together the bars grow, and the tighter our confinement becomes.

In love relationships, this restricting phenomenon is even more prevalent. Both partners, human, limited, and flawed, collectively share twice as many limits as does each partner individually. When combined, the limiting factors multiply. The imprisoning effect seems to accelerate as relationships age and the bond of the union deepens. In line with prevalent but cynical humor, the bad reputation of love and marriage is well deserved.

What are some of these limits? The primary limit is in the capacity to love, potentially expressed by being able to maintain complete openness and acceptance of everything in the present moment, regardless of whether it is experienced as good or bad. Desire for something different invents a limit. Of course, it is very hard to love that which we seem to naturally dislike, such as the limits imposed upon us in all aspects of life. Limits on health, finances and education, limits created by laws and regulations, and limits imposed by death all show that we live in a finite world in which most everything is restricted.

The bars of our cages are made of personal intention. The more closed and angry your intention, the denser the bars become, stronger than steel, harder than diamond. The warmer your intention of love and acceptance, the more the bars can soften and melt, removing restrictions. You can choose, because the bars are none other than an expression of your very self. Be in the space of love, where you are accepting of your very human self, and your cage loves you back by offering freedom.

When in a relationship with another, as you can see, the likelihood of imprisonment is high. The limits that get revealed most in love relationships are limits on the capacity to love. A partner who loves too little, too much, confuses love with need, or loves in the wrong way can drive a mate crazy. We are easily provoked to anger, causing the bars of our jail cell to remain locked in place. Many prevent themselves from receiving love, and are self-confined because the bars of self-hate are particularly impenetrable. A partner's love is human love; always limited and imperfect, less than the perfectly complete love that most crave.

For both partners to simultaneously remain open and loving is a tricky balancing act. Imbalance is an easy pit to fall into. Like riding a bicycle, the ride can be lots of fun when you are balanced, but the moment balance is lost, the resulting crash is very unpleasant. Fighting partner limitations is one way to cause imbalance. Magic occurs when we consistently love the good and the bad, both individually and as a couple. When partners love each other simultaneously in the right way, human failings included, all the bars seem to disappear. It's not that they are gone, but they no longer have an imprisoning effect. Their significance melts away when we practice acceptance, a form of love. Love does that.

11-10. The Blind Spot

As the evening grew long, the gathering was winding down. Some couples had left, but many still talked enthusiastically so that a chorus of voices filled the house. Michelle was chatting with a small group of her girlfriends. Her husband Steve approached the group, having grown tired of the get-together. Without waiting for a gap in their conversation, he forcefully said to Michelle that he'd be sitting in the car. One friend's face displayed obvious amazement. Another's jaw fell agape. A third, Sarah, watched Steve, who didn't wait for a response, turned, and walk unthinkingly out of the front door. The storm door slammed shut behind him. Sarah looked at Michelle and asked, "What was that about?" Michelle responded in a nonchalant tone, "That's just how he is. He's ready to go," suggesting that his abrupt social insensitivity was just normal. "Wow, that would drive me crazy," Sarah said without hesitation. Michelle explained, "Yeah, a few people have said that to me. Steve doesn't think there's anything wrong with it. I've tried to explain it to him. He just doesn't get it." An ache surfaced in her heart.

We all know someone like Steve, and we are all, to some degree, like Steve. Parts of ourselves, emotions, and behavior patterns, are expressed in automatic and unconscious ways. Their impact, consistently negative, is felt most by our romantic partner, and also by others in our social sphere, though to a lesser degree. These are the behaviors, attitudes, and personality nuances that drive our partners crazy. And just like Steve, such troublesome characteristics are not within our own awareness; they reside in the emotional blind spot. If asked about his social insensitivity, Steve would probably respond, "Michelle complains about it, but she doesn't know what she is talking about," or "People are too sensitive. Why don't they focus on something really important like world hunger!" When a blind spot is threatened with vision, the defensive response includes denial or dismissal. Just like the dangerous spot behind a driver's left shoulder that cannot be seen, this is an emotional place located where its owner cannot see it, and which, therefore, to him or her does not exist.

Most of us have such a blind spot, and few of us are aware of it. Yet this blindness is a large obstacle preventing our love relationships from reaching a higher level. It is an area within our psyche and emotional world about which we don't know that we don't know. It is an area of complete blindness, like an intense darkness that an ordinary flashlight will not penetrate. Unconsciously, we prevent ourselves from becoming aware of our own blind spot, but each one of us is clearly aware of others'. We are an expert about our romantic partner's blind spot, and that particular behavior and attitude tempts us to judge and criticize. In reaction to a behavior that reveals another's blindness, it is easy to comment, "What were they thinking?" Holding back on judgement is wise, just as it is best that people who live in glass houses do not throw stones.

The various subjects of personal blindness all fall within the negative range; the ways we unknowingly negatively affect others. One wife, exasperated by her husband's blindness, which often caused her to feel invisible, puts her socks in the kitchen silverware drawer as a test to see if he will notice that they do not belong there, but he doesn't. A husband complains to his wife that every time they sit down to talk to each other, she emphatically lists her frustrations and complaints, preventing him from having a pleasant conversation with her. She denies it upon being confronted.

An oblivious husband always leaves a trail of used items like dirty socks, empty drinking glasses, and wet towels behind him after he leaves a room, without regard for his wife who prefers an orderly house. A wife regularly but unknowingly speaks too loudly, hurting her husband's ears, despite years of requests for a lower voice. A girlfriend has a pattern of being consistently late for every meeting. A boyfriend unconsciously turns every conversation around to himself. These are all examples of people with little self-awareness.

The behaviors that are performed without awareness are typically minor. If not for their repetitive pattern creating a negative snowballing effect, such unconscious behaviors would matter little. They represent an insensitivity to the social world, just like littering; it may not devastate the environment, but unchecked, it contributes ugliness. No one is more influenced than the romantic partner, whose annoyance is likely to grow into resentment and peak in bitterness, should correction of these blind behaviors not occur. Our blind spot behaviors unconsciously contribute to the gradual decline of passion in our relationships, providing an example of how so many loving connections die by a thousand tiny paper cuts.

A romantic partner who tries to shine light into the other's blind spot risks strong opposition formed of denial, dismissal, invalidation, and possibly counterattack, while coming away with little success of change. Taking off the emotional blinders may be slow to occur, but to rid the blind spot of its blindness requires an emotional awakening. Ultimately each one of us has complete control of our actions and choices. We have the power to limit any behavior pattern we choose, but the momentum of habit and personality make many behavior changes unpalatable. Many only choose to change when circumstances force it. For individuals and partners who are ready, growing aware when previously blind empowers a soul with new eyes and a world of fresh possibilities.

> Understanding reduces anger the way water puts out fire.

11-11. The Angry Lifestyle

Some couples live an angry lifestyle. When anger-provoking problems remain unresolved and romantic partners stop using care in how feelings are expressed, partners generate a hostile environment formed by many shades of anger. Gone are the sweet times of "best behavior" during courtship and the early days during the honeymoon phase. At some forgotten moment, the partners made an unconscious agreement to permit the expression of unfiltered anger at any time, in any way. Efforts to be careful with the other fell away. While it may be convenient in the short-term to be emotionally relaxed, saying whatever we want, the long-term cost is very high. The minutes we spend in misery, we never get back.

Within the relationship of those who live an angry lifestyle, the toxicity of chronic anger is thick and quickly evident to others who come near. You know the couple; when in their company it's just a matter of time before the fireworks begin, a bitter word or cutting sarcastic tone, or a small verbal stab all become the norm. Some are so angry that at normally safe social gatherings, where the widespread expectation of civility prevails, hurtful digs spill awkwardly into public view. Responding to anger with anger intensifies the painful gridlock. These partners are angry all the time. Anger looks ugly.

The relationship between partners forms a system of mutual influence. Upon the tacitly agreed suspension of etiquette, the relationship environment becomes one in which anger begets more anger. It is chronic unless one partner, in an effort of strength and wisdom, chooses to no longer let the emotion of anger dictate mood and behavior. When neither partner makes a positive choice, the negative pattern may degrade the relationship for decades. An intermittent style is one in which partners take turns being angry. The torch of righteous anger is typically passed from one to the other following a hurtful event; no episode of peace arrives, and positive togetherness is rarely achieved.

As a common emotion, anger is obvious to most everyone, but not so obvious is its subtle side, which destroys a loving connection slowly and insidiously. The emotion of anger exists along a spectrum of intensity. The angry feelings at the lower end of the spectrum, such as annoyance, frustration, resentment, and irritation, are typically not identified as anger. Yet when routinely dismissed, or habitually internalized, they gradually accumulate to become a force that annuls a positive and loving connection. "Falling out of love" is the end result. Gold doesn't shine when it is buried in the dirt.

On the more higher intensity end of the anger spectrum are feelings more commonly associated with anger; being mad, heated and enraged. Explosions of anger can lead to violence and the destruction of property. Long-held internalized anger leads to resentment, which is characterized by simmering and smoldering that generates negativity. Passive-aggressive behavior, an expression of trapped, powerless anger is indirect, sometimes covert, and dark.

Within an angry couple, in addition to moments of intense anger, the partners have become angry people. For an emotionally healthy person, anger is a normal, temporary response to a momentary hurt, or an obstacle that blocks the way forward. Once an anger-provoking incident has ended, after appropriate action, the anger is allowed to pass. For one who has become an angry person, so much anger has been held onto that he or she is continuously angry; the toxic emotion has become integrated into the individual's personality. Such is the case with toxic people who are just mean, negative, and hurtful.

Relationships can induce anger and interactions between

partners bring differences into their awareness. Because most people are not very good at loving, their insensitivities and poor-quality love quickly inflict hurts from which anger is sparked. Without generously applying a balm of understanding, compassion, and forgiveness, a former bond of love is rapidly transformed into a bond of anger. Held onto, or expressed ineffectively, anger harms the owner, the partner, and the relationship. But as an expression, anger does not teach a poor lover to love better, or encourage a poor lover to come closer. It pushes him or her away, reducing the chance of relationship improvement. If love is the bright sun, anger is the dark cloud that blocks its light.

For a loving atmosphere to be protected and maintained, problems must regularly be resolved. Couples who live the angry lifestyle do not solve problems. They fail to function as a team to develop solutions and make positive change. Their unresolved problems lie all about, easy to trip over like clutter in an untidy house.

Anger will never make your relationship better; it is the wrong tool for the job. However, the energy within anger, if channeled in a loving way, can fix the relationship. The emotionally strong and self-aware partner takes notice of angry feelings and intentionally directs the energy towards quickly solving the problem. Ineffectively expressing anger makes problems worse and makes more of them. Any way you look at it, anger makes a terrible lifestyle.

> Don't let dreams of perfection stop you from being good enough.

11-12. The Dangerous Allure of Perfection

There is no crime in wanting a good life or a good love life. It is normal to want the best. From this facet of human nature arises an emotional trap that ensnares many good people and complicates many love relationships. People who are emotionally compelled to achieve perfect results are called perfectionists. Perfectionism, a condition stubborn to healing, is an emotional imbalance which strongly interferes with romantic satisfaction. An amazing paradox is formed, in which good intentions consistently produce bad results.

At first sight, the label "perfectionism" sounds like it may be positive. When a student gets a perfect "100" on a test, the accomplishment is celebrated, and why not? When any challenging task is attempted and the results are superior and flawless, it is a good thing. But perfectionists expect themselves to achieve perfect results in everything they do, all the time. For the perfectionist, any performance that does not produce perfect results is seen as a failure. In their world only two outcomes exist: perfection or failure. It is a rigged game in which failure seems to occur most of the time. For the perfectionist whose being is only validated by perfect outcomes, his or her being seems to be repeatedly confirmed as a failure. Because the world is not a perfect place, the perfectionist is emotionally set-up for continuous torture.

The critical eye of the perfectionist scrutinizes the romantic partner as readily as it does every other endeavor. The human partner, from the perfectionist's perspective, repeatedly fails; his or her shortcomings blanch the love out of the partner's loving gestures by judging everything and comparing it to imagined perfection. A perfectionist is likely to critically point out the ways in which other's efforts fail to be perfect. Love, instead of being received and appreciated, is diluted by judgement and rejected as imperfect and insufficient. Some perfectionists try to be the perfect partner or perfect lover. The results, however, are enacted in a way that appears more like a performance than a loving presence which feels easy, natural, and comfortable.

From the partner's perspective, the perfectionist is

impossible to please. A perfectionist can be highly specific in their needs, desires and preferences; only the exact thing, done the right way, in the precise amount, in the right size, color and kind will do. Hence the chances of satisfying his or her very narrow conditions are extremely low. Loving the perfectionist can just seem too hard. He or she is too highly calibrated. The partner may constantly feel like a disappointment in the perfectionist's eyes, and their unrealistic, inhuman goals of perfection imprison the partner as much as they do the perfectionist. Judgement and critical tendencies always block love.

Perfectionism is an anxiety-based emotional condition usually occurring in conjunction with other anxiety-based disorders such as Obsessive/Compulsive Disorder, Panic Disorder or Generalized Anxiety Disorder. At its core lies an unconscious fear of inadequacy. The dynamic in perfectionism is the struggle to experience oneself as good enough. In the developmental years, an individual's feelings and needs were frequently criticized, dismissed or invalidated. As a result, he or she neither experienced the possibility of acceptance, nor praise for accomplishments. In an attempt to succeed at being acceptable, the perfectionist developed a strategy to avoid criticism by eliminating all risk of being found at fault. Performing perfectly provided the optimal way to reduce the risk of exposure to hurtful criticism. An automatic devotion to achieving perfection or perfect performance produces inflexible choices which may, at times, be obsessive and compulsive.

Typically highly intelligent and dedicated to hard work, the perfectionist routinely achieves excellence in all that is attempted. Of the many paradoxes that rule in the world of perfectionism, one of them is that the perfectionist gains little or no satisfaction from their accomplishments. Instead they view themselves as only marginally successful, despite abundant evidence of significant achievements. For the individual saddled with perfectionist tendencies, excellence is a failure and only perfection is acceptable. Chronic disappointment results from unrealistic expectations, a facet of the perfectionist's make-up that causes this kind of individual to be among the most chronically miserable. Little will please them. Little can make them happy, although they produce achievements most can only dream about. Typically, trying to love or be loved by a perfectionist is distressing.

The goal of perfection, either regarding yourself, your performance or achievements, creates a bind in which self-acceptance is unobtainable. People who hold tightly to that goal, and the people who love them, stay jailed in a box into which love cannot shine. The way out of the perfectionist trap is found through acceptance of the concept of "good enough," a general level of sufficiency that allows for functionality. To the perfectionist, good enough looks a lot like failure, but in actuality good enough can be very efficient, while also possessing the magic that is gained from allowing life to be what it is. Trying to be perfect, which sounds great in theory, rejects our natural human possession of limits and imperfections. Paradoxically, perfect love does not include perfection; it embraces such virtues as forgiveness and acceptance, which allow for the natural state of imperfection.

11-13. The People-pleasers

They are among the most good-hearted people. They routinely go out of their way to be kind, generous and helpful to others. They also unintentionally leave a trail of destruction in their romantic relationships and family lives. They are the "people-pleasers." Publicly, the people-pleasers possess a purely good reputation. Others say, "S/he is the nicest person!" In stark contrast is the private reputation the pleaser has earned with the romantic partner, who grows resentful, bitter and malnourished by getting only the dregs of the pleaser's time, energy and attention. Those in their group of friends and the community cannot understand why the spouse is so ungrateful. Many others would love to have a romantic partner who seems so thoughtful.

Within each one of us are many "personas," a grouping of personality characteristics that function in some situations but not in others. The most common and well known of these are the workplace persona which our co-workers see and our home persona which our romantic partners and family members see. The public or social persona is another distinct sub-personality. For some, the social persona exhibits discomfort and fear, manifesting as social anxiety, whereas for others the social persona is outgoing, expressive and joyful. People pleasing behaviors are an aspect of the social persona.

At the core of people-pleasing is a desire to be liked, to look good in the eyes of others, to avoid rejection, and to avoid conflict. The fastest route to succeeding at earning others' acceptance is by pleasing them. The moment a request is made, the people-pleaser quickly and automatically responds by saying yes. He or she is willing to offer time, attention, or support without any consideration for the impact on their life or loved ones. An example is a husband who has just joined his fifth committee, even though in a recent discussion with his wife he admitted already being overwhelmed. Another is a wife who just agreed to let her friend stay at the house temporarily, despite the husband's chronic complaints that their house is already too small.

People-pleasers, male or female, are "yes men." When confronted with a request, the pleaser is flooded with fear and anxiety at the prospect of saying "no." Disappointing another provokes strong feelings of shame and of being a bad person. Refusing another is viewed as risking a conflict, a situation people-pleasers desperately wish to avoid, and a behavior pattern that results over time in damage to love relationships. Instead, they seek to validate their value through others' approval. Disappointing others triggers a cascade of self-hate in reaction to the experience of emotionally becoming nobody, something people-pleasers repeatedly felt as a child. Pleasing others is a chronic attempt to matter; so at the moment when they are presented with a request, all other considerations, important or not, disappear. Faced with a decision-making moment, the pleaser is rendered weak and disabled from assertiveness.

For the pleaser type, his or her needs go unmet time and

time again, deferred in favor of gaining someone else's approval. Ignoring their own needs both chronically restates the experience of non-existence and simultaneously ensures its future continuity. Emotionally, the spouse becomes an extension of the pleaser's self, so while the pleaser's needs fall into the bottomless pit of low self-esteem, the romantic partner's needs follow suit. With an objective perspective, the partner, witnessing the dysfunctional nature of the people-pleasing dynamic, grows bitter and resentful about the fact that his or her own needs are regularly ignored. The partner loses respect for the pleaser, who functions from a place of chronic weakness.

People-pleasers view themselves as kind and generous, therefore the romantic partner's bitterness seems confusing and inconsistent. Every time the pleaser impulsively gives away time, money, or attention, the spouse's needs for these same resources are rejected and devalued, risking highly charged conflict, if not smoldering resentment. Because the pleaser has personal well-being at stake, he or she is resistant to changing behaviors. It is hard to stop a bad habit, but even harder to eliminate what seems to be a good one.

Selflessness is a high spiritual value. Being of service to others is also universally lauded. The distinction between selflessness and service on the one hand, and the unintentional hurtfulness of people-pleasing on the other, is lost in an emotional blind-spot for the people-pleaser; the two appear too similar to the pleaser's undiscerning eye. Hence an obstacle to eliminating the people-pleasing dynamic forms, because the pleaser believes that he or she is doing good. When the pleaser's partner, who may make more balanced decisions, tries to point out the problematic pattern, he or she is labeled by the defensive pleaser as selfish.

Saying no to another's request does not risk conflict, as the pleaser fears. Gentle and diplomatic ways of saying "no" exist which do not hurt the other person. In fact, saying “no” neither provokes conflict, nor results in dislike. With gentle assertiveness, a well-worded refusal gains respect from others, because doing so demonstrates confidence and strength, justifying the paraphrased John Bytheway saying, "It is better to be respected than liked."

Love requires balance. Truly loving actions do not carry a dark side-effect of hurt and destruction. Selflessness, when combined with low self-esteem and dysfunction, carry with them the danger of destructive imbalance. The well-worn saying, "Charity begins at home," holds true. Generally, nothing is wrong with pleasing others, so long as it is an effort balanced with first taking good care of one's own needs, and the needs of loved ones. This may be easily practiced by use of the simple word, "no."

11-14. Strength is a Turn-On

What happens in the bedroom is strongly influenced by what happens outside the bedroom. A lack of heat and passion is a common complaint among married couples, yet keeping sexual excitement alive in a long-term love relationship is essential to its survival. The strengths partners possess are a major component in succeeding at doing so. Simply put, strength is a turn on. Our strengths keep our partners interested and invested in us. Partner strengths are a relationship asset, but when they are diminished by weaknesses or hurtfulness, their effectiveness as turn-ons is eliminated.

The trouble is that in a long-term relationship, partners' faults, flaws, and weaknesses grab the greater attention, and can easily upstage strengths, especially because they are chronically on display and because they cause hurt. As romantic partners get to know each other more deeply over time, character flaws grow more apparent than they were in the relationship's beginning. In long-term relationships, since togetherness is of a marathon-like duration, partners' repetitive, weakness-based choices, habits and behaviors have a cumulative negative and deleterious effect. Often invisible in the beginning, our partners' human fallibility and limitations grow annoyingly obvious.

Failures and problems get attention. Look in the newspaper where good news is unusual. That is our challenge as partners, spouses and lovers; to make the effort of growth so that our strengths outweigh our failings and protect our partner, and our failings don't cause hurt and inconvenience. Hiding our flaws to appear strong will not work, but growing so that our weaknesses are transformed into strengths will.

Just like light, which is invisible as it travels through space but visible once it reflects off an object, strength alone is nothing without being colored by a quality of effort or action. Examples of such efforts are love, integrity, sense of humor, intellect, compassion, power, morality; the list is long. Each of these strengths is a likely turn-on for someone. When many strengths combine, they collectively become strength of character.

The most common pattern in long-term love relationships is that passion fades over time. Is it a coincidence that the shine of mutual admiration dulls in equal measure as familiarity with each other's human failings increases? It takes two strong people to make one strong love relationship. Being found sexy and attractive depends upon your strengths. Notice that when anyone points out that someone turns them on, at the root of the attraction is some kind of strength that the attractive person possesses, usually beyond just a pleasing appearance. If we no longer get turned on by our partner, it is certain that we are experiencing our partner's limitations as greater than their strengths. Conversely, if our partner is no longer turned on by us, what are our limitations that are muting our strengths?

When first meeting another whom we find attractive, our tendency is to accentuate our strengths, our positive attributes, because we all instinctively know that strengths are a turn-on. Strength attracts, and does so well beyond making a good first impression. Maintaining passion within your long-term relationship, or resurrecting it, depends upon growing by transforming your limitations into strengths.

> For every minute you are angry, you lose sixty seconds of happiness. *-Mark Twain*

11-15. Handling Anger While in Love

Typically, everyday something or someone makes us angry. Romantic partners are better at angering us than most. In reaction to feeling hurt, blocked or diminished, anger is aroused, the emotion-laden energy mobilized to cope with challenging, usually unpleasant situations. Anger is the intense, direction-oriented energy required to protect, assert or negotiate for our well-being. Anger-based emotions fall along an intensity spectrum from low, including annoyance and frustration, to high, including aggression and rage. Anger expressed in any one of its forms is a sign that a problem is demanding an immediate fix.

Countless rules, laws and inner "shoulds" dictate our choices, and are often at odds with the way our aroused anger would have us behave. As children many of us were trained to avoid expressing anger because of its disrespectful and destructive ways. Many of us witnessed our parents frighteningly lose control of their anger, and as a result we developed negative associations with power. Among all our emotions, anger is just as healthy and necessary as the others, but we are collectively cautious about it. The complexity of this intense emotion makes its balanced use very difficult.

Within a romantic partnership we expect to be loved, a reality that rarely lives up to our fantasies. In addition, within relationships hurts are inevitable, and old, unresolved hurts are reactivated. Commonly the anger felt by partners is misused to punish the other. The only proper use for angry energy is to resolve problems.

To create positive and strong love relationships, the skilled and successful use of anger is essential; its mishandling is a chief cause of relationship dysfunction. Mishandled anger results in many problems, and renders stable, healthy relationships impossible. Angry energy, which is our unrefined individual power, is required to make our lives the way we want them to be. When withheld, also called repression, anger does not dissipate, but instead accumulates within and may result in depression or anxiety, often displayed as fearfulness, bitterness, negativity and explosive rage. Unceasing repression of anger may also lead to panic attacks. Some who withhold anger grow into "angry people," those whose anger has infected their entire personhood. Such individuals are closed and highly defended. A saying of the Buddha highlights repression's self-destructive tendencies: "Holding onto anger is like grabbing a hot coal with the intention of throwing it at someone, you are the one getting burned."

Angry energy expressed without a filter causes harm to others. Acting impulsively from anger results in being an unsafe person and partner. Of all those having contact with an explosive individual, the intimate partner is the one most often hurt. Intense anger impairs judgement, leading to harmful, irrational choices. At the extreme, uncontrolled anger may lead to self-medication, addiction and the involvement of law enforcement.

When handled improperly, the effects of anger have a direct and negative impact on a marriage and a long-term relationship. Emotional habits that reinforce imbalance result in accumulating harm. A partner who habitually withholds anger becomes a depressed, bitter, or non-communicative mate, causing harm to the relationship slowly over the long-term. On the other end of the spectrum, a partner who habitually fails to control their anger is unsafe and not to be trusted. If not corrected, mishandled anger will quickly destroy what is most precious in a relationship.

Two analogies offer greater clarity regarding the nature of angry energy: a knife and an electrical grid transformer. One aspect of anger functions like a knife; it cuts for the purpose of ending or stopping something. Hence the expression "Cut it out!" While a knife is a useful tool for cutting, it is the wrong tool for loving another. Anger can cut and stab a partner emotionally if handled insensitively. The cutting potential of anger must be used with the skill and care of a surgeon to delicately set limits and define boundaries while minimizing harm.

A second useful analogy is that of an electric grid transformer. The high-voltage electricity which flows through high-tension lines must be reduced by transformers so it may be consumed by houses without frying the residential electrical systems. Similarly, high-intensity raw anger must be reduced properly to be constructively applied where change is needed. Harnessing intense anger can be difficult. Each situation requires an appropriate use of force...in some moments a tiny jeweler's hammer gets the job done where a sledgehammer would destroy the opportunity. The force in anger has no regard for consequences. Each partner must develop the capacity, like a transformer, to reduce raw angry energy to the right intensity for a specific situation and thus avoid harm and regret.

A fragile emotional connection is formed between two lovers, which is easily damaged by toxic emotion. Mishandled anger quickly damages and destroys the love and trust partners build. Expressing anger in a constructive fashion is done through assertiveness, a balanced approach that supports self-respect and the need for safety from harm. Balance requires the strength to contain anger's intensity and to overcome fear of conflict. The presence of anger indicates a problem requiring immediate repair, which if done quickly prevents anger from accumulating to disruptive proportions. To keep love present demands that anger is used in a balanced way, delicately using the "knife" of anger to cut out problems, with just the right amount of anger's power to be effective.

11-16. Living with Passion

Passion! I know it when I feel it. Beyond that, it can be incredibly difficult to explain. This is most true when it is missing. Passion is a highly desirable quality in marriages and love relationships and an essential ingredient in the ideal that most hope and yearn for when forming a love relationship. However, within the rigors of long-term love relationships, it can be elusive.

Passion is the expression of an eagerness to merge; to unite, hence it is the interaction of two parts where the quality of that interaction is attraction and merging into oneness. At its best, the desire to merge is mutual. It is a highly dynamic relationship between the two parts, whether it is a person having passion for life, or two people having passion for each other. One aspect of merging is enacted through being sexual when our bodies unite, but more importantly our very being merges if we surrender completely. Our love relationships function as practice for a greater merging, which is the ultimate union between each of us and life. The presence of passion signals that this practice is going well; that partners are alive and vital.

Passion can only exist within the mystery of life in which we are simultaneously a complete individual and a part of a greater whole. For passion to exist, each of these states must be honored and celebrated. We cannot fully merge until we have fully embraced and realized our complete individuality. It is an essential contradiction, since we cannot fully merge until we have become fully separate.

To realize our individuality and celebrate our separateness means being who we are completely in our relationship by being true to ourselves. Emotional strength, a clear sense of who we are and what we are about, must be present to accomplish this. Loving ourselves is only valuable if it is balanced with the giving of ourselves to our partner.

The impediments to passion are common fare. We are challenged to be the best we can be by life itself, but the challenge is steep. When we are not true to ourselves, our sense of self becomes unclear, causing a reduction in our ability to celebrate our individuality, our uniqueness. If we do not have a clear sense of ourselves, then the potential merging in our relationships, and especially during sex, becomes uncomfortable, anxiety-provoking, or frightening, a factor for many who avoid intimacy or sex.

Passion is the fire that brightens our relationships when both partners mutually succeed at honoring themselves.

11-17. Our Disruptive Inner Three-Year-Old

When partners behave badly; this is him. When wives are out of control with anger; this is her. When husbands are manipulative; this is him. When a wife gets intensely jealous without a legitimate reason; this is her. When a husband expresses big anger, seemingly in reaction to nothing; this is him. The him and her about which I write is the inner three-year-old. So if you or your partner behave in troubling ways, consider this inner part to be the likely culprit.

Love relationships are unique among all the relationships we form, because romantic love activates the inner three-year-old like no other relationship. Marriages and love relationships can be incredibly difficult for this reason. The deep emotional connection that can only exist between long-term romantic partners awakens this deep, powerful part, causing us to behave like three-year-olds instead of like mature adults. Three-year-olds can be very unreasonable and disruptive.

If you or your partner is behaving in a way that makes little sense, an angry, hurt, sad or frightened inner three-year-old is taking control. In the same way that a little one may cause great chaos and dominate a family, similarly, our inner counterpart will dominate a relationship by causing lots of trouble. It does so by avoiding or acting out. Sudden, impulsive behavior is a characteristic of this unconscious inner part.

What was life like when you were three? You probably cannot remember. As newborns, we were ready to be loved perfectly, but our humanly imperfect parents were unable to deliver perfect love. Most of us are wounded by this. The pain of this disappointment is beyond memory, but emotional evidence of it lingers in the inner three-year old's behavior. The more intense the challenges in our early lives were, the greater the negative influence this inner part will exert over our partner choices and our emotional struggles in our intimate relationships. As we grow and mature, we leave behind our three-year-old challenges and focus on older developmental needs. The three-year-old troubles get covered over and remain unresolved, only to surface later, awakened when secure love is present once a stable relationship is formed.

Our personalities were built up by the many impressions forged by early life experiences. Within many of our childhood histories were experiences of control, domination or disregard, delivered in the name of love, but these were really distortions of love. Such experiences caused our inner three-year-old to be imperfectly developed relative to love. Self-doubt, self-hate, and insecurities are some of the forms of low self-esteem which result.

Bad behavior signals that the inner three-year-old is active. These are the feelings and behaviors that seem to be beyond our personal control. This little one, when reacting to a perceived hurt, will respond in very immature ways such as sulking, throwing a tantrum, or creative avoidance. In social situations, when the adult is firmly in control, he or she shows the world maturity and restraint. At home, however, behind closed doors and in the more emotional marital environment, the inner three-year-old may assert his or her will by acting in surprisingly irrational ways.

How do you soothe and heal an angry and hurt three-year-old so that he or she doesn't wreak havoc in your life? It took years for your personality to develop, so it may take years of effort to make your inner three-year-old healthier and happier. Forming a loving, patient attitude towards this inner part is the beginning. Even if not by elegant methods, the little one is doing his or her best to inform you that healing and growing changes are necessary. Underneath the three-year-old's bad attitude is the capacity to both give and receive great love, offering the potential for a deeply intimate love connection.

QUOTATIONS

Each quote is preceded by the page number where it will be found. If the quote is not assigned to an author, it was first expressed by Andrew Aaron, LICSW.

16. The more intimately you know someone, the more clearly you will see their flaws. — *Anonymous*

21. Sex is both a way of expressing a close connection and of building a close connection.

22. Loving doesn't start until all the hurtfulness has stopped.

26. It takes two emotionally strong partners to make one strong relationship.

28. Consistent strong effort at first becomes easy and natural effort later.

29. The natural you...is the attainable and healthy perfection.

34. I love myself...I'm not perfect, I'm human.

36. No amount of negativity will ever create a positive relationship.

39. In a relationship, you can do little good until you have learned to do little harm.

41. There's only one corner of the universe you can be certain of improving, and that's your own self.
—Aldous Huxley

47. The way to a woman's heart is through her ears.
—Anonymous

49. Worrying is the least productive activity and a great waste of time and energy.

51. On each side of the scale: one pound makes balance, a thousand pounds crushes the scale.

53. There is no pillow so soft as a clear conscience.
—French Proverb

71. Drugs and alcohol make you feel real good...while they destroy your life.

75. In a love relationship, being strong is not how much you can lift, it is how much you can love.

76. In our fantasies we choose to exclude realistic limitations and negative factors.

86. We grow a little bit we don't take advantage of another's weakness.

56. Whether you think you can, or that you can't, you are usually right. *-Henry Ford*

114. Change is constant. Growth is a choice.
—a variant of John C. Maxwell

117. Criticism is to love what acid is to metal.

128. Relax! Good enough really is good enough.

136. A partner's highest obligation is to protect the partner from being or negatively effected by him or her.

150. Making effort is not the same as producing results.

154. Each gender views the other as childish in areas of its own strengths.

196. Relationships: act how you feel like acting and your relationship will be like a train wreck.

200. Falling in love is easy. Staying in love is not.

204. Feeling hurt is no excuse for bad behavior.

208. Hold yourselves to a high standard of love. You will suffer less this way.

210. Where love rules, there is no will to power; where power predominates, there love is lacking. One is the shadow of the other. *-Carl Jung*

215. Love is: action and effort which supports and nourishes another's well-being and growth while also protecting him or her from harm.

220. One hurtful actions destroys the positive effect of a dozen loving gestures.

222. Police yourselves and your partner will not have to or want to.

233. If you are going through hell, keep going.
-Winston Churchill

243. Blame: among the best ways to not solve a problem.

245. Focus on positive solutions instead of negative problems.

247. Care about people's approval and you will always be their prisoner.

248. Know your partner better than you know your assumptions.

253. We must be less hurtful, but also be less easily hurt.

260. Loving another is rarely wrong, but more importantly hurting another is rarely right.

267. We can often do more for others by trying to correct our own faults than by trying to correct theirs.
— *François Fenelon*

270. Criticism is to love what acid is to metal.

272. Nothing that you do matters...It only matters that you do it. —*Mahatma Ghandi*

278. When arguing about who is right and who is wrong, the relationship always loses.

287. There is no love without pain.

290. Most injuries are not caused by malice, but instead by ignorance. —*Anonymous*

292. Beware of making permanent choices when reacting to temporary emotions. — *Buddha*

302. MARRIAGE: Do it well and it is up lifting. Do it poorly and it is bondage.

310. The present moment is where life actually happens. Stay in the present to fully live it.

313. Hold onto the past and your NOW will be

contaminated by it.

326. You do not have the power to change your partner, but you do have he power to change yourselves.

339. Choose to be angry or choose to fix the problem. You cannot do both.

351. Avoid avoidance.

364. Loving with sensitivity dictates that if a choice or action will impact the partner, he or she must be consulted.

366. The aim of an argument or discussion should not be victory but progress. — *Joseph Joubert*

380. If you allow fear to control you, you will never have a good life.

388. Understanding reduces anger the way water puts out fire.

390. Don't let dreams of perfection stop you from being good enough.

398. For every minute you are angry, you lose sixty seconds of happiness. — *Mark Twain*

Printed in Dunstable, United Kingdom

71678001R00234